CW01456564

Obstetric Anesthesiology

Obstetric Anesthesiology

An Illustrated Case-Based Approach

Edited by

Tauqeer Husain
Ashford and St. Peter's Hospitals NHS Foundation Trust, Surrey, UK

Roshan Fernando
Women's Wellness and Research Centre, Hamad Medical Corporation, Doha, Qatar

Scott Segal
Wake Forest University, Raleigh, NC, USA

CAMBRIDGE
UNIVERSITY PRESS

CAMBRIDGE
UNIVERSITY PRESS

University Printing House, Cambridge CB2 8BS, United Kingdom

One Liberty Plaza, 20th Floor, New York, NY 10006, USA

477 Williamstown Road, Port Melbourne, VIC 3207, Australia

314–321, 3rd Floor, Plot 3, Splendor Forum, Jasola District Centre, New Delhi – 110025, India

79 Anson Road, #06–04/06, Singapore 079906

Cambridge University Press is part of the University of Cambridge.

It furthers the University's mission by disseminating knowledge in the pursuit of education, learning, and research at the highest international levels of excellence.

www.cambridge.org
Information on this title: www.cambridge.org/9781107095649
DOI: 10.1017/9781316155479

© Cambridge Univeristy Press 2019

This publication is in copyright. Subject to statutory exception and to the provisions of relevant collective licensing agreements, no reproduction of any part may take place without the written permission of Cambridge University Press.

First published 2019

Printed and bound in Great Britain by Clays Ltd, Elcograf S.p.A.

A catalogue record for this publication is available from the British Library.

ISBN 978-1-107-09564-9 Hardback

Cambridge University Press has no responsibility for the persistence or accuracy of URLs for external or third-party internet websites referred to in this publication and does not guarantee that any content on such websites is, or will remain, accurate or appropriate.

....

Every effort has been made in preparing this book to provide accurate and up-to-date information that is in accord with accepted standards and practice at the time of publication. Although case histories are drawn from actual cases, every effort has been made to disguise the identities of the individuals involved. Nevertheless, the authors, editors, and publishers can make no warranties that the information contained herein is totally free from error, not least because clinical standards are constantly changing through research and regulation. The authors, editors, and publishers therefore disclaim all liability for direct or consequential damages resulting from the use of material contained in this book. Readers are strongly advised to pay careful attention to information provided by the manufacturer of any drugs or equipment that they plan to use.

Chapter 12 is dedicated to Dr. J. T. "Bill" Parer, who dedicated his life to mentoring, teaching, and most importantly caring for pregnant women. He leaves a legacy in the numerous healthcare providers he has trained over the course of his illustrious career.

Contents

Contributors

Rasha Abouelmagd, FRCA
Northern Schools of Anaesthesia, Royal Victoria
Infirmary, Newcastle-Upon-Tyne, UK

Samantha Allen, BSc, MB BS, FRCA
Department of Anaesthesia, University Hospital
Southampton NHS Foundation Trust, Southampton,
UK

Neil Amison, MB ChB, MD, BSc (Hons)
Bath Department of General Practice, Royal United
Hospital Bath, Somerset, UK

Sarah Armstrong, MB BS, MA, FRCA
Department of Anaesthetics, Frimley Park Hospital,
Surrey, UK

Mrinalini Balki, MB BS, MD
Department of Anesthesia & Pain Management, and
Department of Obstetrics & Gynaecology, University
of Toronto, Mount Sinai, Lunenfeld-Tanenbaum
Research Institute, University of Toronto, Toronto,
ON, Canada

Philip Barclay, MB ChB, FRCA
Chelsea and Westminster Hospital NHS Foundation
Trust, Imperial College London, and Anaesthetic
Department, West Middlesex University Hospital,
Isleworth, UK

Sohail Bampoe, BSc, MSc, MB BS, FRCA
Centre for Anaesthesia and Perioperative
Medicine, University College London, and
Department of Anaesthesia and Perioperative
Medicine, University College London Hospitals NHS
Foundation Trust, London, UK

Yaakov Beilin, MD
Departments of Anesthesiology, Perioperative and
Pain Medicine and OB/GYN. Obstetric
Anesthesiology and Obstetric Anesthesia Fellowship,
Icahn School of Medicine at Mount Sinai, New York,
NY, USA

Jessica Booth, MD
Department of Anesthesiology, Wake Forest School
of Medicine, Raleigh, NC, USA

William Camann, MD
Department of Anesthesia and Pain Management,
Harvard Medical School, Boston, MA, USA

Christopher R. Cambic, MD
Department of Anesthesiology, Northwestern
University Feinberg School of Medicine, Chicago, IL,
USA

Alison Carter, MB BS, BSc, FRCA
University Hospital Southampton NHS Trust
Southampton, Hampshire, UK

Jose C. A. Carvalho, MD, PhD, FANZCA, FRCPC
Department of Anesthesia, Mount Sinai Hospital,
Toronto, ON, Canada

Anthony Chau, MD, MMSc, FRCPC
Department of Anesthesia, BC Women's Hospital and
Health Centre, and Department of Anesthesiology,
Pharmacology and Therapeutics, University of British
Columbia, Vancouver, BC, Canada

Rachel Collis, FRCA
Department of Anaesthesia, University Hospital of
Wales, Cardiff, South Wales, UK

Jean M. Connors, MD
Anticoagulation Management Services, Hematology
Division, Brigham and Women's Hospital, Harvard
Medical School, Boston, MA, USA

Claire Daly, MB BS, BSc
Department of Anaesthetics, Guys and St. Thomas'
NHS Hospital Trust, London, UK

Anna David, MD
Obstetrics and Maternal-Fetal Medicine, Institute for Women's Health, University College London, UK

Carlos Delgado, MD
Obstetric Anesthesia Division, Department of Anesthesiology and Pain Medicine, University of Washington, Seattle, WA, USA

Alicia T. Dennis, MB BS, PhD, MPH, PGDipEcho, FANZCA
Departments Pharmacology and Obstetrics and Gynaecology, Department of Anaesthesia, The Royal Women's Hospital, Melbourne, Australia

Daryl Dob, BSc (Hons), MB BS, FRCA
Magill Department of Anaesthesia, Chelsea and Westminster Hospital, London, UK

Robert A. Dyer, BSc (Hons), MB ChB (UCT), FFA (SA), FCA, PhD (UCT)
Department of Anaesthesia and Perioperative Medicine, University of Cape Town, South Africa

Zara Edwards, MB ChB, BSc, FRCA
Magill Department of Anaesthesia, Chelsea and Westminster Hospital, London, UK

William John Fawcett, FRCA, FFPMRCA
Department of Anaesthesia and Pain Management, Royal Surrey County Hospital and Postgraduate Medical School, University of Surrey, Guildford, Surrey, UK

Roshan Fernando, MB ChB, FRCA
Women's Wellness and Research Centre, Hamad Medical Corporation, Doha, Qatar

Gabriela Frunza, FRCA
Chelsea and Westminster Hospital, Imperial College London, and Chelsea and Westminster Hospital, London, UK

Thierry Girard, MD
Department of Anesthesiology, University Hospital of Basel, Switzerland

Stephanie R. Goodman, MD
Department of Anesthesiology, Columbia University Medical Center and New York Presbyterian Hospital, New York, NY, USA

David L. Hepner, MD, MPH
Weiner Center for Preoperative Evaluation, Department of Anesthesiology, Perioperative and Pain Medicine, Brigham and Women's Hospital, Harvard Medical School, Boston, MA, USA

Rachel Hignett, MA, MB BChir, MRCP, FRCA
Department of Anaesthesia, Royal Infirmary of Edinburgh, Scotland, UK

David Hill, MD, FCARCSI, FFPMRCSI
South Eastern Health and Social Care Trust, Ulster Hospital, Belfast, Northern Ireland, UK

Ross Hofmeyr, MB ChB (Stell), DipPEC, DA, MMed (Anaes) (UCT), FAWM, FCA (SA)
Department of Anaesthesia and Perioperative Medicine, University of Cape Town, South Africa

Tom Hurst, FRCA, FFICM
Intensive Care and Major Trauma, King's College Hospital, London, UK

Tauqeer Husain, MB BS, BSc (Hons), FRCA, MAcadMEd
Ashford and St. Peter's Hospitals NHS Foundation Trust, Surrey, UK

Richard Isaacs, MB B Chir, FRCA
Department of Anaesthesia, University Hospital Southampton NHS Foundation Trust, Southampton, UK

Doron Kabiri, MD
Department of Obstetrics and Gynecology, Hadassah-Hebrew University Medical Center, Jerusalem, Israel

Fatima Khatoon, MB BS, MD
Women's Wellness and Research Centre, Hamad Medical Corporation, Doha, Qatar

Stephen Michael Kinsella, MB BS, FCAI
Department of Anaesthesia, St. Michael's Hospital, Bristol, UK

Nakiyah Knibbs, MD
Department of Anesthesiology, Perioperative and Pain Medicine, Icahn School of Medicine at Mount Sinai, New York, NY, USA

Mitko Kocarev, MD, DESA
Women's Wellness and Research Centre, Hamad Medical Corporation, Doha, Qatar

Alison Gar-Pui Koo, MB BS, FHKCA, FHKAM
Department of Anaesthesia and Intensive Care, Chinese University of Hong Kong, and Prince of Wales Hospital, Hong Kong, China

Katherine Kosman, MD
Department of Psychiatry, Beth Israel Deaconess Medical Center, Boston, MA, USA

Ruth Landau, MD
Columbia University Medical Center, and Department of Anesthesiology, Columbia University College of Physicians and Surgeons, New York, NY, USA

Lucy de Lloyd, MB BCh, FRCA
Department of Anaesthesia, University Hospital of Wales, Cardiff, South Wales, UK

Lisa Leffert, MD
Obstetric Anesthesia Division, Massachusetts General Hospital, and Harvard Medical School, Boston, MA, USA

Nuala Lucas, MB BS, FRCA
Department of Anaesthesia, London North West Healthcare NHS Trust, Northwick Park Hospital, Harrow, UK

Jennifer Lucero, MD
Department of Anesthesia and Perioperative Care and Department of Obstetrics, Gynecology and Reproductive Sciences, University of California, San Francisco, CA, USA

Shubha Mallaiah FRCA
Liverpool Women's Hospital, Liverpool, UK

John C. Markley, MD, PhD
Department of Anesthesia and Perioperative Care, University of California, San Francisco, and Zuckerberg San Francisco General Hospital and Trauma Center, San Francisco, CA, USA

Grace McClune, MB BCh, BAO, FCARCSI, DIP-PG
Ulster Hospital and Dundonald, South Eastern Health and Social Care Trust, Northern Ireland, UK

Kate McCombe, MB BS, MRCP, FRCS, MA
Mediclinic City Hospital, and Mohammed Bin Rashid University of Medicine and Healthcare Sciences, Dubai, UAE

Tim Meek, FRCA
Department of Anaesthesia, James Cook University Hospital, Middlesbrough, UK

Marie-Louise Meng, MD
Department of Anesthesiology, Columbia University Medical Center and New York Presbyterian Hospital, New York, NY, USA

Rebecca D. Minehart, MD MSHPEd
Department of Anesthesia, Critical Care, and Pain Medicine, Massachusetts General Hospital, Boston, MA, USA

E. Lindsay Moore, MD
Matrix Anesthesia, Signature Healthcare Brockton Hospital, Brockton, MA, USA

Ruth E. Murphy, BM BCh, BA (Oxon)
Department of Anaesthesia, University Hospitals Bristol NHS Foundation Trust, Bristol, UK

Mary C. Mushambi, MB ChB, FRCA, LLM
Department of Anaesthesia, University Hospitals of Leicester and Royal Infirmary, Leicester, UK

Shobana Murugan, MD
US Anesthesia Partners Pavilion for Women at Texas Children's Hospital Houston, TX, USA

Warwick D. Ngan Kee, BHB, MB ChB, MD, FANZCA, FHKCA, FHKAM (Anaesth)
Department of Anesthesiology, Sidra Medicine, Doha, Qatar

James Noblet, BSc, MB BS (Hons), FRCA
Department of Anaesthesia, Royal London Hospital and Barts Health NHS Trust, London, UK

Errol R. Norwitz, MD, PhD, MBA
Tufts Medical Center and Tufts University School of Medicine, Boston, MA, USA

Elena Olearo, MD
University College London Hospital, UK

Michael J. Paech, MB BS, DRCOG, FRCA, FANZCA, FFPMANZCA, FRANZCOG (Hons), DM (Pharm)
Department of Anaesthesia and Pain Medicine, King Edward Memorial Hospital, University of Western Australia, Perth, Australia, and Division of Maternal-Fetal Medicine, Department of Obstetrics, Gynecology and Reproductive Sciences, University of California, San Francisco, CA, USA

Julian T. Parer, MD, PhD (deceased)
Division of Maternal-Fetal Medicine, Department of Obstetrics, Gynecology and Reproductive Sciences, University of California, San Francisco, CA, USA

Selina Patel, BMedSci, BMBS, FRCA
Department of Anesthesiology, Perioperative and Pain Medicine, University of Miami, Miller School of Medicine, Miami, FL, USA

Linzi Peacock, BSc (Hons), MB ChB (Hons), MRCP, FRCA
Department of Anaesthesia, Royal Infirmary of Edinburgh, Scotland, UK

Sioned Phillips, MB BS, MRCP, MCEM, FRCA, EDRA
Department of Anaesthesia, Frimley Park Hospital, Surrey, UK

Melissa Potisek, MD
Department of Anesthesiology, Wake Forest School of Medicine, Raleigh, NC, USA

Ellile Pushpanathan, BMedSci, BM BS, FRCA, MSc CRA
Guys and St Thomas' NHS Foundation Trust, London, UK

Karunakaran Ramaswamy DA FRCA MBA
Sidra Medicine, Doha, and Wiell Cornell Medical College, Qatar

Alexandra Reeve, MB BCh, BAO, LRCPI & SI (NUI) Hons, FCAI
Royal Berkshire NHS Foundation Trust, Reading, Berkshire, UK

Ian Renfrew, MB BS (Hons), MCRP, FRCR
Department of Interventional Radiology, Royal London Hospital, Whitechapel, London, UK

Neeti Sadana, MD
Obstetric Anesthesia, Department of Anesthesiology and Pain Management, University of Oklahoma Health Sciences Center, Oklahoma City, OK, USA

Frank Schroeder, MD, DEAA, FRCA, FFICM
St. George's University Hospitals NHS Foundation Trust, London, UK

Scott Segal, MD, MHCM
Wake Forest School of Medicine, Winston-Salem, NC, USA

Thunga Setty, MB ChB, FRCA
Department of Anaesthesia, Queens Medical Centre, Nottingham, UK

Andrew Shennan, OBE, MB BS, MD, FRCOG
Department of Women and Children's Health, School of Life Course Sciences, FoLSM, Kings College, London, UK

Simon Slinn, BSc, MB BCh (Hons), FRCA
Department of Anaesthesia, University Hospital of Wales, Cardiff, UK

Denis Snegovskikh, MD
Warren Alpert Medical School, Brown University, Providence, RI, USA

Adrienne Stewart, FRCA
Department of Anaesthesia and Perioperative Medicine, University College Hospital, London, UK

Gary Stocks, MB BS, BSc, FRCA
Department of Anaesthesia, Queen Charlotte's and Chelsea Hospital, Imperial College Healthcare NHS Trust, London, UK

Pervez Sultan, MB ChB, FRCA, MD (Res)
University College London Hospital and University College London

Lorna Swan, MB ChB, MD, FRCP
Department of Adult Congenital Heart Disease, Royal Brompton Hospital, London, UK

Chiraag Talati, BSc (Hons), MB BS, FRCA
Department of Anaesthesia, Homerton University Hospital NHS Foundation Trust, London, UK

Roulhac D. Toledano, MD, PhD
Department of Obstetric Anesthesia, Lutheran Medical Center, SUNY Downstate, Brooklyn, NY, USA

Han T. Truong, MB ChB, FANZCA
Department of Anaesthesia and Acute Pain Management, Hutt Valley District Health Board, Lower Hutt, New Zealand

Lawrence C. Tsen, MD
Division of Obstetric Anesthesia, Department of Anesthesiology, Perioperative and Pain Medicine, Brigham and Women's Hospital, Harvard Medical School, Boston, MA, USA

Sikha Shastham Valappil, MB BS, MD
Department of Anesthesia and Perioperative Medicine, Women's Wellness and Research Center, Hamad Medical Corporation, Doha, Qatar

Marc Van de Velde, MD, PhD, EDRA
Department of Cardiovascular Sciences KU Leuven, Department of Anesthesiology, University Hospitals Leuven, Belgium

Andre Vercueil, MB ChB, MRCP, FRCA, EDIC, FFICM
Christine Brown Critical Care Unit, King's College Hospital, London, UK

Nicola Vousden, MB BS, BSc
King's College London, and Department of Women's and Children's Health, St. Thomas' Hospital, London, UK

Michael Y. K. Wee, BSc (Hons), MB ChB, FRCA
Department of Anaesthesia, Poole Hospital NHS Foundation Trust, Poole, Dorset, UK

Carolyn F. Weiniger, MB ChB
Division of Anesthesia and Critical Care and Pain, Tel Aviv Sourasky Medical Center, Tel Aviv, Israel

Samantha Wilson, BSc, BMBCh, FRCA
Department of Anaesthesia, Basingstoke and North Hampshire Hospital, Hampshire Hospitals NHS Foundation Trust, Basingstoke, Hampshire, UK

Steve Yentis, BSc, MB BS, FRCA, MD, MA
Chelsea and Westminster Hospital, and Imperial College London, UK

Eating and Drinking in Labor

Risks versus Benefits

Nicola Vousden, Claire Daly, and Andrew Shennan

Case Study

A low-risk nulliparous patient was admitted for induction of labor at 40 + 5 weeks of gestation following spontaneous rupture of membranes 24 hours previously. She was given a prostaglandin pessary and encouraged to rest. She began to have mildly painful contractions, but after 1 g paracetamol (acetaminophen), she was comfortable and ate a light meal. Throughout the following 6 hours she became increasingly distressed and tearful. She was only 1 cm dilated, so she was given 5 mg IM diamorphine. This provided good analgesia but caused vomiting. Despite having 10 mg IM cyclizine, she continued to be nauseous and had little oral intake for the subsequent 6 hours. The fetal heart rate was normal.

Four hours later she complained that she was hungry, and her partner gave her soup and toast. She was reexamined but had not made any progress, so an oxytocin intravenous (IV) infusion was started and fetal monitoring using a cardiotocograph (CTG) was commenced. With the onset of contractions, there was a sudden fetal bradycardia lasting 3.5 minutes. A vaginal examination was performed at this time, and she was found to be only 2 cm dilated. The patient was moved into the left lateral position, and IV fluids were commenced. The fetal heart rate returned to baseline, but the fetus continued to show signs of distress for a further 40 minutes despite a further change in maternal position. The decision was made for the patient to have an emergency cesarean delivery. As per hospital protocol, she was given ranitidine 150 mg orally prior to transfer to operating theater.

The anesthetic trainee on duty tried twice to site her spinal anesthetic, but it proved very difficult. He called a colleague to attend from the main theater who also struggled to place the spinal and had two further unsuccessful attempts. The CTG remained a concern, and the obstetric team stressed the urgency for delivering by cesarean delivery because 40 minutes had

passed. In the circumstances, the patient's partner was asked to leave the theater, and the patient was given a general anesthetic using a technique that included a rapid-sequence induction. The patient was successfully intubated, and the surgery was commenced. A baby boy was delivered 2 minutes later and was initially pale with poor tone and an Apgar score of 4 at 1 minute. He was stimulated and given three inflation breaths before crying, and his Apgar score was 9 at 5 minutes. The cesarean delivery was complicated by uterine atony, resulting in a measured blood loss of 900 ml. This was managed with an additional oxytocin bolus of 5 units alongside an ongoing oxytocin infusion. The patient was transferred to an obstetric high-dependency bed for recovery, which was uncomplicated.

Key Points

- This patient initially had an uneventful induction of labor and was eating small amounts at her discretion. She started vomiting after IM diamorphine injection and had no oral intake for several hours.
- After feeling better, she requested to eat and was provided with a light meal but then unexpectedly required an emergency general anesthetic for fetal compromise. She routinely had received ranitidine preoperatively.
- The general anesthetic was conducted successfully without complication.
- This case illustrates that many women will have eaten to some degree in labor and, in spite of no risk factors, will commonly receive opioid-based drugs that may influence gastric emptying and the risk of aspiration.
- It also demonstrates that women needing operative delivery and anesthesia cannot be easily identified in early labor.

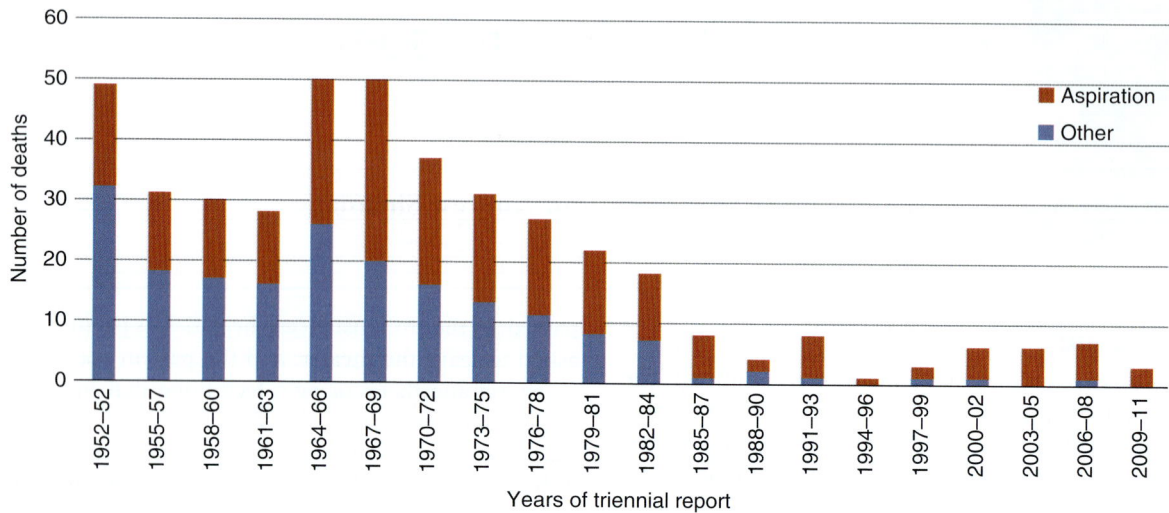

Figure 1.1 Graph showing triennial rates of maternal death from aspiration compared with other anesthetic causes. Source: Data collated from Confidential Enquiry into Maternal and Child Health from 1952 to 2011.

Discussion

Historically, oral intake during labor was widely acknowledged as a risk for pulmonary aspiration. This was following publication of a now-classic observational study by Mendelson in 1946 in which an association was made between aspiration during general anesthesia and feeding during labor.[1] This lead to the introduction of nil by mouth (NPO) policies being used during labor with the aim of reducing the risk of aspiration should a general anesthetic be required. Obstetric anesthesia practice has developed considerably since then with increased use of regional anesthesia and safer general anesthetic practice. This, in addition to concern that fasting may be detrimental to labor, has lead to considerable research in this field. Several authorities have relaxed their recommendations, but practice varies widely. The NICE intrapartum care guideline (2014) recommends that women can drink during established labor and may eat a light diet unless they have received opioids or they develop risk factors that make a general anesthetic more likely.[2] The American Congress of Obstetricians and Gynecologists made a recommendation to allow intake of only clear liquids in 2009 (reaffirmed in 2015).[3] Despite this increase in oral intake, there has been a dramatic decline in pulmonary aspiration in obstetrics over the last 60 years,[4,5] as demonstrated in Figure 1.1. This chapter aims to discuss the risks versus benefits of eating in labor given the current anesthetic practices.

Is There Any Value to Eating in Labor?

Labor can be prolonged, and considerable caloric expenditure may be involved. There is belief by some clinicians and midwives that calorific intake in labor may be beneficial to the mother, fetus, and the labor process. Evidence regarding required nutrition during labor is limited.

Labor has been shown to cause maternal ketosis, which is improved with isotonic drink consumption, but the impact of this on maternal and fetal well-being is unknown.[6] It may be more appropriate to consider whether important clinical outcomes are affected by oral intake in labor, rather than metabolic disturbance. A Cochrane review undertaken in 2013[7] included five studies on restriction of oral intake compared with eating during active labor and found little evidence of clinical benefit, even though there were sufficient numbers to detect important clinical differences. There was no significant difference in the rates of cesarean delivery, duration of labor, operative vaginal deliveries, Apgar scores, admission to neonatal special care, and maternal nausea or vomiting.[8] Therefore, it is unlikely that any physiologic changes resulting from fasting or indeed eating during labor have a significant impact on maternal or fetal outcome.

Labor can be a stressful time, and restrictions on oral intake may be an additional distress for some women. Additionally, nausea and vomiting occur frequently in labor, and therefore many women may not wish to eat. Nevertheless, clinicians should be sensitive to patient requests.

Is There Any Harm in Eating in Labor?

The most serious risk of oral intake during labor is of aspiration should a general anesthetic be required. This is exceptionally rare. There have been approximately 10 million deliveries over the last 15 years in the United Kingdom, during which time only four fatal cases of aspiration have been reported.[4] This is despite an overall increase in the rate of cesarean deliveries and operative deliveries and a significantly more relaxed approach to oral intake during labor. The reasons for this are likely to be multifactorial. A possible factor is the reduction in the number of general anesthetics for cesarean deliveries in favor of regional anesthesia. However, the number of cesarean deliveries performed has increased, and thus the absolute decrease in the number of general anesthetics is marginal.[8] What is clear is that the increase in oral intake has had little impact on severe morbidity and mortality.

The Cochrane review of eating in labor did not have sufficient evidence to detect differences in rates of pulmonary aspiration.[7] It was the opinion of the Cochrane authors that because there is no evidence of benefit or harm, there is no justification for restriction of fluids and food in labor for low- or high-risk women. However, pulmonary aspiration is so rare that it is a challenging endpoint to investigate. Even large multicenter trials will not have adequate power to detect differences in aspiration risk, and the current meta-analysis cannot provide evidence of safety. Therefore, it should really be argued that there is insufficient evidence to determine whether it is safe to eat, given that it is accepted practice to avoid oral intake prior to anesthesia.

Who Should Eat, What to Eat, and When to Eat?

The commonly recognized patient factors for aspiration are obesity and airway management problems, which can cause air to inflate the stomach and potentially increase gastroesophageal reflux.[8] However, the volume and nature of gastric contents are likely to be equally, if not more, important.[8]

Normally, gastric emptying depends on the pressure gradient between the stomach and the duodenum, as well as the volume, caloric density, and pH of the gastric fluid. Clear liquids are emptied from the stomach very quickly (mean half-time of ~10 minutes[9]), which means that 95 percent of the contents are emptied within 1 hour.[10,11] Solids are much slower to empty, with a mean half-time of 2 hours depending on the caloric density of the food,[12] meaning that between 10 and 30 percent will remain in the stomach 6 hours after ingestion.[13] Gastric emptying is also delayed following opioid administration and in diabetic patients. In the pregnant population, gastric emptying is not delayed in healthy, term, nonlaboring patients.[12–14] This is true for women with both a normal[14] and a raised body mass index (BMI).[15] Therefore, the obstetric anesthesia guideline approved by the American Society of Anesthesiologists' (ASA) House of Delegates in 2006 is that uncomplicated pregnant women undergoing elective cesarean delivery should adhere to the same preoperative fasting plan as nonpregnant women.[16] This is to be fasted for 6 hours prior to an elective procedure with clear fluids up until 2 hours before.[17]

While the rate of gastric emptying in pregnancy is the same, several studies report that it is delayed in labor, as confirmed by bedside ultrasonography of the cross-sectional antral area,[18] as shown in Figure 1.2, and acetaminophen absorption rates after delivery.[12] There is limited evidence on the recommended duration of fasting prior to emergency cesarean delivery, and given the unpredictable nature of labor, it would not be feasible to make guidelines for this. A more pragmatic approach would be to identify patients at greatest risk of requiring operative delivery and advise them on an individual basis.

Preoperative medications such as histamine-2 receptor antagonists are used frequently to increase gastric pH and reduce gastric volumes. In the nonpregnant adult population, they have been shown to significantly reduce gastric volume and increase gastric pH.[19] However, their routine use for elective surgery in the healthy population is not recommended because they are not effective in all patients and are relatively slow acting and expensive.[19] Pregnant women are thought, however, to be at high risk of aspiration because progesterone reduces the competency of the lower esophageal sphincter in the presence of increased intra-abdominal pressure from an enlarged uterus. A meta-analysis of 2,658 pregnant patients demonstrate that antacids, proton pump inhibitors, and histamine-2 receptor antagonists all significantly reduced the risk of gastric pH less than 2.5.[20] While these agents have not been proven to

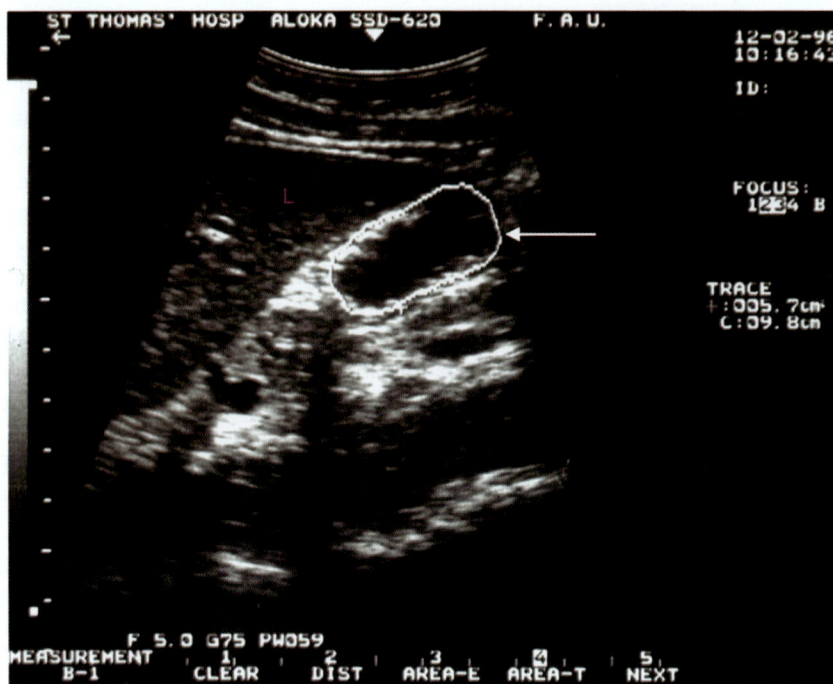

Figure 1.2 Gastric antral ultrasound demonstrating gastric volume in pregnancy

reduce morbidity or mortality, physiologically, their use seems justifiable. The NICE guideline for cesarean delivery (2011) recommends that women be given antacids and medications to reduce gastric acid prior to cesarean delivery.[21]

What Should Women Be Told?

Women should be informed that they have a choice whether to have food or drink in labor. They should be warned that labor itself or drugs given for analgesia may influence their appetite. It is not necessary to consume calories if they do not wish to because there is no proven benefit in doing so. Labor and/or the drugs given may also increase the risk of nausea and vomiting. If patients do wish to drink, they should be advised to take isotonic calorific fluids. If they wish to eat, they should be advised to choose low-residue foods. They can be informed that the risks of oral intake in labor are extremely low. If the risk of operative delivery increases due to circumstances of labor, patients may be advised to go NPO and be given interventions such as antacids to reduce the risk of aspiration. Women can be informed that the risk of aspiration is related to having general anesthetics, which are rarely given in labor because most procedures can be performed using regional anesthesia.

Summary

In summary, fasting in labor is not known to be harmful to mother or baby. Aspiration is an extremely rare event, but whether this justifies the risk of relaxing recommendations on oral intake in low-risk laboring women remains unknown. As in this case, it is probably justifiable to allow normal, low-risk women to eat a light diet if they are informed of the risks and they wish to do so. However, close attention is required because this risk may change throughout labor. In this case, the patient received diamorphine, and there were signs of fetal compromise. Therefore, she should have been advised not to eat. Practices that reduce this risk, such as optimal premedication, ranitidine in this case, and senior clinician involvement, should be encouraged. In the absence of evidence demonstrating that eating in labor is safe, it would be prudent for patients at higher risk of requiring a general anesthetic, such as patients with a high BMI or anticipated difficulty with regional anesthesia, to be advised not to eat. Carbohydrate drinks may be a suitable alternative to provide some maternal comfort.

Learning Points

- Feeding or fasting during labor is not known to be harmful to mother or baby in normal labor.
- Aspiration is an extremely rare event; this probably justifies relaxing recommendations on oral intake in low-risk laboring women.
- Steps to reduce risk such as preoperative medication to reduce gastric pH and volume and senior clinician involvement are encouraged in women with risk factors including the risk of anesthesia.

References

1. Mendelson CL. The aspiration of stomach contents into the lungs during obstetric anesthesia. *Am J Obstet Gynecol* 1946; **52**:191–206.

2. National Institute for Health and Care Excellence. *Intrapartum Care for Healthy Women and Babies* (NICE Clinical Guideline 190). London: National Institute for Health and Care Excellence; 2014. Available at www.nice.org.uk/guidance/cg190/chapter/1-recommendations#care-throughout-labour (accessed August 24, 2016).

3. Committee on Obstetric Practice, American College of Obstetricians and Gynecologists. Oral intake during labor (ACOG Committee Opinion No. 441). *Obstet Gynecol* 2009; **114**(3):714.

4. Department of Health, Welsh Office, Scottish Home and Health Department, and Department of Health and Social Services, Northern Ireland. *Report on Confidential Enquiries into Maternal Deaths in the United Kingdom 1988–1990*. London: HMSO; 1994.

5. Lewis G, ed. *Saving Mothers' Lives: Reviewing Maternal Deaths to Make Motherhood Safer, 2003–2005. The Seventh Report on Confidential Enquiries into Maternal Deaths in the United Kingdom*. London: CEMACH; 2007.

6. Kubli M, Scrutton MJ, Seed PT, O'Sullivan G. An evaluation of isotonic "sport drinks" during labor. *Obstet Anesth* 2002; **94**:404–8.

7. Singata M, Tranmer J, Gyte GML. Restricting oral fluid and food intake during labour. *Cochrane Database Syst Rev* 2013; **8**:CD003930. DOI: 10.1002/14651858. CD003930.pub3

8. O'Sullivan G, Liu B, Shennan AH. Oral intake during labor. *Int Anesthesiol Clin* 2007; **45**(1):133–47.

9. Soreide E, Eriksson LI, Hirlekar G, et al. Pre-operative fasting guidelines: an update. *Acta Anaesthesiol Scand* 2005; **49**:1041–47.

10. Meakin G, Murat I. Immediate preoperative preparation, in Sumner E, Hatch DJ (eds.), *Paediatric Anaesthesia*. London: Arnold; 1999, pp. 71–93.

11. Read NW, Houghton LA. Physiology of gastric emptying and pathophysiology of gastroparesis. *Gastroenterol Clin North Am* 1989; **18**: 359–73.

12. Whitehead EM, Smith M, Dean Y, O'Sullivan G. An evaluation of gastric emptying times in pregnancy and the puerperium. *Anaesthesia* 1993; **48**(1):53–57.

13. Phillips S, Daborn AK, Hatch DJ. Preoperative fasting for paediatric anaesthesia, *Br J Anaesth* 1994; **73**: 529–36.

14. Wong CA, Loffredi M, Ganchiff JN, et al. Gastric emptying of water in term pregnancy. *Anesthesiology* 2002; **96**:1395–40.

15. Wong CA, McCarthy RJ, Fitzgerald PC, Raikoff K, Avram MJ. Gastric emptying of water in obese pregnant women at term. *Anaesth Analg* 2007; **105**(3): 761–65.

16. American Society of Anesthesiologists Task Force on Obstetric Anesthesia. Practice guidelines for obstetric anesthesia. *Anesthesiology* 2007; **106**:843–63.

17. Verma R, Kwee MYK, Hartle A, et al. AAGBI Safety Guideline: Pre-operative Assessment and Patient Preparation, the Role of the Anaesthetist, 2010. Available at www.aagbi.org/sites/default/files/preop2010.pdf (accessed August 13, 2015).

18. Bataille A, Rousset J, Marret E, Bonnet F. Ultrasonographic evaluation of gastric content during labour under epidural analgesia: a prospective cohort study. *Br J Anaesth* 2014; **112**(4):703–7.

19. Westby M, Bullock I, Gray W, Lardner-Browne C, Rashid R. Clinical Practice Guidelines: Preoperative Fasting in Adults and Children, a Royal College of Nursing Guideline for the Multidisciplinary Team, 2005. Available at www.rcn.org.uk/__data/assets/pdf_file/0009/78678/002800.pdf (accessed August 13, 2015).

20. Paranjothy S, Griffiths JD, Broughton HK, et al. Interventions at caesarean section for reducing the risk of aspiration pneumonitis. *Int J Obstet Anesth* 2010; **20**(2):142–48.

21. National Institute for Health and Care Excellence. *Caesarean Section* (NICE Clinical Guideline No. 132). London: National Institute for Health and Care Excellence; 2005. Available at www.nice.org.uk/guidance/cg132/resources/guidance-caesarean-section-pdf (accessed August 13, 2015).

Epidural Analgesia Maintenance

Thierry Girard

Case Study

A primiparous 24-year-old parturient with 38 + 4 weeks of gestation requires labor analgesia at 11 P.M. The cervical dilation is minimal. An 18-gauge multi-orifice epidural catheter was inserted at the L3–L4 interspace with a loss of resistance at 4.5 cm. Depth of insertion was 9.5 cm from the skin, which corresponds to 5 cm of catheter within the epidural space. After negative aspiration, an initial epidural loading dose of 15 ml of a mixture containing bupivacaine 0.1% (1 mg/ml) with 2 µg fentanyl per milliliter was administered. At 11.45 P.M., the pain score decreased from an initial 90/100 to 30/100. The parturient's blood pressure remained stable, and she retained full motor strength of her lower extremities. Thereafter, patient-controlled epidural analgesia (PCEA) was started with the same epidural solution, allowing the parturient a 5-ml PCEA bolus with a lockout time of 20 minutes. At 1 A.M., the anesthesiologist was called to address breakthrough pain with a pain score of 60/100. Cervical dilation was 3 cm. Sensory level was at T11 bilaterally, and lower extremity motor function remained unaffected. Fifteen minutes following a manual bolus of 8 ml of the epidural solution, the parturient reported a pain score of 30/100. At 3 A.M. the anesthesiologist applied another manual bolus to address breakthrough pain. Thereafter, he decided to run an epidural background infusion of 7 ml/h bupivacaine 0.1% with fentanyl 2 µg/ml. No further intervention was requested to address breakthrough pain. At 11 A.M., a healthy 3.5-kg male baby was delivered via ventouse. At removal of the epidural catheter, the patient was very happy with her pain control and somewhat disappointed about her inability to bend both of her knees during the last 2 hours before delivery.

Key Points

- Labor epidural analgesia was established with patient-controlled epidural analgesia (PCEA).
- Following breakthrough pain, a background infusion was added to the analgesia regime.
- The patient experienced improved analgesia but additional lower extremity motor block.

Discussion

Local Anesthetic Solutions for Maintenance of Labor Epidural Analgesia

The synergistic effect of local anesthetics and lipophilic opioid allows the use of solutions with low concentrations of local anesthetics. Typical mixtures use bupivacaine ≤ 0.1% (1 mg/ml) or ropivacaine ≤ 0.125% (1.25 mg/ml) combined with either fentanyl 2 µg/ml or sufentanil 0.5–1 µg/ml. This results in a reduction in total dose of local anesthetic, although the injected volume has been shown to be more important than the dose.[1,2] When compared with higher concentrations, low-dose epidural analgesia has the advantage of less motor block, more ambulation, less urinary retention, higher patient satisfaction, and fewer instrumental deliveries.[2–5]

Bupivacaine versus Ropivacaine

"Differential blockade" with substantially less motor block was believed to be a particular property of ropivacaine. Ropivacaine is an S-enantiomer that has approximately 75 percent of the potency of bupivacaine. If this reduced potency is taken into account, then there is little or no difference in the occurrence of motor block between these two local anesthetics.[2,4] Ropivacaine is associated with a lower risk of serious cardiotoxicity compared with bupivacaine.[6] The IV dose causing CNS symptoms in healthy (nonpregnant) volunteers was 99 and 124 mg with bupivacaine and ropivacaine, respectively.[6] However, with the current practice of using low concentrations of local anesthetics in labor analgesia, there is no clinically relevant difference in safety between bupivacaine and ropivacaine.

Patient-Controlled Epidural Analgesia

There are different options for maintaining epidural labor analgesia. The "low-tech" solution is a manual injection either by the midwife or by the anesthesiologist. This manual injection can be on a regular basis (e.g., every hour) or on maternal request. The downside is the potential time lag between request and delivery of the drug, as well as dependence on physical presence. Another potential limitation is the frequent manipulation at the epidural filter with the risks of infection and drug errors. These disadvantages can be overcome with an infusion pump or syringe pump for PCEA. A predefined volume is triggered by the parturient with a defined lockout period. Addition of a background infusion – usually between 3 and 8 ml/h of the epidural solution – reduces the number of interventions by the physician.[2,5]

Breakthrough Pain

Breakthrough pain might be due to the epidural catheter or to obstetrical reasons, such as dystocia. Lack of adequate sensory blockade can be a sign of intravascular catheter migration, which is even possible after several hours of fully functional epidural labor analgesia.[7] Unilateral analgesia can be due to anatomic barriers in the epidural space but is more likely to be due to lateral deviation of the catheter. Frequently, the catheter is withdrawn by 0.5–1 cm to resolve this issue, but this is not very likely to be successful[8] unless the catheter is at more than 5 cm epidural depth.[9]

Inadequate analgesia is less frequent with multiorifice catheters.[10] Frequently, a manual bolus of 5–10 ml of the solution used for PCEA can significantly improve analgesia. The substantially higher pressure generated by a manual bolus results in wider spread in the epidural space.[11] In fact, the number of activated catheter orifices depends on the speed of injection.[12] If a manual bolus does not improve analgesia and the extension of sensory block is adequate, a bolus of local anesthetic in higher concentrations, such as lignocaine 1% or bupivacaine 0.25%, might be helpful. The issue with the latter solution is that it might well result in motor block. Lower extremity motor block despite inadequate analgesia most likely represents epidural maldistribution. A manually injected bolus might improve analgesia.

Table 2.1 Modified Bromage Score

Score	Extent of motor block
1	Complete block (unable to move feet or knees)
2	Almost complete block (able to move feet only)
3	Partial block (just able to move knees)
4	Detectable weakness of hip flexion while supine (between scores 3 and 5)
5	No detectable weakness of hip flexion while supine (full flexion of knees)
6	Able to stand and to perform partial knee bend

Source: Breen et al.[13]

Generally inadequate analgesia should be resolved in a timely manner. If simple measures are unsuccessful, then the best solution is probably to replace the epidural catheter.

Lower Extremity Motor Block

Lower extremity motor function should be quantified in order to compare the effect of different modes of epidural labor analgesia on motor function. The most frequently used scoring system is the modified Bromage score[13] (Table 2.1).

The use of low-dose epidural solutions has substantially decreased the incidence of lower extremity motor block. Maintenance of lower extremity muscle strength is not only important for ambulation. In fact, not many women opt for ambulation, but retaining their normal motor function increases satisfaction.[2-4] There might be an association between the occurrence of lower extremity motor block and an increased rate of assisted vaginal deliveries.[4,14] The problem with continuous infusion of local anesthetics is a concentration effect at the site of administration, which intensifies the block in a limited area and thus leads to development of motor block over time.[15]

Novel Concepts for Maintenance of Labor Analgesia

As mentioned earlier, the spread of local anesthetics depends on the speed of injection. The addition of a background infusion to a PCEA reduces the need for interventions by clinicians. If a background infusion is not given continuously (e.g., 5 ml/h) but as a timed bolus (e.g., 5 ml every hour), then this can lead to a wider epidural spread of local anesthetics. This effect depends on the speed of injection, as well as on the resistance of the catheter and the pressure generated by the pump.[15] It has been shown that injection speeds of 280 ml/h or more are needed to activate all three orifices of 20-gauge epidural catheters.[12] Theoretical advantages of an intermittent boluses are improved analgesia and a reduction in lower extremity motor block.

Programmed Intermittent Epidural Boluses

With a programmed intermittent epidural bolus (PIEB), the background infusion is replaced with a programmed bolus at predefined intervals. The parturient is still allowed to request PCEA boluses. Several variations of bolus volumes and different time intervals have been investigated.[16] Larger boluses of up to 10 ml bupivacaine 0.0625% with longer intervals of up to 60 minutes proved to be most efficient.[16] In a recent clinical study comparing PIEB and PCEA with background infusion, the PIEB group had significantly less lower extremity motor block and a significant reduction in assisted vaginal delivery, from 20 to 7 percent.[14] At present, this remains the only study with such favorable results.[17] While the study was performed with interconnected pumps and different concentrations of local anesthetics, modern pumps are able to deliver a PIEB protocol in a single pump. There are two intervals to be set: the PIEB interval and the PCEA lockout time. If a PIEB bolus is to be delivered within a PCEA lockout interval, then the PIEB bolus is postponed accordingly (Figure 2.1). The optimal protocol for timing and volume of the bolus has not yet been determined. This most probably depends on the size of the epidural catheter and the speed of injection. In our institution, we use a 20-gauge multiorifice epidural catheter with bupivacaine 0.1% and fentanyl 2 μg/ml with the following settings: PIEB bolus 5 ml, PIEB interval 60 minutes, injection speed 250 ml/h.

Variable-Frequency Automated Mandatory Boluses

Another modification of intermittent boluses was presented by Sia et al.[18] Following initiation of labor analgesia with a combined spinal epidural (CSE), patients were randomly assigned to either PCEA and background infusion (5 ml/h) or PCEA and variable-frequency automated mandatory boluses. The authors used ropivacaine 0.1% with fentanyl 2 μg/ml. Delivery of a variable-frequency mandatory bolus depends on

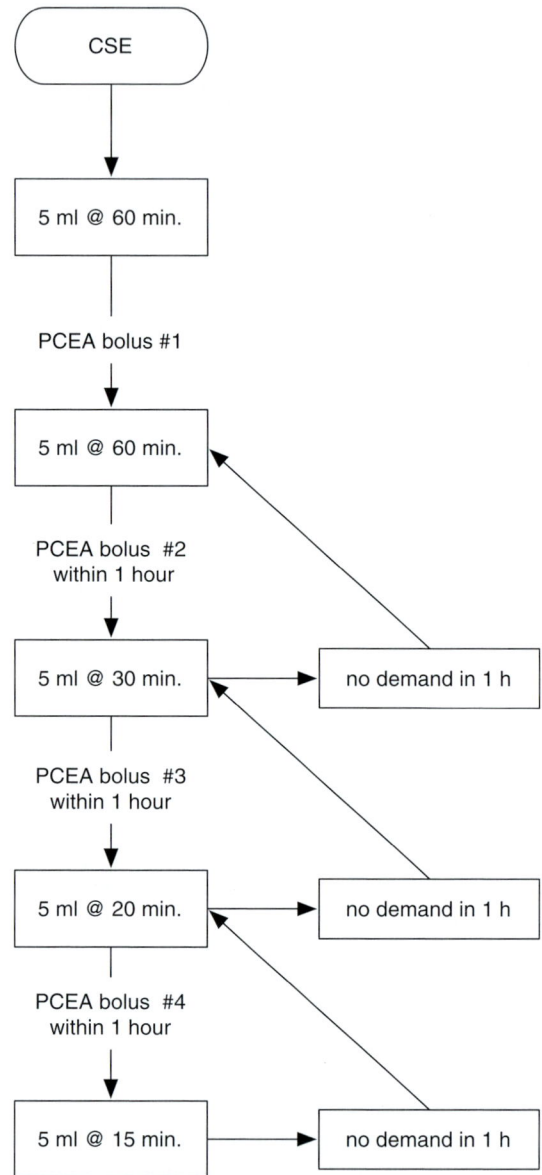

Figure 2.1 Schematic of the variable-frequency automated mandatory bolus regimen

the history of PCEA bolus requests. The initial interval is 60 minutes. If the parturient requires two boluses within 60 minutes, then the interval is shortened to 30 minutes. In case of a third demand within 60 minutes, mandatory boluses are delivered every 20 minutes, and if the parturient demands four PCEA boluses per hour, then the mandatory interval is decreased to 15 minutes. If no PCEA bolus is requested during 60 minutes, then the interval of mandatory boluses is prolonged by 15 minutes[18] (Figure 2.1). This schema leads to a significant reduction in breakthrough pain and increased patient satisfaction compared with the PCEA group. Duration of the second stage of labor and total local anesthetic consumption were not different between the groups. However, the number of machine-delivered boluses during the second stage of labor was approximately doubled in the variable-frequency mandatory bolus group.

Variable-frequency automated mandatory boluses seem to be an exciting (although not yet commercially available) new method to provide epidural labor analgesia.

Learning Points

- Low-dose solutions (i.e., mixtures of low-concentrated local anesthetics with lipophilic opioids) are the standard for maintenance of epidural labor analgesia.
- PCEA with or without a background infusion is the most frequently used method for maintenance of epidural labor analgesia.
- Breakthrough pain frequently can be treated with a manual bolus. Timely replacement of the epidural should be considered if simple measures are unsuccessful.
- Speed of injection determines the number of catheter orifices to be activated and the spread of local anesthetics in the epidural space.
- Avoidance of lower extremity motor block increases patient satisfaction.
- Substituting a background infusion with automated intermittent boluses has the potential to further reduce lower extremity motor block and influence the mode of delivery.

References

1. Lyons GR, Kocarev MG, Wilson RC, et al. A comparison of minimum local anesthetic volumes and doses of epidural bupivacaine (0.125% w/v and 0.25% w/v) for analgesia in labor. *Anesth Analg* 2007; **104**:412–15.

2. Halpern SH, Carvalho B. Patient-controlled epidural analgesia for labor. *Anesth Analg* 2009; **108**:921–28.

3. Sultan P, Murphy C, Halpern S, Carvalho B. The effect of low concentrations versus high concentrations of local anesthetics for labour analgesia on obstetric and anesthetic outcomes: a meta-analysis. *Can J Anesth* 2013; **60**:840–54.

4. Stewart A, Fernando R. Maternal ambulation during labor. *Curr Opin Anaesthesiol* 2011; **24**:268–73.

5. Loubert C, Hinova A, Fernando R. Update on modern neuraxial analgesia in labour: a review of the literature of the last 5 years. *Anaesthesia* 2011; **66**:191–212.

6. Mather LE, Chang DH. Cardiotoxicity with modern local anaesthetics: is there a safer choice? *Drugs* 2001; **61**: 333–42.

7. Norris MC. Are combined spinal-epidural catheters reliable? *Int J Obstet Anesth* 2000; **9**:3–6.

8. Beilin Y, Zahn J, Bernstein HH, et al. Treatment of incomplete analgesia after placement of an epidural catheter and administration of local anesthetic for women in labor. *Anesthesiology* 1998; **88**:1502–6.

9. Beilin Y, Bernstein HH, Zucker-Pinchoff B. The optimal distance that a multiorifice epidural catheter should be threaded into the epidural space. *Anesth Analg* 1995; **81**:301–4.

10. Segal S, Eappen S, Datta S. Superiority of multi-orifice over single-orifice epidural catheters for labor analgesia and cesarean delivery. *J Clin Anesth* 1997; **9**:109–12.

11. Hogan Q. Epidural catheter tip position and distribution of injectate evaluated by computed tomography. *Anesthesiology* 1999; **90**:964–70.

12. Fegley AJ, Lerman J, Wissler R. Epidural multiorifice catheters function as single-orifice catheters: an in vitro study. *Anesth Analg* 2008; **107**:1079–81.

13. Breen TW, Shapiro T, Glass B, Foster-Payne D, Oriol NE. Epidural anesthesia for labor in an ambulatory patient. *Anesth Analg* 1993; 77:919–24.

14. Capogna G, Camorcia M, Stirparo S, Farcomeni A. Programmed intermittent epidural bolus versus continuous epidural infusion for labor analgesia: the effects on maternal motor function and labor outcome. A randomized double-blind study in nulliparous women. *Anesth Analg* 2011; **113**:826–31.

15. Capogna G, Stirparo S. Techniques for the maintenance of epidural labor analgesia. *Curr Opin Anaesthesiol* 2013; **26**:261–67.

16. Wong CA, McCarthy RJ, Hewlett B. The effect of manipulation of the programmed intermittent bolus time interval and injection volume on total drug use for labor epidural analgesia: a randomized controlled trial. *Anesth Analg* 2011; **112**:904–11.

17. George RB, Allen TK, Habib AS. Intermittent epidural bolus compared with continuous epidural infusions for labor analgesia: a systematic review and meta-analysis. *Anesth Analg* 2013; **116**:133–44.

18. Sia ATH, Leo S, Ocampo CE. A randomised comparison of variable-frequency automated mandatory boluses with a basal infusion for patient-controlled epidural analgesia during labour and delivery. *Anaesthesia* 2013; **68**:267–75.

Breakthrough Pain after Labor Epidural Analgesia

Nakiyah Knibbs and Yaakov Beilin

Case Study

An otherwise healthy nulliparous 26-year-old woman at 40 weeks' gestation presented to the labor and delivery unit. She was scheduled for induction of labor and was not experiencing uterine contractions at that time. On vaginal examination, her cervix was closed and not effaced.

She requested labor analgesia prior to the start of labor induction. An epidural catheter was placed by the anesthesiologist using the loss of resistance to air technique without complications. The catheter was threaded 5 cm into the epidural space. Patient-controlled epidural analgesia was started with a 15-ml bolus of bupivacaine 0.0625% and fentanyl 2 μg/ml and then maintained with a 10 ml/h basal infusion of the same solution.

Four hours later, the patient complained of numbness on her left side and increasing discomfort on her right side. On physical examination, she was unable to move her left leg but had complete range of motion of her right leg.

The patient was positioned laterally with her right (painful) side in the dependent position, and a bolus of 5 ml of bupivacaine 0.25% was administered through the epidural catheter. Over the next 15 minutes, her pain was reassessed, and no difference was observed. The epidural catheter was pulled back 1 cm, and a dose of 10 ml of lidocaine 2% was given. After an additional 10 minutes, the patient felt some relief on the right side but was still visibly uncomfortable.

The decision was made to replace her epidural catheter using the combined spinal epidural technique. She received 25 μg of intrathecal fentanyl prior to insertion of an epidural catheter. The maintenance infusion of bupivacaine and fentanyl was restarted. She remained comfortable until delivery 5 hours later.

Key Points

- This patient experienced inadequate labor analgesia, specifically a unilateral or patchy block.

- Multiple interventions were used to correct her incomplete analgesia without success.
- Ultimately, the procedure was repeated employing the combined spinal-epidural technique.

Discussion

Neuraxial analgesia is commonly used to mitigate the pain associated with labor. Its popularity has increased secondary to both its efficacy and its safety. From the anesthesiologist's perspective, the epidural catheter provides a means not only of labor analgesia but also of surgical anesthesia if an operative procedure such as cesarean delivery is required. During progressive stages of labor, the volume and/or concentration of local anesthetic administered through the epidural catheter can be altered to maintain adequate analgesia. Also, an adjunct, such as an opioid, can be added to the local anesthetic to minimize side effects (e.g., hypotension and motor block). The catheter is used to maintain a low dermatomal level of analgesia for labor; T10–L1 for the first stage of labor and additionally S2–S4 for the second stage. If necessary, the dermatomal level can be raised to T4 for cesarean delivery.

Although epidural analgesia is considered the "gold standard" for labor analgesia, inadequate analgesia can occur in up to 15 percent of epidural catheter placements.[1] Pan et al.[2] reviewed approximately 19,259 deliveries, of which 12,590 had neuraxial analgesia. The overall failure rate was 12 percent, with a 14 percent failure rate with epidural techniques and 10 percent with the combined spinal epidural (CSE) technique. Even when adequate analgesia was established initially, 6.8 percent still required epidural catheter replacement due to the development of inadequate analgesia as labor progressed. During cesarean delivery, 7 percent of the epidural catheters placed failed. In another study, Eappen et al.[3] found that 13.1 percent of all epidural catheters required replacement. Inadequate labor analgesia not only

Table 3.1 Factors Associated with Inadequate Labor Epidural Analgesia

Advanced age
Morbid obesity
Scoliosis
Spinal disc surgery
Multiparity
History of prior failed epidural catheter
Cervical dilatation > 7 cm

leads to a dissatisfied patient but can also be more serious if an urgent cesarean delivery is required and an adequate level of anesthesia cannot be readily achieved. It may also lead to legal action.[4]

Risk Factors

Many patient factors can influence the rate of inadequate labor epidural analgesia (Table 3.1). These include advanced age,[3] morbid obesity, scoliosis (whether corrected or not), and a history of spinal disc surgery. Additionally, multiparity, history of a previous failure of epidural analgesia, and cervical dilatation greater than 7 cm at insertion are associated with inadequate epidural analgesia.[5]

Tonidandel et al.[6] retrospectively examined the differences in obstetric and anesthetic outcomes, including failed epidural rate, between 230 morbidly obese parturients (weight > 136 kg) and their matched controls (weight < 113 kg). The rate of repeat procedures due to inadequate pain control or failure to achieve bilateral dermatomal sensory levels was significantly greater in the morbidly obese group (17 versus 3 percent).

In a literature review of neuraxial procedures in parturients with scoliosis, Ko and Leffert[7] found that patchy, asymmetric or unilateral blocks were seen in 8% of patients without surgical correction. Failed placement or multiple attempts at placement occurred 4% of the time. Patients who had undergone surgical scoliosis correction had greater rates of neuraxial anesthesia complications than those without correction, including failed placement (22 percent) and multiple placement attempts (13 percent).

Patients are often concerned that their history of lumbar spine surgery, unrelated to scoliosis, will preclude them from receiving labor neuraxial analgesia. Bauchat et al.[8] found no difference in time to epidural placement or local anesthetic consumption in patients with a history of lumbar discectomy compared with

control individuals. However, the number of interspaces attempted prior to successful placement was greater in the discectomy group (more than one interspace attempted, 17 versus 2 percent).

Preventing or Avoiding Inadequate Analgesia

It is best if one can avoid or reduce the occurrence of inadequate analgesia in the first place, and this requires attention to detail during placement of the block and an understanding of the anatomy of the neuraxis.

Placement Techniques

The key to successful placement of an epidural or combined spinal epidural (CSE) is finding the midline. This is accomplished by palpating the spinous processes and rolling the fingers in both medial-to-lateral and cephalad-to-caudad directions. At times, the spinous processes cannot be felt, and an approximation of the midline can be achieved by drawing a line from the seventh cervical vertebral (C7) spinous process, which is generally prominent even in the morbidly obese, and the gluteal cleft.

Some clinicians also use ultrasound to assist in finding the midline. In a randomized trial, Grau et al.[9] found fewer insertion attempts were required when using spinal ultrasound prior to epidural placement than with palpation alone (2.6 ± 1.4 attempts in the ultrasound group versus 1.5 ± 0.9 attempts in the palpation group). However, Arzola et al.[10] found no difference in the number of attempts or median epidural insertion time in a study that randomized patients with easily palpated landmarks to either pre-epidural spinal ultrasound or palpation only. For a complete discussion of the role of ultrasound in obstetric anesthesia, see Chapter 6.

After the midline is found and the skin is adequately anesthetized, the epidural needle is advanced into the space using a loss of resistance to air or saline technique. In a randomized study, Beilin et al.[11] found that the saline technique was superior to the air technique with regard to the ultimate success of the block as well as fewer complications. However, others have questioned this finding, particularly if it requires the practitioner to use a technique he or she may not otherwise use.[12] In a meta-analysis of seven studies involving over 800 patients undergoing epidural placement, Antibas et al.[13] found that there was no difference in identification of the epidural space or reduction of complications when using either an air or saline loss-of-resistance technique.

The distance the catheter is threaded is important to increase the likelihood that the catheter will remain in the midline within the epidural space. Beilin et al.[14] found that threading a multiorifice catheter 5 cm into the epidural space, compared with 3 or 7 cm, is associated with a greater analgesic success rate. The use of multiorifice catheters is associated with a more even distribution of local anesthetic and a lower incidence of a "patchy" block – requiring less manipulation than single-orifice catheters.[15] Additionally, wire-reinforced flexible catheters demonstrate a lower incidence of intravascular cannulation, paresthesia, and inadequate analgesia than stiffer catheters.[16]

Combined Spinal-Epidural versus Epidural Technique

The CSE technique is associated with both better initial analgesia and fewer subsequent failures. The difference in success rate with CSE versus epidural has been reported in many studies. Pan et al.[2] reported a significantly lower incidence of inadequate analgesia when using the CSE technique compared with epidural analgesia (4.2 versus 8.4 percent). In another study, Norris[17] found that epidural catheters were more likely to fail, defined as lack of analgesia or sensory change, compared with those inserted as part of the CSE technique (1.3 versus 0.2 percent). Eappen et al.[3] reported a lower epidural catheter replacement rate with CSE than with the epidural technique. However, the replacement rate appeared to be inversely proportional to the experience of the anesthesia provider. The mechanisms by which CSE provides these advantages may include the presence of a confirmatory endpoint (i.e., the presence of spinal fluid), in addition to loss of resistance, to gauge success. Additionally, transarachnoid passage of local anesthetic and synergism between spinally and epidurally administered drugs may contribute to better analgesia. Some have questioned this advantage, particularly in comparison with modern, high-volume, low-concentration epidural analgesia.[18]

Anatomic Considerations

Even with meticulous insertion technique, it is possible the catheter will not be placed in the epidural space and may in fact be elsewhere, including the subdural,

intradural,[19] or subarachnoid space. Subarachnoid placement is usually easy to identify because aspiration of the catheter may produce CSF or a higher than expected level of anesthesia if a test dose of medication is given. However, if the catheter is placed in the subdural or intradural space, aspiration of the catheter will not produce any fluid (e.g., blood or CSF), but the block may be asymmetric or may take longer than expected to achieve adequate analgesia.

Even if the catheter is in the epidural space, there may be anatomic barriers to adequate spread of the local anesthetic. Collier[20] studied the etiology of failed epidural catheters by injecting radio-opaque dye through the catheters and performing lumbar radiographs in 35 parturients with atypical blocks. The two major causes of inadequate block were found to be transforaminal passage of the catheter tip and obstructive barriers in the epidural space.

The epidural space can be divided into a larger posterior space and a smaller anterior space. Even when placed in the epidural space, the catheter should be in the posterior space, remain in the midline, and not deviate to one side or the other. If an excessive length of epidural catheter is left in the space, it can possibly migrate to the anterior space. Usubiaga et al.[21] discovered that due to trabeculations in the midline of the anterior epidural space, it is much more difficult for the anesthetic solution to spread bilaterally, leading to a greater incidence of inadequate analgesia.

Management of Inadequate Analgesia

If an epidural catheter is placed and analgesia is not adequate, a systematic approach should be taken to improve the analgesia. First, one should evaluate the patient's labor progress and the description (e.g., pressure versus sharp pain) and location of their pain. Next, one should assess the dermatomal level of the sensory block in the caudad and cephalad directions. During the first stage of labor, a T10–L1 level is necessary for adequate analgesia, and during the second stage of labor, the patient will need an anesthetic level extending down to S2–S4. If there is no demonstrable anesthetic level after an appropriate dose, the epidural catheter should be replaced at this time.

During early labor, with an appropriate T10–L1 anesthetic level, injection of a more concentrated local anesthetic solution or an epidural opioid (e.g., fentanyl) should be administered for denser analgesia.

Conversely, if the block does not extend to the sacral level during late labor, injection of a large volume of a local anesthetic solution (e.g., 15 ml of 0.0625% bupivacaine) may improve spread.

If the block is unilateral or there are missed segments, the patient can be turned so that the painful side is in the dependent position, and the catheter can be withdrawn 1–2 cm and then redosed.[1] We prefer to use a concentrated local anesthetic for redosing (e.g., 5–10 ml of lidocaine 2%). This allows for quick determination of whether the catheter is working and removes any doubt as to whether the local anesthetic concentration is adequate. If the patient still does not have adequate analgesia, then the epidural catheter should be replaced.

Learning Points

- Inadequate labor epidural analgesia is common and is a cause of dissatisfaction for patients.
- The epidural catheter can be inadvertently threaded into many different spaces, including the subarachnoid, subdural, and intradural spaces.
- Use of multiorifice flexible epidural catheters as well as employing a combined spinal-epidural technique may decrease the incidence of inadequate analgesia.
- With a systematic approach, almost all cases of inadequate analgesia can be corrected. If not, the catheter should be replaced.

References

1. Beilin Y, Zahn J, Bernstein HH, et al. Treatment of incomplete analgesia after placement of an epidural catheter and administration of local anesthetic for women in labor. *Anesthesiology* 1998; **88**:1502–6.

2. Pan PH, Bogard TD, Owen MD. Incidence and characteristics of failures in obstetric neuraxial analgesia and anesthesia: a retrospective analysis of 19,259 deliveries. *Int J Obstet Anesth* 2004; **13**:227–33.

3. Eappen S, Blinn A, Segal S. Incidence of epidural catheter replacement in parturients: a retrospective chart review. *Int J Obstet Anesth* 1998; **7**:220–25.

4. Chadwick HS, Posner K, Caplan RA, Ward RJ, Cheney FW. A comparison of obstetric and nonobstetric anesthesia malpractice claims. *Anesthesiology* 1991; **74**:242–49.

5. Agaram R, Douglas MJ, McTaggart RA, Gunka V. Inadequate pain relief with labor epidurals: a multivariate analysis of associated factors. *Int J Obstet Anesth* 2009; **18**:10–14.

6. Tonidandel A, Booth J, D'Angelo R, Harris L, Tonidandel S. Anesthetic and obstetric outcomes in morbidly obese parturients: a 20-year follow-up retrospective cohort study. *Int J Obstet Anesth* 2014; **23**:357–64.

7. Ko JY, Leffert LR. Clinical implications of neuraxial anesthesia in the parturient with scoliosis. *Anesth Analg* 2009; **109**:1930–34.

8. Bauchat JR, McCarthy RJ, Koski TR, et al. Prior lumbar discectomy surgery does not alter the efficacy of neuraxial labor analgesia. *Anesth Analg* 2012; **115**:348–53.

9. Grau T, Leipold RW, Conradi R, Martin E. Ultrasound control for presumed difficult epidural puncture. *Acta Anaesthesiol Scand* 2001; **45**:766–71.

10. Arzola C, Mikhael R, Margarido C, Carvalho JC. Spinal ultrasound versus palpation for epidural catheter insertion in labour: a randomised controlled trial. *Eur J Anaesthesiol* 2014; **31**:1–7.

11. Beilin Y, Arnold I, Telfeyan C, Bernstein HH, Hossain S. Quality of analgesia when air versus saline is used for identification of the epidural space in the parturient. *Reg Anesth Pain Med* 2000; **25**:596–99.

12. Segal S, Arendt KW. A retrospective effectiveness study of loss of resistance to air or saline for identification of the epidural space. *Anesth Analg* 2010; **110**:558–63.

13. Antibas PL, do Nascimento Junior P, Braz LG, et al. Air versus saline in the loss of resistance technique for identification of the epidural space. *Cochrane Database Syst Rev* 2014; **7**:CD008938.

14. Beilin Y, Bernstein HH, Zucker-Pinchoff B. The optimal distance that a multiorifice epidural catheter should be threaded into the epidural space. *Anesth Analg* 1995; **81**:301–4.

15. D'Angelo R, Foss ML, Livesay CH. A comparison of multiport and uniport epidural catheters in laboring patients. *Anesth Analg* 1997; **84**:1276–79.

16. Jaime F, Mandell GL, Vallejo MC, Ramanathan S. Uniport soft-tip, open-ended catheters versus multiport firm-tipped close-ended catheters for epidural labor analgesia: a quality assurance study. *J Clin Anesth* 2000; **12**:89–93.

17. Norris MC. Are spinal-epidural catheters reliable? *Int J Obstet Anesth* 2000; **9**:3–6.

18. Simmons SW, Taghizadeh N, Dennis AT, Hughes D, Cyna AM. Combined spinal-epidural versus epidural

analgesia in labour. *Cochrane Database Syst Rev* 2012; **10**:CD003401.

19. Collier CB. The intradural space: the fourth place to go astray during epidural block. *Int J Obstet Anesth* 2010; **19**:133–41.

20. Collier CB. Why obstetric epidurals fail: a study of epidurograms. *Int J of Obstet Anesth* 1996; **5**:19–31.

21. Usubiaga JE, dos Reis A, Jr, Usubiaga LE. Epidural misplacement of catheters and mechanisms of unilateral blockade. *Anesthesiology* 1970; **32**:158–61.

Epidural Analgesia and Intrapartum Fever

Scott Segal

Case Study

A healthy nulliparous patient at term entered labor spontaneously and was admitted to the labor floor. At 3 cm of cervical dilation, an uncomplicated labor epidural was initiated to successfully provide analgesia with a patient-controlled regimen of 0.1% bupivacaine with fentanyl 2 µg/ml. The patient's membranes were ruptured artificially 2 hours later, and oxytocin augmentation of labor was begun. Six hours after initiation of epidural analgesia, the patient was dilated 6 cm. Her temperature measured orally was increased to 38.0°C (100.4°F), after having been admitted with a normal temperature of 37.0°C (98.6°F). Antibiotics were started by her obstetrician. Two hours later, she was still 6 cm dilated, and she was taken to the operating room for cesarean delivery. A male infant was delivered with Apgar scores of 5 and 9 at 1 and 5 minutes, respectively. He required brief bag-mask ventilation for treatment of a low heart rate immediately after delivery but recovered promptly and was discharged home with the mother on postdelivery day 4.

Key Points

- This patient experienced an increase in temperature during administration of epidural labor analgesia.
- While the etiology of intrapartum fever is diverse, neuraxial analgesia has emerged as a leading cause of predominately noninfectious but inflammatory fever.
- Her slow labor progress and fever led her obstetrician to deliver her by cesarean, and her baby experienced transient respiratory depression after birth.
- The precise etiology and consequences of epidural-associated fever remain incompletely characterized but are a concern for the obstetric anesthetist, obstetrician, and neonatologist.

Discussion

Women receiving labor epidural analgesia experience a greater incidence of clinical fever. Two decades ago, observational studies demonstrated a gradual rise in temperature in women receiving epidurals compared with those receiving no analgesia or systemic opioids alone.[1,2] Although originally ascribed to altered thermoregulation, it is now evident that this represents an artifact from averaging afebrile women's temperatures and those developing clinical fever.[3,4] Substantial evidence suggests that true clinical fever develops more often in women with epidurals than in those without. The data come from retrospective observations (which attempt to statistically control for confounding factors such as longer labors, prolonged rupture of membranes, and number of cervical examinations), sentinel event studies (in which epidural analgesia suddenly becomes available to a population), and randomized, controlled trials.[5-7] Once dismissed as a physiologic curiosity or artifact of selection bias, this phenomenon can no longer be ignored.

The mechanism of epidural-associated fever remains unclear. Earlier, investigators noting the very slow gradual rise in temperature *on average* hypothesized that thermoregulation might be altered in laboring women with epidurals. For example, by inhibiting sweating and hyperventilation, the neuraxial block might impair heat dissipation. Other investigators suggested that opioids given to women without epidurals might be suppressing temperature elevation rather than epidurals causing it. There is some evidence from nonlaboring volunteers to support each of these mechanisms. However, the observation that "epidural fever" is actually clinical fever in some women averaged with normal temperature in others leads to a search for an explanation of more frequent overt fever in some women with epidural analgesia. Some evidence suggests that placental inflammation (chorioamnionitis) is more common in febrile women with epidural analgesia.[8] Importantly, in a nonrandomized comparison, bacterial infection in the placenta was not found to be associated with epidural analgesia, although inflammation.[9] Furthermore, prophylactic treatment with broad-spectrum antibiotics did not inhibit maternal fever or placental inflammation.[10] Moreover, high-dose methylprednisolone (but not acetaminophen) given to laboring women with epidurals blocks the febrile response.[11] Unfortunately, this treatment also leads to a substantial increase in asymptomatic bacteremia in the exposed babies, making it untenable as a clinical strategy. Thus the mechanism of epidural-associated fever is most likely sterile inflammation. Recently, some have suggested that bupivacaine itself may trigger noninfectious inflammation.[12] However, epidural-related fever has been observed with similar frequency when other drugs are used or even when solely intrathecal opioids are used, making this explanation incomplete.

Variations in epidural technique do not appear to have an important effect on the phenomenon. Increased fever has been observed with a variety of local anesthetics and opioid adjuncts, with the combined spinal-epidural technique as well as conventional epidurals, with intermittent versus continuous administration of local anesthetics, and even with continuous intrathecal opioid with no local anesthetic.[13]

Epidural-associated fever may have significant effects on the fetus and newborn. One of the earliest recognized effects was an indirect one, namely an influence on the practice of neonatologists. Lieberman[5] demonstrated that babies born to mothers with epidurals underwent evaluation for sepsis four times more often than babies born to mothers electing for natural childbirth or systemic opioids. Actual sepsis was vanishingly rare and did not differ between epidural and no-epidural groups. This phenomenon may be a function of neonatology practice style, however, because other institutions have reported different results.[8] Other adverse effects related to intrapartum maternal fever include increased need for bag-mask ventilation and increased incidence of otherwise unexplained neonatal seizures.[14] Obstetricians may also be more likely to perform operative delivery in the setting of fever,[15] although it is unclear whether this reflects an effect on the labor process itself or an effect on obstetrical decision making.

A far more worrisome possibility is that maternal fever may cause neonatal brain injury. Over 50 years ago, an association between cerebral palsy and maternal fever was first noted, but the observation was not investigated further until recently. Substantial epidemiologic evidence now confirms a four- to nine-fold increase in the risk of otherwise unexplained cerebral palsy in term and near-term infants exposed to maternal fever or clinical or pathologically diagnosed chorioamnionitis.[16,17] Other neonatal brain injuries have likewise been associated with maternal fever, including neonatal encephalopathy (which often has devastating lifelong neurologic consequences for the infant).[18] Even babies not manifesting these profound impairments may nonetheless experience neurologic injury. Dammann[19] found that cognitive deficits at age nine, as measured by the Kaufman Assessment Battery for Children, were four times as common in children whose mothers had fever at the time of delivery compared with control individuals.

The link between maternal fever and neurologic injury in the newborn is most likely inflammation. In experimental pregnant animal preparations, bacterial intrauterine infection causes white matter lesions in the fetuses. Yoon[20] injected *Eschericia coli* or saline into the cervix of pregnant rabbits. Thirty-six percent of infected dams delivered fetuses with white matter lesions (6 percent of all fetuses of infected mothers had such lesions) compared with 0 percent in the saline control group. Similarly, Rodts-Palenik[21] demonstrated white matter lesions and enlarged cerebral ventricles in pups of infected pregnant rats more frequently than in saline-treated rats. Importantly, these lesions were not seen if the mothers were treated with the anti-inflammatory interleukin 10 (IL-10). Although such experiments do not definitively demonstrate that maternal intrapartum fever causes neonatal brain injury via fetal inflammation in humans, Yoon[22] has documented increased IL-6 and IL-8 (pro-inflammatory cytokines) in amniotic fluid in a cohort of pregnancies resulting in babies with cerebral palsy compared with controls with normal brain development. In our own laboratory, we have demonstrated similar brain injury in fetuses of mothers exposed to a noninfectious inflammatory stimulus (IL-6) injected for a few hours before delivery, mimicking the clinical situation of epidural fever.[23]

Many questions remain. First, it is far from clear how epidural analgesia is associated with maternal inflammatory fever. If the neuraxial block itself causes inflammation, the mechanism would be unique and startling. Conversely, if neuraxial analgesia blocks pathways that might otherwise oppose inflammation in susceptible mothers, then it may be possible to block inflammation in selected women. Second, it is not clear yet whether fever itself can cause injury or whether inflammation causes both fever and brain injury. Hyperthermia itself can worsen the effects of other brain-injuring stimuli, so the two effects may be additive. Third, it is not known whether epidural-associated fever is specifically associated with brain injury. Fourth, it is unknown whether epidural-associated fever can be safely blocked. Trials of various anti-inflammatory strategies are ongoing. These questions will likely be the subject of intense investigation in the near future.

Learning Points

- Epidural analgesia is associated with a significant increase in the incidence of maternal intrapartum fever. Variations in technique and drug do not appear to have an important effect on the incidence, which is approximately 20 percent.
- The most likely mechanism is noninfectious inflammation.
- Antibiotics and antipyretics (acetaminophen) are ineffective in blocking fever.
- Maternal intrapartum fever may have significant adverse effects on the fetus.

References

1. Camann WR, Hortvet LA, Hughes N, Bader AM, Datta S. Maternal temperature regulation during extradural analgesia for labour. *Br J Anaesth* 1991; **67**(5): 565–68.

2. Fusi L, Steer PJ, Maresh MJ, Beard RW. Maternal pyrexia associated with the use of epidural analgesia in labour. *Lancet* 1989; **1**(8649):1250–52.

3. Goetzl L, Rivers J, Zighelboim I, et al. Intrapartum epidural analgesia and maternal temperature regulation. *Obstet Gynecol* 2007; **109**(3):687–90.

4. Gelfand T, Palanisamy A, Tsen LC, Segal S. Warming in parturients with epidurals is an averaging artifact. *Anesthesiology* 2007; **106**:A5.

5. Lieberman E, Lang JM, Frigoletto F Jr, et al. Epidural analgesia, intrapartum fever, and neonatal sepsis evaluation. *Pediatrics* 1997; **99**(3):415–19.

6. Yancey MK, Zhang J, Schwarz J, Dietrich CS 3rd, Klebanoff M. Labor epidural analgesia and intrapartum maternal hyperthermia. *Obstet Gynecol* 2001; **98**(5 Pt 1):763–70.

7. Segal S. Labor epidural analgesia and maternal fever. *Anesth Analg* 2010; **111**(6):1467–75.

8. Vallejo MC, Kaul B, Adler LJ, et al. Chorioamnionitis, not epidural analgesia, is associated with maternal fever during labour. *Can J Anaesth* 2001; **48**(11):1122–26.

9. Riley LE, Celi AC, Onderdonk AB, et al. Association of epidural-related fever and noninfectious inflammation in term labor. *Obstet Gynecol* 2011; **117**(3):588–95.

10. Sharma SK, Rogers BB, Alexander JM, McIntire DD, Leveno KJ. A randomized trial of the effects of antibiotic prophylaxis on epidural-related fever in labor. *Anesth Analg* 2014; **118**(3):604–10.

11. Goetzl L, Zighelboim I, Badell M, et al. Maternal corticosteroids to prevent intrauterine exposure to hyperthermia and inflammation: a randomized, double-blind, placebo-controlled trial. *Am J Obstet Gynecol* 2006; **195**(4):1031–37.

12. Sultan P, David AL, Fernando R, Ackland GL. Inflammation and epidural-related maternal fever: proposed mechanisms. *Anesth Analg* 2016; **122**(5): 1546–53.

13. Arendt KW, Segal BS. The association between epidural labor analgesia and maternal fever. *Clin Perinatol* 2013; **40**(3):385–98.

14. Lieberman E, Lang J, Richardson DK, et al. Intrapartum maternal fever and neonatal outcome. *Pediatrics* 2000; **105**(1 Pt 1):8–13.

15. Sharpe EE, Arendt KW. Epidural labor analgesia and maternal fever. *Clin Obstet Gynecol* 2017; **60**(2):365–74.

16. Grether JK, Nelson KB. Maternal infection and cerebral palsy in infants of normal birth weight. *JAMA* 1997; **278**(3):207–11.

17. Wu YW, Escobar GJ, Grether JK, et al. Chorioamnionitis and cerebral palsy in term and near-term infants. *JAMA* 2003; **290**(20):2677–84.

18. Impey L, Greenwood C, MacQuillan K, Reynolds M, Sheil O. Fever in labour and neonatal encephalopathy: a prospective cohort study. *BJOG* 2001; **108**(6):594–97.

19. Dammann O, Drescher J, Veelken N. Maternal fever at birth and non-verbal intelligence at age 9 years in preterm infants. *Dev Med Child Neurol* 2003; **45**(3):148–51.

20. Yoon BH, Kim CJ, Romero R, et al. Experimentally induced intrauterine infection causes fetal brain white matter lesions in rabbits. *Am J Obstet Gynecol* 1997; **177**(4):797–802.

21. Rodts-Palenik S, Wyatt-Ashmead J, Pang Y, et al. Maternal infection-induced white matter injury is reduced by treatment with interleukin-10. *Am J Obstet Gynecol* 2004; **191**(4):1387–92.

22. Yoon BH, Romero R, Park JS, et al. Fetal exposure to an intra-amniotic inflammation and the development of cerebral palsy at the age of three years. *Am J Obstet Gynecol* 2000; **182**(3): 675–81.

23. Segal S, Pancaro C, Bonney I, Marchand JE. Noninfectious fever in the near-term pregnant rat induces fetal brain inflammation: a model for the consequences of epidural-associated maternal fever. *Anesth Analg* 2017 Dec; **125** (6):2134–40.

Tips and Tricks for Labor Neuraxial Block

Sikha Shastham Valappil, Gary Stocks, and Roshan Fernando

Case Study

A 28-year-old primigravida at 39 weeks of gestational age with 5 cm of cervical dilation in labor requested epidural analgesia for painful contractions. She was noted to be obese by the obstetric team with a body mass index (BMI) of 40 kg/m^2 but no other comorbidities .The anesthesiologist arrived and assessed the patient, after which he explained the procedure and took informed consent. He started the procedure using a 16-gauge epidural needle with a loss of resistance to saline technique with the patient in the left lateral position. After multiple attempts, he was unable to identify the epidural space and therefore tried again with the patient in the sitting position. After two attempts, he successfully identified the epidural space at 7 cm from the skin at the L3–L4 level using a midline approach. He then threaded a multiorifice epidural catheter, leaving 5 cm within the epidural space (12 cm at the skin surface). He went on to confirm the epidural catheter position with a negative aspiration to CSF or blood. He then asked the patient to sit upright and then to lie down in the left lateral position so that he could securely fix the epidural catheter with a clear sterile dressing. A patient-controlled epidural analgesia (PCEA) pump was started using 0.1% levobupivacaine with 2 μg/ml fentanyl (basal rate of 5 ml/h and a PCEA demand dose of 10 ml with a lockout time 20 minutes). The patient became comfortable within 20 minutes. Unfortunately, after 3 hours, she started complaining of pain in her right lower abdomen. The anesthesiologist assessed her and decided to give her a bolus dose with 10 ml 0.125% levobupivacaine manually. He advised her to lie down in the right lateral position for approximately 20 minutes. Her pain was relieved after 15 minutes. The patient continued to be comfortable and extremely happy with her pain relief and used the PCEA for additional analgesia until the delivery of her baby several hours later.

Key Points

- Proper positioning of the patient during an epidural procedure is important.
- Securing the epidural catheter after the procedure can prevent catheter movement within the epidural space, which sometimes results in suboptimal analgesia.
- Breakthrough pain can be managed occasionally by changing the patient's position, withdrawing the epidural catheter, and delivering a manual bolus of low-dose epidural local anesthetic mixture such as 0.1% levobupivacaine with 2 μg/ml fentanyl.
- Follow-up of patients with epidurals in the delivery suite is advisable at regular intervals during labor so that timely interventions can be made if needed for inadequate analgesia.

Discussion

It is not uncommon to have a failed epidural that has previously been administered for labor analgesia. In the literature, the largest case series, which was published in 2004 by Pan et al.,[1] reports an overall failure rate of 12 percent, with 6.8 percent of patients requiring reinsertion of the epidural catheter. Other studies by Paech et al.,[2] Eappen et al.,[3] and Crawford[4] show failure rates of 4.7, 13.1, and 15.5 percent, respectively

There can be different reasons for failed epidural analgesia.

Predicting Epidurals that May Become Suboptimal or Fail

A study by Lecoq et al.[5] in 456 labor epidurals showed that a lack of effect of the first epidural drug dose, posterior presentation of the fetus, radicular pain during catheter insertion, and a duration of labor of more than 6 hours are risk factors for inadequate analgesia. Another trial by Agaram et al.[6] identified a cervical dilation of more than 7 cm, epidural insertion by a trainee, history of opioid tolerance, and a previous failed epidural were risk factors. A systematic review and meta-analysis of observational studies by Bauer et al.[7] regarding risk factors for failed conversion of labor epidural analgesia to provide anesthesia for cesarean delivery showed that an increased number of epidural drug boluses, care provided by a non-obstetric anesthetist, and an enhanced urgency for cesarean delivery are predictors of failed conversion. In 2006, Orbach-Zinger et al.[8] showed that the chances of a failed epidural top-up for cesarean delivery is higher in younger, more obese parturients with a greater gestational age. These patients also required more epidural top-ups during labor and had high Visual Analogue Scale (VAS) scores 2 hours before their cesarean delivery.

Improving Techniques for Labor Epidural Analgesia

Maternal Position during an Epidural Procedure: Sitting versus Lateral

There is no conclusive evidence in the literature that patient positioning affects the efficacy of subsequent epidural analgesia. Although the sitting position makes it much easier to identify the midline and epidural space, it may not be comfortable for patients experiencing labor pain. The sitting position may increase the chance for orthostatic hypotension. The epidural venous plexus is also thought to be more engorged in this position, leading to a higher rate of venous puncture with the epidural catheter. Although the lateral position may be more comfortable for the patient, it is often technically difficult for the obstetric anesthetist, especially in obese patients, to locate the midline and the epidural space.

Loss-of-Resistance Technique: Air versus Saline

There are controversies regarding the loss-of-resistance (LOR) technique with saline or air and the subsequent success of epidural analgesia. A 2011 meta-analysis suggested an increased risk of unblocked segments when loss of resistance to air (LORA) was used due to air bubbles in the intervertebral foramina.[9] However, another study by Segal and Arendt[10] showed that there was no significant difference in neuraxial block success whether you use loss of resistance to air or saline. These days, the consensus appears to be that anesthetists should always use a technique (LORA or LORS) that is familiar to them.

There are other devices such as the Epidrum or Episure that have been used to identify the epidural space. A trial comparing the Epidrum with a standard LOR technique for inserting an epidural for labor analgesia did not show any difference in success or complication rate.[11] A 2008 pilot study of 325 patients compared the Episure Auto Detect syringe with a glass syringe.[12] Eight residents performed 291 procedures (90 percent) and two consultants performed 34 procedures (10 percent). Overall, epidural analgesia failed in five subjects in the glass syringe group, whereas there were no failures in the spring-loaded Episure Auto Detect syringe group ($P = 0.025$).

Type of Epidural Catheter

There is evidence in the literature that polyurethane multiorifice catheters have a lower risk of inadequate analgesia.[13] Segal et al.[14] showed that replacement rates were less when multiorifice catheters were used with fewer episodes of paresthesia when compared with single-orifice catheters.

Wire-reinforced epidural catheters are available that are designed with fewer coils in the distal tip, which reportedly confers greater flexibility to minimize paresthesias and perforations of the dura mater and epidural blood vessels. There are in addition distal and proximal flashback windows for visualization of CSF or blood. A few studies have compared traditional multiport catheters and the newer wire-reinforced catheters in terms of both analgesic efficacy and the incidence of complications. In a prospective quality assurance study, Jaime et al.[15] compared clinical complications in 2,612 obstetric patients who received epidural analgesia with either a 20-gauge closed-tipped multiport (three lateral ports) nylon catheter or a 19-gauge open-end uniport spring-wound polyurethane catheter. Although the incidence of unsatisfactory block was similar in both groups, the incidence of paresthesias, venous cannulation, and reinsertion related to venipuncture was significantly higher in the patients who received the non-wire-reinforced nylon catheters.

Combined Spinal-Epidural (CSE) or Epidural

There is good evidence that a CSE technique provides more rapid and reliable analgesia initially than an epidural technqiue[16] (see Chapter 7). However, this initial benefit in terms of analgesia may not apply for the duration of labor. Many studies demonstrate lower VAS scores for labor pain with CSE compared with epidural. There are many, mainly retrospective trials that show that the reliability of epidural catheters following CSE is significantly increased compared with an epidural technique alone. Interestingly, a recent Cochrane review[16] found no difference in overall maternal satisfaction despite a slightly faster onset time with a CSE technique. Fetal bradycardia is often reported to be a significant drawback after a CSE for labor analgesia. Following a meta-analysis of 24 trials demonstrated an increase in the incidence of fetal bradycardia in patients receiving intrathecal opioids, some clinicians recommended avoiding intrathecal opioids when a nonreassuring fetal status is present before performing a CSE technique for labor analgesia.[17] However, a 2014 study by Patel et al.[18] showed no significant difference in fetal heart rate changes, Apgar scores, or umbilical artery and vein acid-base status between epidural and CSE groups.

Epidural Catheter Length to Be Left within the Epidural Space

Berlin et al.[19] found that leaving 5 cm of a multiorifice catheter within the epidural space provided superior analgesia compared with 3 and 7 cm. A nonobstetric study by Afsan et al.[20] showed no change in postoperative pain scores in patients who underwent abdominal hysterectomy between groups with 3, 5, or 7cm of epidural catheter left in the epidural space. A patient in the 7-cm group had unilateral sensory analgesia. Of note, there was a much higher rate of epidural catheter dislodgement in the 3-cm group. It seems that the most appropriate length should be 5 cm.

Fixation of the Epidural Catheter

The position of the patient during fixation of an epidural catheter is important. The evidence from the literature[21] shows that the epidural catheter position within the epidural space can change significantly with patient movement. If the epidural catheter is secured while the patient is sitting up in a flexed position, the catheter may be pulled outward later once the patient straightens her back because there is no space for soft tissue movement. Therefore, it is important to keep the patient in a neutral position (whether the patient is sitting or lying down in a

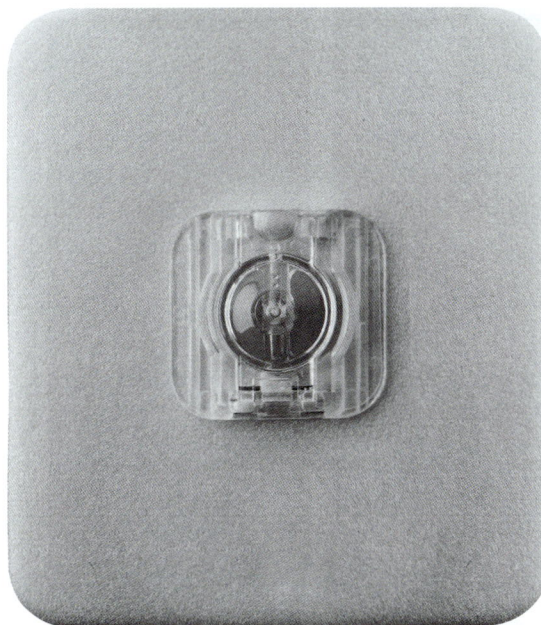

Figure 5.1 LockIt Plus epidural fixation device

lateral position for her initial epidural procedure) before fixing the epidural catheter to prevent dislodgement. This may be more important in obese patients.

A randomized, controlled trial investigated the efficacy of Epi-Fix, LockIt Plus (Figure 5.1), and Tegaderm as fixation devices for intrapartum epidural catheters and showed that those secured with the LockIt Plus device exhibited less epidural catheter migration compared with fixation using either Epi-Fix and Tegaderm clear adhesive dressing.[22]

Inadequate Pain Relief/Unilateral Block/Patchy Block

It's not uncommon for the obstetric anesthesiologist on duty within the delivery area to be asked to review a patient who is still complaining of pain following an epidural. We believe that a pragmatic approach to resolving such issues should involve the following:

- Obtain a proper history about the timing and efficacy of the epidural block.
- Is the pain unilateral/bilateral?
- Pain scores: What was the VAS score before and after the neuraxial block?
- Technique: CSE or epidural
- Evaluate the block: both sensory (e.g., using ethyl chloride spray) and motor components.

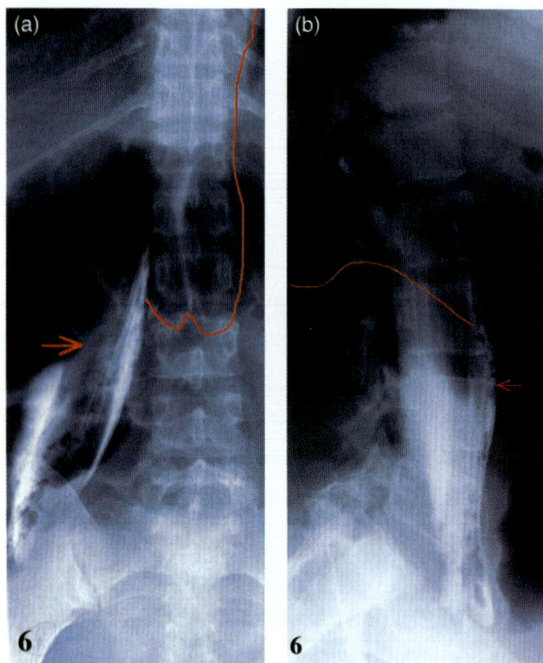

Figure 5.2 (A) Anteroposterior (AP) epidurogram following catheter escape through the right L2–L3 intervertebral foramen, with contrast material outlining the right psoas muscle (arrowed). (B) Lateral epidurogram showing the escaping catheter, with contrast material collecting anterior and lateral to the right psoas muscle (arrowed).
Source: Reproduced with the permission from Wolters et al. *Anesthesiology* 2017; 102:112–18.

- Fetal evaluation (is the fetal head in an occipitoposterior [OP] position?)
- Epidural catheter check (has your epidural catheter been dislodged?)

In some cases, a unilateral or "patchy" block may be due to the epidural catheter becoming dislodged or having migrated through an intervertebral foramina (Figure 5.2; see also Chapter 3).

Volume or Dose: Which Is More Important for Epidural Analgesia?

Lyons et al.[23] attempted to determine and compare the minimum local anesthetic volumes (MLAVs) and minimum local anesthetic doses (MLADs) of two concentrations of bupivacaine for epidural pain relief in labor and to quantify the effect on dose. Bupivacaine 0.125% (weight/volume), when compared with bupivacaine 0.25% (weight/volume), produced equivalent analgesia with a 50 percent increase in volume but with a 25 percent reduction in dose. Therefore, the analgesic efficacy of 13.6 ml of 0.125%

bupivacaine (17 mg) is equivalent to 9.2 ml of 0.25% bupivacaine (23.1 mg). Any reduction in dose, without loss of efficacy, reduces the risk of toxicity and improves safety. Christiaens et al.[24] showed that the number of dermatomes blocked using epidural analgesia is associated with volume first and then concentration of local anesthesia.

Ultrasound Guidance

Ultrasound may help to localize the midline of the back and the epidural space correctly and avoid multiple attempts at epidural insertion[25] (see Chapter 6). In a 2013 systematic review and meta-analysis, 14 studies were evaluated, of which nine studies were on epidural catheterization and concluded that ultrasound imaging can reduce the risk of failed or traumatic lumbar puncture and epidural catheterizations as well as the number of needle insertions and redirections.[26] Many clinicians claim that it may be useful in difficult cases, including its use in obese patients and those with scoliosis, in terms of improving identification of the epidural space and the midline.

Learning Points

- Proper positioning of the patient is important while doing a neuraxial block. The sitting position is technically easier.
- Fix the epidural catheter in a deflexed, position to avoid pulling out the catheter.
- The volume of local anesthetic mixture is more important than the dose for epidural analgesia.
- Breakthrough pain can be managed with an additional bolus dose or withdrawing the catheter by 1 cm and then giving an epidural bolus with the patient lying down on her painful side in case of a unilateral block.
- Ultrasound may be useful to avoid multiple attempts by identifying the midline of the back as well as the epidural space.
- If there is no pain relief using epidural top-ups and catheter manipulation, early resiting of the catheter is recommended.
- Regular review of existing epidural blocks within the delivery area is important.

References

1. Pan PH, Bogard TD, Owen MD. Incidence and characteristics of failures in obstetric neuraxial analgesia and anesthesia: a retrospective analysis of 19,259 deliveries. *Int J Obstet Anesth* 2004; **13**:227–33.

2. Paech MJ, Godkin R, Webster S. Complications of obstetric epidural analgesia and anaesthesia: a prospective analysis of 10995 cases. *Int J Obstet Anesth* 1998; 7:5–11.

3. Eappen S, Blinn A, Segal S. Incidence of epidural catheter replacement in parturients: a retrospective chart review. *Int J Obstet Anesth* 1998; 7:220–25.

4. Crawford JS. The second thousand epidural blocks in an obstetric hospital practice. *Br J Anaesth* 1972; **44**:1277–86.

5. LeCoq G, Ducot B, Benhamou D. Risk factors of inadequate pain relief during epidural analgesia for labor and delivery. *Can J Anaesth* 1998; **45**:719–23.

6. Agaram R, Douglas MJ, McTaggart RA, Gunka V. Inadequate pain relief with labor epidurals: a multivariate analysis of associated factors. *Int J Obstet Anesth* 2009; **18**:10–14.

7. Bauer ME, Kountanis JA, Tsen LC, Greenfield ML, Mhyrea JM. Risk factors for failed conversion of labor epidural analgesia to cesarean delivery anesthesia: a systematic review and meta-analysis of observational trials. *Int J Obstet Anesth* 2012; **21**:294–309.

8. Orbach-Zinger S, Friedman L, Avramovich A, et al. Risk factors for failure to extend labor epidural analgesia to epidural anesthesia for cesarean section. *Acta Anaesthesiol Scand* 2006; **50**(8):1014–18.

9. Murphy JD, Ouanes J-PP, Togioka BM, et al. Comparison of air and liquid for use in loss-of-resistance technique during labor epidurals: a meta-analysis. *J Anesth Clin Res* 2011; **2**:175.

10. Segal S, Arendt KW. A retrospective effectiveness study of loss of resistance to air or saline for identification of the epidural space. *Anesth Analg* 2010; **110**:558–63.

11. Deighan M, Briain DO, Shakeban H, et al. A randomised controlled trial using the Epidrum for labour epidurals. *Irish Med J* 2015; 73–75.

12. Habib AS, George RB, Allen TK, Olufolabi AJ. A pilot study to compare the Episure Auto Detect syringe with the glass syringe for identification of the epidural space in parturients. *Anesth Analg* 2008; **106**(2):541–43.

13. D'Angelo R, Foss ML, Livesay CH. A comparison of multiport and uniport epidural catheters in laboring patients. *Anesth Analg* 1997; **84**:1276–79.

14. Segal S, Eappen S, Datta S. Superiority of multi-orifice over single-orifice epidural catheters for labor analgesia and cesarean delivery. *J Clin Anesth* 1997; **9**(2):109–12.

15. Jaime F, Mandell GL, Vallejo MC, Ramanathan S. Uniport soft-tip, open-ended catheters versus multiport firm-tipped close-ended catheters for epidural labor analgesia: a quality assurance study. *J Clin Anesth* 2000; **12**:89–93.

16. Simmons SW, Taghizadeh N, Dennis AT, Hughes D, Cyna AM. Combined spinal-epidural versus epidural analgesia in labour. *Cochrane Database Syst Rev* 2012; (10):CD003401.

17. Mardirossof C, Dumont L, Boulvain M, Tramer MR. Fetal bradycardia due to intrathecal opioids for labour analgesia: a systematic review. *Br J Obstet Gynaecol* 2002; **109**:274–81.

18. Patel NP, El-Wahab N, Fernando R, et al. Fetal effects of combined spinal-epidural vs epidural labour analgesia: a prospective, randomised double-blind study. *Anaesthesia* 2014; **69**(5):458–67.

19. Beilin Y, Bernstein HH, Zucker-Pinchoff B. The optimal distance that a multiorifice epidural catheter should be threaded into the epidural space. *Anesth Analg* 1995; **81**:3014.

20. Afshan G, Chohan U, Khan FA, et al. Appropriate length of epidural catheter in the epidural space for postoperative analgesia: evaluation by epidurography. *Anaesthesia* 2011; **66**(10):913–18.

21. Hamilton CL, Riley ET, Cohen SE. Changes in the position of epidural catheters associated with patient movement. *Anesthesiology* 1997; **86**:778–84.

22. Odor PM, Bampoe S, Hayward J, Ster C, Evans E. Intrapartum epidural fixation methods: a randomised controlled trial of three different epidural catheter securement devices. *Anaesthesia* 2016; **71**(3):298–305.

23. Lyons GR, Kocarev MG, Wilson RC, Columb MO. A comparison of minimum local anesthetic volumes and doses of epidural bupivacaine (0.125% w/v and 0.25% w/v) for analgesia in labor. *Anesth Analg* 2007; **104**:412–15.

24. Christiaens F, Verbourgh C, Dierick A, Camu F. Effects of diluent volume of a single dose of epidural bupivacaine in parturients during the first stage of labor. *Reg Anesth* 1998; **23**:134–41.

25. Vallejo MC, Phelps AL, Singh S, Orebaugh SL, Sah N. Ultrasound decreases the failed labor epidural rate in resident trainees. *Int J Obstet Anesth* 2010; **19**:373–78.

26. Shaikh F, Brzezinski J, Alexander S, et al. Ultrasound imaging for lumbar punctures and epidural catheterisations: systematic review and meta-analysis. *BMJ* 2013; **346**:f1720.

Spinal Ultrasound for Neuraxial Anesthesia Placement

Chiraag Talati and Jose C. A. Carvalho

Case Study

A multiparous woman (gravida 3, para 2) was admitted to the delivery suite at 39 weeks' gestation following the onset of labor. She described a pain score of 5/10 and requested labor analgesia prior to the initiation of oxytocin for labor augmentation.

Her medical history was positive for severe obesity. On further questioning, the previous obstetric history revealed two spontaneous vaginal deliveries with several problems related to her epidural analgesia. On both occasions, multiple attempts were required to site the epidural. Furthermore, the first epidural provided a unilateral block that could not be optimized, and the second epidural "did not work."

On physical examination, the patient weighed 145 kg and measured 160 cm in height to give a body mass index (BMI) of 57 kg/m^2. It was impossible to palpate bony landmarks on examination of her spine.

The patient adopted the sitting position, and a preprocedure spinal ultrasound assessment was performed. Successful identification of the L3–L4 interspace was achieved. The ideal insertion point for the epidural puncture was marked based on the identification of the midline and interspace, and the depth to the epidural space was estimated at 9.5 cm. Following this, the back was cleaned and draped, and the procedure was undertaken with a 17-gauge, 11.5-cm Tuohy needle. Loss of resistance to saline was achieved at approximately 9.75 cm, and an epidural catheter was sited uneventfully at the first attempt.

A test dose of 3 ml bupivacaine 0.125 percent was negative, and the epidural was loaded with a further 12 ml bupivacaine 0.125 percent plus fentanyl 50 µg. Satisfactory analgesia was achieved. The patient remained comfortable during labor and delivery with a patient-controlled epidural analgesia pump administering bupivacaine 0.0625 percent with fentanyl 2 µg/ml (bolus 5 ml, lockout 10 minutes, continuous infusion 10 ml/h, maximum 20 ml/h).

Key Points

- It is not uncommon to encounter patients who have had a previous difficult placement of an epidural, sometimes due to obesity or problems identifying anatomic landmarks.
- Spinal ultrasound imaging performed before the procedure to facilitate epidural insertion may be considered for such patients.

Discussion

Conventional placement of spinal or epidural anesthesia is a blind technique that relies on palpation of anatomic landmarks to identify the optimal puncture point. Typical landmarks that are examined include the iliac crests, tips of the spinous processes, and the intervertebral spaces. It is not unusual to fail to identify these landmarks in the setting of obesity, anatomic spinal variations, or edema.

Furthermore, studies have demonstrated that even when the bony landmarks are easily identified, experienced clinicians often fail to accurately identify the desired interspace. One investigation showed that when compared with MRI, anesthetists were correct in their assessment in only 29 percent of cases, and the error in their assessment could be as much as four interspaces. In 94 percent of the errors, the actual level was higher than assumed.[1] The safety implications of these inaccuracies for central neuraxial blockade are concerning, especially in the context of spinal anesthesia.

Advantages of Spinal Ultrasound Assessment

The use of ultrasound as an adjunct in anesthesia has risen significantly, and ultrasound-assisted nerve blockade, peripheral or central, is no exception. In the United Kingdom, the National Institute for Health and Care Excellence (NICE) has issued guidance regarding the facilitation of epidural space catheterization with the use of spinal ultrasound.[2] A significant source of knowledge can be provided by preprocedural spinal ultrasound to facilitate the placement of neuraxial anesthesia. It assists in the identification of the desired intervertebral space, the optimal insertion point, the angle of needle insertion, and the depth to the epidural space.

A technique that minimizes the number of puncture points and needle redirections can reduce trauma and subsequent infection, bleeding, bruising, back pain, post–dural puncture headache, and nerve damage. In addition, patient satisfaction can be improved and the efficacy of epidural anesthesia can be enhanced.[3] A recent systematic review and meta-analysis concluded that there was a reduction in the number of failed attempts, traumatic attempts, insertion attempts, and needle redirections with the use of ultrasound when performing epidural placements or lumbar punctures.[4] Novice residents have also shown a significantly higher success rate of epidural insertion with the use of ultrasound.[5]

The accuracy of ultrasound in identifying the desired interspace is superior to the conventional palpatory technique. One study showed a success rate of 71 percent in the ultrasound group versus 30 percent in the palpatory group, with errors greater than one space occurring in the palpation group but not in the ultrasound group.[6]

Preprocedural spinal ultrasound prior to spinal or epidural anesthesia can provide the clinician with knowledge that can help select the most appropriate needle length. For example, if the depth of the epidural space is measured on ultrasound to be greater than 8 cm, an extralong needle can be selected from the outset. This can reduce unnecessary multiple passes and trauma, as well as the risk of infection.

One may predict difficult neuraxial anesthesia in certain patient groups. Assessment of surface landmarks in obesity can be challenging, and identification of the intervertebral space and midline can prove problematic. In scoliosis, spinal anatomy is distorted and associated with lateral curvatures of the spine along the longitudinal plane but also with varying degrees of rotation around the longitudinal axis. Therefore, determining the optimal puncture site in either of these clinical scenarios may be impossible by palpation, and preprocedural spinal ultrasound certainly can facilitate success in these settings. Chin et al.[7] demonstrated a twice-as-high first-attempt success rate and a twofold difference in the number of needle insertion attempts and number of needle passes for spinal anesthesia with ultrasound compared with the conventional landmark technique in patients with difficult predicted spines (body mass index > 35 kg/m^2, moderate to severe lumbar scoliosis, or previous lumbar spine surgery).

Technique

Spinal ultrasound assessment can prove to be challenging for two reasons. First, the spinal structures are protected by a complex encasement of bones that provides only a narrow acoustic window for the ultrasound beam. Second, the desired structures to be imaged are deeper than those imaged for peripheral nerve blocks or placement of central vascular catheters. Therefore, a low-frequency (5–2 MHz) curved ultrasound probe is used, which allows deeper penetration, albeit at the expense of a lower resolution.

Spinal sonoanatomy can be assessed via two useful acoustic windows: the longitudinal paramedian oblique approach and the transverse midline approach, both providing invaluable information.[8]

Longitudinal Paramedian Oblique Approach

The probe is held vertically over the sacral area, parallel to the long axis of the spine, and initially placed 2–3 cm to the left or to the right of the midline and angled slightly to target the center of the spinal canal (Figure 6.1a). The sacrum is visualized as a continuous hyperechoic (bright) line. Slowly, the probe is moved cephalad until a hyperechoic sawlike image is visualized (Figure 6.1b). The teeth of the saw represent the lamina of each vertebrae, and the spaces between the teeth indicate the intervertebral spaces. One can then mark on the skin the exact level of each interspace from L5–S1 to L1–L2.

At a given intervertebral space (Figure 6.1c), one can identify the *posterior unit* (ligamentum flavum and posterior dura mater), intrathecal space, and *anterior unit* (anterior dura mater, posterior longitudinal ligament, and vertebral body; Figure 6.1d).

Transverse Midline Approach

Once the desired interspaces are determined, transverse scanning of one or more interspaces can be performed. The ultrasound probe is positioned horizontally at the marked levels, perpendicular to the long axis of the spine (Figure 6.2a). Therefore, the midline of the spine is determined by visualizing the tip of the spinous process, a small hyperechoic signal

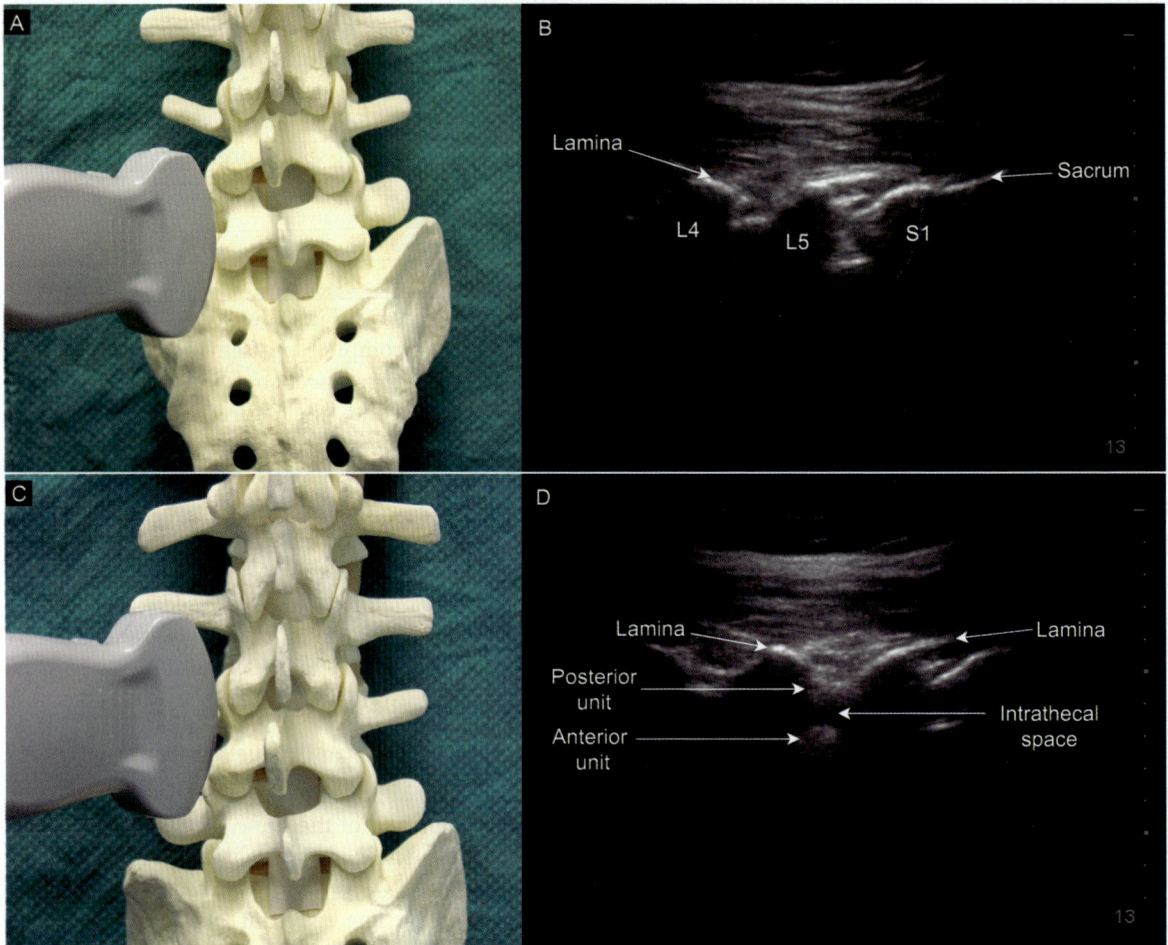

Figure 6.1 Longitudinal paramedian oblique approach. (a) Orientation of the ultrasound probe over the sacrum and lower lumbar spine. (b) Corresponding sonogram to a. Hyperechoic image of the sacrum and of the saw sign, the teeth of which represent the laminae of the lumbar vertebrae and the gaps of which indicate the interspaces. (c) Orientation of the ultrasound probe more cephalad on the lumbar spine. (d) Corresponding sonogram to c. Laminae of two adjacent vertebrae and elements of an interspace; from superficial to deep, there is visualization of the posterior unit, the intrathecal space, and the anterior unit. (Posterior unit: ligamentum flavum and posterior dura mater; anterior unit: anterior dura mater, posterior longitudinal ligament, and vertebral body.)

immediately under the skin that continues as a long triangular hypoechoic (dark) shadow (Figure 6.2b). The probe is then moved slightly caudad or cephalad to capture a good view of the desired interspace (Figure 6.2c). This view will typically show the "flying bat" pattern and allows visualization of the posterior unit, intrathecal space, anterior unit, and paramedian structures such as the articular and transverse processes (Figure 6.2d).

On visualizing a clear image of the interspace ("flying bat" pattern), the image is frozen. The probe is held steady, and two points are marked on the skin: one coinciding with the center of the upper horizontal surface of the probe (midline) and the other with the middle point of the right lateral surface of the probe (interspace). At the intersection of extensions of these two points, the puncture site is determined (Figure 6.3).

Once the optimal insertion point has been determined, the key to successful puncture is to insert the needle at an angle that reproduces the same angle at which the best image of the "flying bat" was acquired. The ultrasound beam penetrated the interspace without being distorted, and theoretically, the needle, likewise, should follow an uninterrupted path.

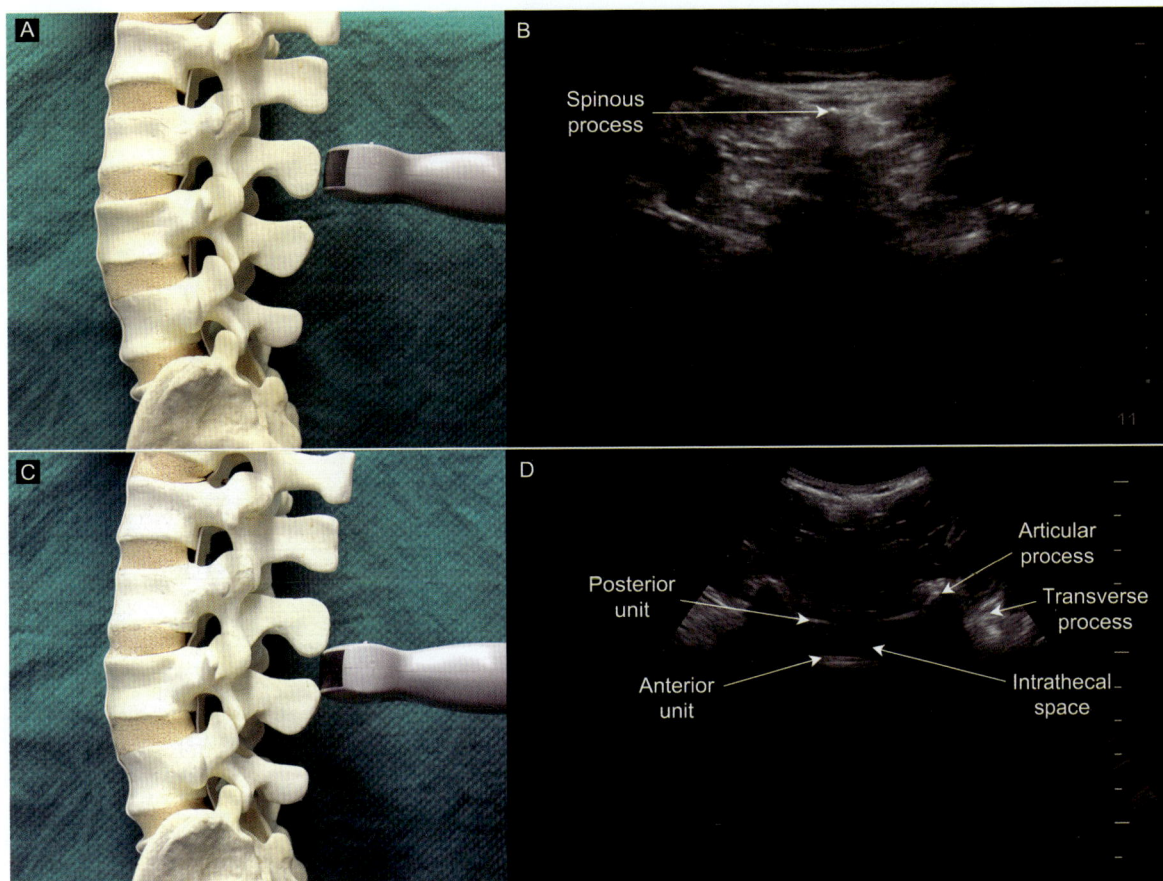

Figure 6.2 Transverse midline approach. (a) Orientation of the ultrasound probe at the tip of a lumbar spinous process. (b) Corresponding sonogram to a. The tip of the spinous process appears as a small hyperechoic structure immediately beneath the skin and determines a long vertical black hypoechoic shadow. (c) Orientation of the ultrasound probe at a lumbar interspace. (d) Corresponding sonogram to c. Typical interspace depicting the "flying bat" sign. Within the interspace, from superficial to deep, there is visualization of the posterior unit, the intrathecal space, and the anterior unit. Paramedian structures such as the articular and transverse processes can also be visualized. (Posterior unit: ligamentum flavum and posterior dura mater; anterior unit: anterior dura mater, posterior longitudinal ligament, and vertebral body.)

The depth to the epidural space can be accurately estimated from the frozen image of the interspace displaying the "flying bat" pattern. The captured image will display the ligamentum flavum and posterior dura mater as a single unit (posterior unit). On the ultrasound machine, built-in calipers can be used to measure the distance from the skin to the inner side of the posterior unit. It is important to keep the degree of compression of the subcutaneous tissue by the ultrasound transducer to a minimum while capturing the image because any degree of compression will lead to considerable underestimation of the depth to the epidural space. This is especially important in obese patients. Obese patients may have poorer image quality on spinal ultrasound, especially in the transverse plane ("flying bat" pattern). In this group of patients, the longitudinal paramedian oblique plane usually provides better images, with clear visualization of the posterior dura mater, which offers a very precise landmark for measurement of the depth to the epidural space. Furthermore the images can be obtained with much less compression of the subcutaneous tissue, which increases the accuracy of the assessment. Recent evidence has indicated that assessment of the depth to the epidural space in the longitudinal paramedian oblique plane is comparable with that obtained in the transverse midline plane

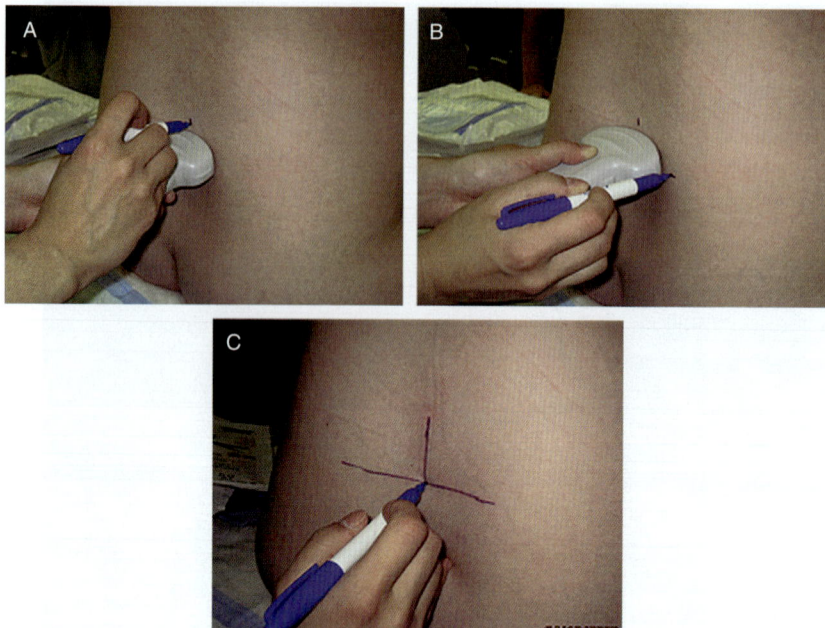

Figure 6.3 Determination of the puncture point. On visualizing a clear image of the interspace, the image is frozen. (a) A point at the center of the upper horizontal surface is marked. (b) A point at the middle point of the right lateral surface of the probe is marked. (c) At the intersection of the extensions of these two points, the puncture site is determined.

Source: Reprinted from JCA Carvalho, Ultrasound-facilitated epidural and spinals in obstetrics. *Anesthesiol Clin* 2008; 26:153.

and that both these measurements can be used interchangeably while performing midline punctures.[9]

Current Controversies and Future Directions

Most of the studies showing the benefits of spinal ultrasound have been conducted by individuals with a high level of experience and a special interest in performing spinal ultrasound. The level and type of training required to teach a novice spinal ultrasound and achieve competence are controversial. Margarido et al.[10] concluded that despite teaching experienced anesthetists spinal ultrasound using reading and video material, a lecture, and live demonstrations, this remained insufficient for full knowledge transfer. A cohort of trainees taught spinal ultrasound showed no improvement in the ease of insertion of epidural catheters with preprocedural ultrasound.[11] Therefore, extrapolating the benefits of spinal ultrasound from the current evidence base may not be directly applicable to the novice in spinal ultrasound. This supports the requirement for more comprehensive teaching in spinal ultrasound for complete acquisition of skills.

Blind palpatory landmark techniques for epidural or spinal anesthesia do not provide the clinician with the ability to predict a technically difficult needle insertion. However, visualization of the spinal anatomy with the aid of ultrasound may allow the user to anticipate technical difficulties. Chin et al.[12] demonstrated the association between a good transverse midline view on preprocedural ultrasound and subsequent ease of spinal anesthesia. Similarly, an association between the ultrasonographic identification of the posterior longitudinal ligament (a component of the anterior unit) in the longitudinal paramedian oblique view and technical ease of spinal injection has been shown.[13] Therefore, spinal ultrasound has a role in predicting difficult neuraxial anesthesia. Although suggestions for *predicted difficult spinal scores* exist,[12,13] there is no validated universal score in current practice.

Another area of future interest is real-time ultrasound imaging and epidural or spinal insertion. This provides the advantage of observing the passage of the needle into the desired space under real-time ultrasound vision. Of course, the challenges of this are clear and include the need for an assistant to perform either the ultrasound or the loss-of-resistance component, advanced training with higher interventional skills and manual dexterity, and meticulous preparation and care to maintain sterility. Feasibility studies have been undertaken with a single operator and the use of a loss-of-resistance syringe with an internal compression spring allowing automatic detection of the epidural space.[14] However, the technique of real-time ultrasound and epidural anesthesia currently remains a novel practice.

Learning Points

- Preprocedural spinal ultrasound reduces the risk of failed epidural or spinal anesthesia. Furthermore, it decreases the number of traumatic procedures, puncture attempts, and needle redirections.
- There is the theoretical benefit of added safety with spinal ultrasound. Confirmation of the lower lumbar interspaces when breaches of the dura are planned (i.e., in spinal anesthesia) is imperative in minimizing the risk of spinal cord trauma.
- Spinal ultrasound can improve the success rate of neuraxial blockade in predicted difficult subpopulations, such as patients with obesity or scoliosis.
- Other benefits may include selection of appropriate needle length from the outset, improved patient satisfaction, and the prediction of a technically difficult spine based on the ultrasound image.
- The transfer of full knowledge of spinal ultrasound and the ability to achieve competence require comprehensive teaching, the exact nature of which is yet to be determined. To undertake preprocedural ultrasound in predicted difficult cases such as obesity or scoliosis, you must first practice and develop proficiency in patients with normal spinal sonoanatomy.

References

1. Broadbent CR, Maxwell WB, Ferrie R, et al. Ability of anaesthetists to identify a marked lumbar interspace. *Anaesthesia* 2000; **55**:1122–26.

2. National Institute for Health and Clinical Excellence. Ultrasound guided catheterisation of the epidural space: understanding NICE guidance, January 2008.

Available at www.nice.org.uk (accessed November 11, 2014).

3. Grau T, Leipold RW, Conradi R, et al. Efficacy of ultrasound imaging in obstetric epidural anesthesia. *J Clin Anesth* 2002; **14**:169–75.

4. Shaikh F, Brzezinski J, Alexander S, et al. Ultrasound imaging for lumbar punctures and epidural catheterisations: systematic review and meta-analysis. *BMJ* 2013; **346**:f1720.

5. Grau T, Bartusseck E, Conradi R, et al. Ultrasound imaging improves learning curves in obstetric epidural anesthesia: a preliminary study. *Can J Anesth* 2003; **50**: 1047–50.

6. Furness G, Reilly MP, Kuchi S. An evaluation of ultrasound imaging for identification of lumbar intervertebral level. *Anaesthesia* 2002; **57**:277–80.

7. Chin KJ, Perlas A, Chan V, et al. Ultrasound imaging facilitates spinal anesthesia in adults with difficult surface anatomic landmarks. *Anesthesiology* 2011; **115**:94–101.

8. Carvalho JCA. Ultrasound-facilitated epidurals and spinals in obstetrics. *Anesthesiol Clin* 2008; **26**:145–58.

9. Sahota JS, Carvalho JCA, Balki M, et al. Ultrasound estimates for midline epidural punctures in the obese parturient: paramedian sagittal oblique is comparable to transverse median plane. *Anesth Analg* 2013; **116**: 829–35.

10. Margarido CB, Arzola C, Balki M, et al. Anesthesiologists' learning curves for ultrasound assessment of the lumbar spine. *Can J Anesth* 2010; **57**: 120–26.

11. Arzola C, Mikhael R, Margarido C, et al. Spinal ultrasound versus palpation for epidural catheter insertion in labor: a randomised controlled trial. *Eur J Anaesthesiol* 2014; **31**:1–7.

12. Chin KJ, Ramlogan R, Arzola C, et al. The utility of ultrasound imaging in predicting ease of performance of spinal anesthesia in an orthopedic patient population. *Reg Anesth Pain Med* 2013; **38**:34–38.

13. Weed JT, Taenzer AH, Finkel KJ, et al. Evaluation of pre-procedure ultrasound examination as a screening tool for difficult spinal anaesthesia. *Anaesthesia* 2011; **66**:925–30.

14. Karmakar MK, Li X, Ho AMH, et al. Real-time ultrasound guided paramedian epidural access: evaluation of a novel in-plane technique. *Br J Anaesth* 2009; **102**:845–54.

Combined Spinal-Epidural Anesthesia/Analgesia

Marc Van de Velde

Case Study

A healthy primigravidous patient with an uncomplicated pregnancy was induced at 41 weeks' gestation. Her booking blood pressure was 125/75 mmHg. Following cervical ripening with prostaglandins, artificial rupture of membranes, and initiation of an oxytocin infusion, the patient requested neuraxial analgesia when at 5 cm of cervical dilation and in active labor. A combined spinal-epidural (CSE) was performed at the L3–L4 interspace using the loss of resistance to saline needle-through-needle technique. The spinal injectate consisted of ropivacaine 4.5 mg and sufentanil 2.25 µg. Following threading of the epidural catheter, patient-controlled epidural analgesia (PCEA) with a bolus of 4 ml and a 15-minute lockout was started immediately, combined with programmed intermittent boluses (PIEBs) of 10 ml hourly as a fixed maintenance regimen. The fixed bolus was administered 30 minutes after the initial spinal dose. The epidural solution was ropivacaine 0.1% with sufentanil 0.5 µg/ml.

The patient reported visual analogue scores (VAS) for pain of 0 within minutes and of below 20 mm throughout labor and delivery. The patient was positioned in the supine position with left lateral tilt by the anesthesiology trainee immediately after the CSE had been placed. Seven minutes after the spinal injection, a sustained fetal bradycardia (70 beats/min) was recorded on the cardiotocogram (CTG). Simultaneously, uterine hypertonicity was noted. Maternal blood pressure was 110/65 mmHg. A consultant anesthesiologist was called while the midwife administered 5 mg ephedrine as per standing order. The patient was turned to the full left lateral position, and the oxytocin infusion was temporarily stopped. Six minutes into the fetal bradycardia, the fetal heart rate improved and returned to normal. Gradually, oxytocin was restarted. Three hours later the patient delivered a healthy baby with good Apgar scores and umbilical artery blood gases. She was discharged home 24 hours after delivery.

Key Points

- CSE combines the fast onset of a single-shot spinal with the flexibility of an epidural technique.
- The use of CSE remains a topic of controversy owing to the perceived imbalance of risks and benefits
- In this case, fetal bradycardia was associated with administration of intrathecal local anesthetic and opioid while the patient was positioned supine with left lateral tilt.
- Ephedrine and better positioning resolved the fetal bradycardia by improving uteroplacental perfusion and uterine hypertonicity.

Discussion

Combined spinal-epidural anesthesia/analgesia (CSE) has been around for many decades.[1] It combines the fast onset of a single-shot spinal with the flexibility of an epidural technique. The technique has also gained significant popularity in obstetric anesthetic practice both for labor analgesia and for anesthesia for cesarean delivery.[1–3] However, it remains a topic of controversy.[4]

CSE in Labor

Advantages of CSE over Epidurals

Onset Time of Analgesia. The most obvious advantage of the CSE technique is the rapid onset of analgesia.[5–9] Consistently, effective labor analgesia is accomplished within 5 minutes following the intrathecal injection of drugs. With epidurals, analgesia is usually achieved between 15 and 25 minutes **following injection**, but onset time demonstrates a wide **interpatient** variability, depending on factors such as parity and stage of labor.[6–10] Especially in advanced labor, epidural analgesia is often delayed, requiring large doses and volumes of epidural solution. With CSE, onset time is short in most patients irrespective of the stage of labor.

Quality of Pain Relief: VAS Scores, Satisfaction, and Anesthesiology Intervention Rate and Local Anesthetic Consumption. Lower VAS scores for labor pain with CSE compared with epidural analgesia have been consistently reported, especially during the initial period after the spinal injection and up to 120 minutes.[7,8,11] Throughout the entire labor duration, CSE also provides better-quality analgesia. Patients treated with conventional epidural analgesia are more likely to experience recurrent breakthrough pain than CSE-treated women and have more problems with unilateral analgesia.[11,12] The presence of a dural puncture may facilitate the passage of drugs from the epidural space to the CSF.[12] Furthermore, with CSE, local anesthetic requirements are significantly reduced compared with low-dose conventional epidural techniques.[7]

Epidural Catheter Reliability

Various investigators noted that the reliability of epidural catheters following CSE was similar or increased compared with stand-alone epidural catheters,[13] reflected by lower catheter replacement rates, fewer failures when topping up the epidural catheters for cesarean delivery, and less unilateral analgesia. Unfortunately, epidural catheter reliability was never a primary outcome variable, making interpretation of available data difficult. When using a CSE technique, a perfect midline approach is required to identify the subarachnoid space, and consequently, more epidural catheters are reliably positioned in the epidural space. Thomas et al.[14] interestingly noted that when no CSF was obtained following attempted CSE, subsequently many more epidural catheters required replacement compared with those placed when CSF was noted.

Potential Risks of CSEs

Pruritus, Nausea, and Hypotension

Pruritus is the most common side effect of intrathecal and epidural opioids. No difference in the incidence of nausea has between reported when comparing the two techniques. As with any neuraxial technique, hypotension can occur following labor analgesia.

Both CSE and conventional epidural analgesia have been associated with usually mild hypotension, which is easily treated.[6] In routine clinical practice, it is important with CSE to avoid the supine position. In my hospital, patients are positioned in the completely left lateral position immediately after the CSE to avoid any effect of aortocaval compression.

CNS Infections

Some authorities claim that the risk of CNS infections is increased secondary to the breach of the dura. However, at present, there is no scientific evidence supporting this claim. Following 30,000 obstetric CSEs performed in my institution over the last 25 years, no CNS infection has been noted.

Neurologic Complications

As with any regional technique, the potential for nerve damage is present. Several case reports in pregnant women of damage to the conus medullaris when using CSE have been published.[15] Especially with CSE, it is imperative to perform the block as low as possible because the conus medullaris might extend below the L2 vertebral body. Up to 5 percent of parturients can have a conus that extends lower than the L2 vertebral body. To avoid conus damage, careful attention to the correct interspace is required. It is also important to remember that anesthesiologists miss the correct interspace in more than 50 percent of cases when determining the interspace by anatomic landmarks.[16]

Post–Dural Puncture Headache (PDPH)

Because CSE includes a dural puncture, there is a theoretical risk of post–dural puncture headache (PDPH). The incidence is not increased over that with conventional epidural analgesia.[17]

Fetal Heart Rate Changes

Abnormal fetal heart rate recordings and fetal bradycardia are worrisome side effects that may follow any type of effective labor analgesia. More abnormal cardiotocographic readings following CSE than with systemic analgesia are reported.[18] Also compared with conventional epidural analgesia, CSE induces more fetal heart rate abnormalities.[6] It is important to note that neonatal and obstetric outcome is not affected by the use of CSE.

The mechanism of fetal heart rate abnormalities is not completely resolved, but uterine hypertonicity is crucial. As a result of rapid analgesia, an imbalance

31

occurs between norepinephrine and epinephrine levels (due to different half-lives), resulting in a brief higher concentration of norepinephrine, which is a uterine stimulant, resulting in uterine hypertonicity. Potentially also involved are intrathecal opioids, which have been shown to produce more fetal heart rate changes when higher doses are used.[6,19]

CSE for Cesarean Delivery

Spinal anesthesia is the technique of choice for cesarean delivery, but spinal-induced hypotension is also a common problem, with the potential for causing serious maternal and fetal morbidity.[20] In recent years, a shift in understanding of the pathophysiology of spinal-induced hypotension has occurred, with less emphasis on venodilation and more on peripheral vasodilation.[21] Three strategies exist to prevent/treat hypotension: fluid loading, vasopressors and reducing the spinal local anesthetic dose.[22] Strategies to increase fluid loading have minimal success (e.g., left lateral tilt, crystalloid or colloid loading, and leg wrapping). Furthermore, prophylactic volumes of IV fluids increase the risk of iatrogenic pulmonary edema. Vasopressors are more successful in preventing hypotension, but they also have side effects such as myocardial ischemia, fetal acidosis, bradycardia, and hypertension. The third option, to lower the spinal anesthesia dose, is also possible, especially when a CSE technique is used. The goal of lowering the spinal dose is to avoid hypotension while preserving good-quality anesthesia.

Less Hypotension

Studies have demonstrated that lowering the spinal anesthesia dose to less than 9 mg and more than 5 mg bupivacaine can significantly reduce the incidence and severity of hypotension, as was demonstrated by Arzola et al. in a recent meta-analysis.[23] Several additional studies not included in the meta-analysis by Arzola produced similar results.[24–27]

Vercauteren et al.[24–26] published three trials in which they evaluated the incidence of hypotension following CSE anesthesia with 6.6 mg hyperbaric bupivacaine and 3.3 µg sufentanil. Hypotension occurred for both studies combined in only eight of 102 patients (8 percent).

Van de Velde et al.[27] performed a randomized comparison of patients treated with CSE using either 6.5 or 9.5 mg hyperbaric bupivacaine combined in both groups with 2.5 µg sufentanil. Patients in the 9.5-mg group experienced more pronounced and longer hypotensive periods than those in the 6.5-mg group. The mean lowest recorded systolic pressure was higher in the 6.5-mg group (102 ± 16 mmHg versus 88 ± 16 mmHg in the 9.5-mg group; $p < 0.05$). More patients in the 9.5-mg group experienced hypotension than in the 6.5-mg group (68 versus 16 percent; $p < 0.05$). In the 9.5-mg group, 15 patients required pharmacologic treatment for hypotension versus five in the 6.5-mg group.

McNaught and Stocks[28] concluded that epidural saline could extend a spinal block. They also found that the CSE technique itself results in a higher sensory level of the block. This is explained by a change in epidural pressure when the epidural space is identified with the Tuohy needle because negative epidural pressure is neutralized by the open connection to atmospheric pressure, resulting in a reduction in dural sac volume, similar to the injection of fluid.

Quality of Anesthesia

Many anesthetists would worry that lowering the spinal dose would reduce the quality of anesthesia and increase the incidence of pain during cesarean delivery. However, single-shot spinal anesthesia is also associated with inadequate anesthesia in 5–10 percent of patients.[29] Arzola et al.[22] reported a 3.79 relative risk that low-dose spinal anesthesia was associated with intraoperative pain versus high-dose spinal anesthesia. However, Arzola et al.[22] considered it a failure if the epidural was used for a top-up, whereas using the epidural catheter is an integral part of the anesthetic technique and should not be considered a failure. Indeed, a CSE technique could be considered mandatory when low-dose spinal anesthesia is used. In their review of the literature, McNaught and Stocks[28] did conclude that the technique of using low intrathecal doses has an increased risk of intraoperative pain, shorter duration of effective anesthesia, and a slower onset.

In our experience, epidural supplementation is required in approximately 20 percent of patients treated with 6.5 mg bupivacaine versus only 8 percent of patients treated with 9.5 mg bupivacaine. If additional epidural anesthesia was required, this only occurred if surgery was prolonged more than 60 minutes from the start of the spinal injection. Since we are using low spinal doses (5.5–6.5 mg bupivacaine with sufentanil) routinely as part of a CSE technique, we now know that if the uterus is not closed approximately 45 minutes after start of the CSE, epidural supplementation will be required, and an epidural top-up (5–8 ml ropivacaine 0.75% with sufentanil) is given prophylactically. We only very rarely have to supplement the initial spinal dose with epidural local anesthetic within 1 hour of the spinal injection. We also very rarely observe complete motor block. Indeed, many authors report on faster motor recovery.

Learning Points

- CSE is an excellent option for both labor analgesia and anesthesia for cesarean delivery.
- During labor, it provides excellent quality of analgesia with rapid onset and superior epidural catheter reliability.
- During cesarean delivery, low-dose spinal anesthesia can be used, providing better hemodynamic stability with less need for fluid and vasopressors.
- Patient comfort (less nausea and vomiting) is also increased.

References

1. Rawal N, Holmstrom B, Crowhurst JA, Van Zundert A. The combined spinal epidural technique. *Anesth Clin North Am* 2000; **18**:267–95.

2. Camann WR, Mintzer BH, Denney RA, Datta S. Intrathecal sufentanil for labor analgesia. *Anesthesiology* 1993; **78**:870–74.

3. Collis RE, Baxandall ML, Srikantharajah ID, et al. Combined spinal epidural analgesia: technique, management and outcome of 300 mothers. *Int J Obstet Anesth* 1994; **3**:75–81.

4. Preston R. The role of combined spinal epidural analgesia for labour: is there still a question? *Can J Anaesth* 2007; **54**:9–14.

5. Simmons SW, Taghizadeh N, Dennis AT, Hughes D, Cyna AM. Combined spinal-epidural versus epidural analgesia in labour. *Cochrane Database Syst Rev* 2012; **10**:CD003401.

6. Van de Velde M, Teunkens A, Hanssens M, Vandermeersch E, Verhaeghe J. Intrathecal sufentanil and fetal heart rate abnormalities: a double blind, double placebo controlled trial comparing two forms of combined spinal epidural analgesia with epidural analgesia in labor. *Anesth Analg* 2004; **98**:1153–59.

7. Van de Velde M, Mignolet K, Vandermeersch E, Van Assche A. Prospective, randomized comparison of epidural and combined spinal epidural analgesia during labor. *Acta Anaesthesiol Belg* 1999; **50**:129–36.

8. Collis RE, Davies DWL, Aveling W. Randomised comparison of combined spinal epidural and standard epidural analgesia in labour. *Lancet* 1995; **345**:1413–16.

9. Wilson MJ, Cooper G, MacArthur C, Shennan A. Randomized controlled trial comparing traditional with two mobile epidural techniques: anesthetic and analgesic efficiency. *Anesthesiology* 2002; **97**:1567–75.

10. Van de Velde M. Combined spinal epidural analgesia for labor and delivery: a balanced view based on experience and literature. *Acta Anaesthesiol Belg* 2009; **60**(2):109–22.

11. Gambling D, Berkowitz J, Farrell TR, Pue A, Shay D. A randomized controlled comparison of epidural analgesia and combined spinal-epidural analgesia in a private practice setting: pain scores during first and second stages of labor and at delivery. *Anesth Analg* 2013; **116**:636–43.

12. Capiello E, O'Rourke N, Segal S, Tsen LC. A randomized trial of dural puncture epidural technique compared with the standard epidural technique for labor analgesia. *Anesth Analg* 2008; **107**:1646–51.

13. Heesen M, Van de Velde M, Klohr S, et al. Meta-analysis of the success of block following combined spinal-epidural vs epidural analgesia during labour. *Anaesthesia* 2014; **69**:64–71.

14. Thomas JA, Pan PH, Harris LC, Owen MD, D'Angelo R. Dural puncture with a 27-gauge Whitacre needle as part of a combined spinal-epidural technique does not improve labor epidural catheter function. *Anesthesiology* 2005; **103**:1046–51.

15. Reynolds F. Damage to the conus medullaris following spinal anaesthesia. *Anaesthesia* 2001; **56**:238–47.

16. Van Gessel EF, Forster A, Gamulin Z. Continuous spinal anesthesia: where do spinal catheters go? *Anesth Analg* 1993; **76**:1004–7.

17. Van de Velde M, Teunkens A, Hanssens M, van Assche FA, Vandermeersch E. Post dural puncture headache following combined spinal epidural or epidural anaesthesia in obstetric patients. *Anaesth Intensive Care* 2001; **29**:505–99.

18. Mardirosoff C, Dumont L, Boulvain M, Tramer MR. Fetal bradycardia due to intrathecal opioids for labour analgesia: a systematic review. *BJOG* 2002; **109**:274–81.

19. Cheng SL, Bautista D, Leo S, Sia TH. Factors affecting fetal bradycardia following combined spinal epidural for labor analgesia: a matched case-control study. *J Anesth* 2013; **27**:169–74.

20. Reynolds F, Seed PT. Anaesthesia for caesarean section and neonatal acid-base status: a meta-analysis. *Anaesthesia* 2005; **60**:636–53.

21. Langesaeter E, Dyer RA. Maternal haemodynamic changes during spinal anaesthesia for caesarean section. *Curr Opin Anaesthesiol* 2011; **24**:242–48.

22. Roofthooft E, Van de Velde M. Low-dose spinal anaesthesia for caesarean section to prevent spinal-induced hypotension. *Curr Opin Anaesthesiol* 2008; **21**:259–62.

23. Arzola C, Wieczorek PM. Efficacy of low-dose bupivacaine in spinal anaesthesia for caesarean delivery: systematic review and meta-analysis. *Br J Anaesth* 2011; **107**:308–18.

24. Vercauteren MP, Coppejans HC, Hoffman VH, Mertens E, Adriaensen HA. Prevention of hypotension by a single 5-mg dose of ephedrine during small dose spinal anesthesia in prehydrated cesarean delivery patients. *Anesth Analg* 2000; **90**:324–27.

25. Coppejans HC, Hendrickx E, Goossens J, Vercauteren MP. The sitting versus right lateral position during combined spinal-epidural anesthesia for cesarean delivery: block characteristics and severity of hypotension. *Anesth Analg* 2006; **102**: 243–47.

26. Coppejans HC, Vercauteren MP. Low-dose combined spinal-epidural anesthesia for cesarean delivery: a comparison of three plain local anesthetics. *Acta Anaesth Belg* 2006; **57**:39–43.

27. Van de Velde M, Van Schoubroeck D, Jani J, et al. Combined spinal epidural anestehsia for cesarean section: dose dependent effects of hyperbaric bupivacaine on maternal hemodynamics. *Anesth Analg* 2006; **103**:187–90.

28. McNaught AF, Stocks GM. Epidural volume extension and low-dose sequential combined spinal-epidural blockade: two ways to reduce spinal dose requirement for caesarean section (review). *IJOA* 2007; **16**:346–53.

29. Kinsella SM. A prospective audit of regional anaesthesia failure in 5,080 caesarean sections. *Anaesthesia* 2008; **63**:822–32.

Nonpharmacologic Analgesia for Childbirth

E. Lindsay Moore and William Camann

Case Study

A 31-year-old healthy nulliparous patient at 40 + 2 weeks' gestation presented to the Labor & Delivery Unit in spontaneous labor. She was under the care of a midwife and strongly desired natural childbirth. On admission, she was accompanied by her husband and her doula. She presented her nurse with a written birth plan that detailed several requests for her labor experience, including nonpharmacologic pain management. She wanted to begin in the birthing tub and use hypnotherapy techniques during her labor.

Key Points

- Patients may present to labor and delivery with plans to employ several nonpharmacologic methods of relaxation and pain mitigation during their labor.
- Many of these techniques are entirely compatible with neuraxial or pharmacologic analgesia.
- Anesthesiologists should strive to understand the variety of options available, maintain respect for the patient's goals, and facilitate a satisfying and safe labor experience for the patient.

Discussion

This patient's case represents a common clinical scenario encountered on labor and delivery units. Some obstetric patients are motivated to experience labor with little or no medical intervention. As anesthesiologists, it is important for us to acknowledge their goals, recognize alternative methods of analgesia, and appreciate that many of these methods are still compatible with conventional anesthetic interventions. Often the patient's satisfaction with the childbirth process does not necessarily correlate with pain control.[1] The efficacy of these complementary or alternative medicine (CAM) techniques is difficult to evaluate scientifically; nonetheless, they are widely accepted by many patients and incorporated into their birth plans.[2–5]

Water Immersion

The use of birthing tubs or whirlpools has increased in popularity, and many hospitals have this equipment available for laboring patients (Figure 8.1). Women may choose to labor in the tub, and some may also deliver while submerged in water (based on institutional policy). Water immersion provides a warm, soothing environment for the parturient and is thought to increase relaxation and decrease the perception of pain, although the exact mechanism of analgesia is unknown.[6]

Several benefits of water immersion have been identified, in addition to its potential analgesic effects. Parturients who participate in hydrotherapy have been shown to have shorter labors, fewer tears and episiotomies, fewer obstetric interventions (e.g., amniotomy, pharmacologic augmentation), and lower analgesic requirements (pharmacologic or regional).[3] Studies have not shown a decreased incidence of instrumental or operative deliveries in these patients, however. A randomized, controlled trial (RCT) has shown that water immersion may be helpful in early labor to manage labor dystocia.[7] It is difficult to objectively assess the true analgesic effects of water immersion given the inability to provide it in a blinded fashion, and patients who seek water immersion therapy may be highly motivated to undergo natural childbirth.

Laboring with water immersion does not preclude the patient from using other methods of analgesia. Although parturients are generally not permitted to have an epidural while in the tub, they may choose to labor initially using water immersion and then ask for an epidural after they leave the tub. Other laboring techniques also may be used simultaneously with water immersion, such as hypnobirthing and

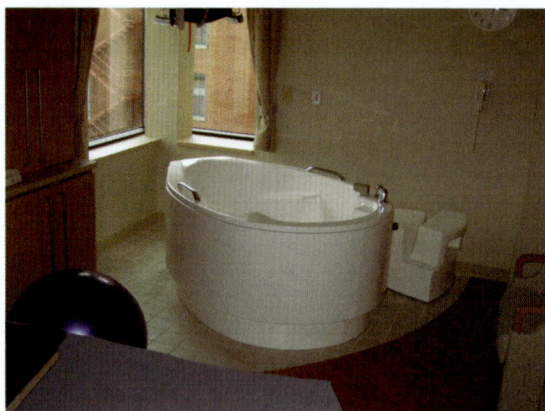

Figure 8.1 A typical labor tub

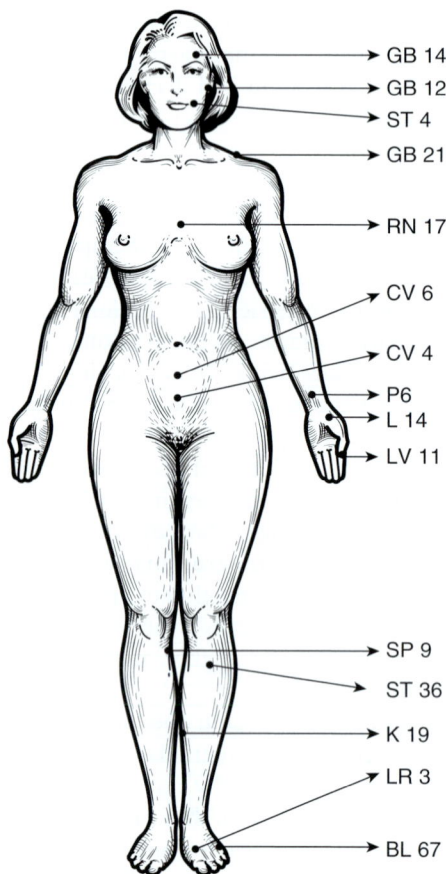

Figure 8.2 Selected acupoint sites relevant to obstetrics and anesthesia
Source: Artwork courtesy of Getty Images.

massage. Water-compatible monitors allow for continuous fetal heart rate monitoring even while the patient is submerged in water.

Certain patients may not be eligible for hydrotherapy. Relative contraindications, based on institutional policy, may include premature labor, ruptured membranes, and the presence of meconium, infection, or vaginal bleeding. Another important consideration is the sanitation of the tub, water, and hose equipment. Bacteria such as *Pseudomonas aeruginosa* and *Klebsiella pneumoniae* have been cultured from these labor whirlpools and pose an infection risk for both the mother and the neonate.[8]

Water immersion is generally considered safe in low-risk parturients undergoing uncomplicated vaginal deliveries.[9] Caregivers who oversee patients laboring with hydrotherapy must be aware of its risks and promote proper sanitation of equipment. Although there is not sufficient data to determine the true analgesic effect of water immersion, many women report great satisfaction while laboring with hydrotherapy.

Acupuncture and Acupressure

Acupuncture is a form of traditional Chinese medicine based on the belief that energy, or *Qi* (pronounced "chi"), flows along channels in the body called *meridians* (Figure 8.2). Acupuncture theory holds that many medical conditions result from the disruption of this energy flow and that the insertion of fine needles along these meridians helps to restore the harmony of *Qi*. No anatomic correlations between the meridians and Western medicine exist, but the efficacy of acupuncture may be related to its interaction with the neuroendocrine system.[3]

Acupuncture has been used to treat a variety of medical conditions, including infertility and hyperemesis gravidarum. Data suggest that acupuncture, in conjunction with moxibustion (the burning of mugwort adjacent to the tip of the fifth toe), may help to convert a breech fetus to vertex.[10] There are also several uses for acupuncture during labor, such as induction of labor and treatment of nausea and pain.[11]

The true efficacy of acupuncture is difficult to assess because of the inability to blind both patients and acupuncturists. A meta-analysis of 10 RCTs showed that acupuncture did not significantly decrease pain scores in comparison with minimal acupuncture (placing needles in areas that are not acupoints).[12] However, other studies using placebo or sham acupuncture (mimics acupuncture without actually inserting needles) demonstrated a decrease in use of pharmacologic or regional analgesia in the patients who received acupuncture.[13] A further study that randomized 36 patients to receive electroacupuncture versus placebo found that the women receiving acupuncture had decreased pain intensity, greater relaxation, and increased levels of B-endorphin and 5-hydroxytryptamine in blood samples.[14]

Acupuncture is considered safe for use in labor with no reported complications. Its success relies on the involvement of an experienced acupuncturist and motivated patient.

Hypnosis

Hypnosis is considered a scientifically accepted method of analgesia. Parturients may opt to practice various forms of hypnosis during labor, including self-hypnosis, instructor-guided hypnosis, and the use of audio recordings. These techniques help to put the patient in a state of focused concentration, in which she is unaware of, although not completely blinded to, her surroundings. Many hypnotic techniques use "softer" words than usual medical terminology to ease the patient into a relaxed state. For example, using the word *release* rather than *rupture, blossom* rather than *dilate*, and *tightening* rather than *pain* can help to comfort patients.[15]

Positron emission tomography (PET) has shown that hypnosis modulates pain by suppression of neural activity in the anterior cingulate gyrus.[16] Hypnosis requires a motivated patient, as well as prenatal preparation. It is generally a well-received practice given its noninvasive nature and compatibility with other analgesic techniques, including regional anesthesia.

Sterile Water Papules and TENS

The intracutaneous injection of sterile water papules is a technique often used by midwives that offers relief for patients suffering from back labor. Laboring patients may experience lower back pain, often due to malpresentation of the fetal head in the occiput posterior position. The injection of four small (0.1 ml) papules of sterile water in a square pattern above the sacrum may provide temporary analgesia for these patients (Figure 8.3). The mechanism of analgesia may be related in part to the gate theory of pain or the distraction technique. Patients reported experiencing less severe back pain after these injections, but the use of intravenous or neuraxial anesthesia did not change.[17] Although its effects are transient, this low-risk technique may be a helpful adjunct for patients experiencing severe back pain during labor.[2]

A transcutaneous electrical nerve stimulation (TENS) unit may be applied to the lower back. Such units deliver low-voltage impulses that are believed to provide pain relief, again also related to the gate theory of pain. Electrical impulses delivered by the TENS unit may interfere with the perception of other painful stimuli simultaneously being transmitted along the same path. TENS has also been postulated to increase endorphin release, distracting the patient and reducing anxiety.[3] A meta-analysis of nine randomized trials found no significant benefit in pain relief or need for additional analgesia but also no adverse effects of TENS in labor.[18]

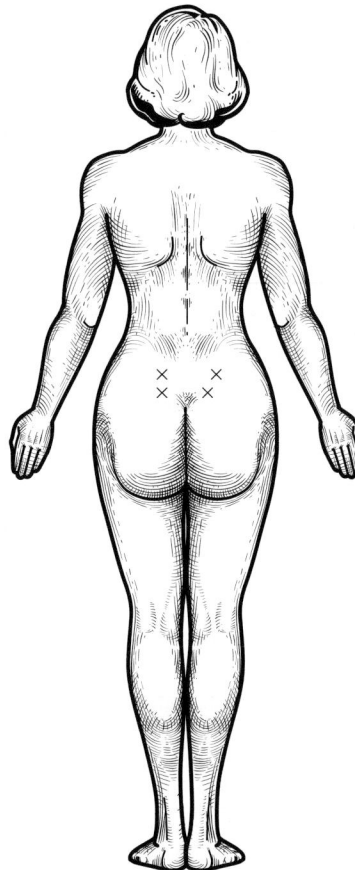

Figure 8.3 Sterile water papule placement
Source: Artwork courtesy of Getty Images.

Adjuvant Therapies

In addition to the methods previously discussed, several adjuvant therapies are available that aid in promoting relaxation and reducing anxiety during labor. Continuous one-on-one labor support, whether through a doula, friend, or partner, has been associated with favorable outcomes for laboring women. Women who receive continuous emotional support have been shown to have shorter labors, fewer instrumental or operative deliveries, request less intrapartum analgesia, and report increased satisfaction with the childbirth experience.[19]

Massage, aromatherapy, music, and biofeedback are additional techniques that promote relaxation. Position changes, ambulation, and the birthing ball are other activities that may be beneficial during labor. Most evidence surrounding these methods is anecdotal, and it is likely that the benefit of these techniques lies in stress relief and a motivated patient rather than analgesia. Nonetheless, these therapies often provide significant comfort and satisfaction for patients and pose little to no risk for the mother and baby.

Learning Points

- Multiple nonpharmacologic adjuvant or alternative therapies are available for labor analgesia.
- For some patients, satisfaction does not necessarily equate to absolute pain relief.
- It is important for anesthesiologists to understand and respect the patient's goals, as well as to shape expectations and facilitate safe labor and delivery.
- Most forms of complementary or alternative medicine (CAM) are entirely compatible with pharmacologic and regional anesthesia.

References

1. Kannan S, Jamison RN, Datta S. Maternal satisfaction and pain control in women electing natural childbirth. *Reg Anesth Pain Med* 2001; **26**(5):468–72.

2. Arendt KW, Camann W. Alternative (nonpharmacologic) methods of labor analgesia, in Suresh MS, Segal BS, Preston RL, et al. (eds.), *Schnider & Levinson's Anesthesia for Obstetrics*, 5th edn. Baltimore, MD: Lippincott Williams & Wilkins; 2013, pp. 81–91.

3. Arendt KW, Tessmer-Tuck JA. Nonpharmacologic labor analgesia. *Clin Perinatol* 2013; **40**(3):351–71.

4. Simkin PP, O'Hara M. Nonpharmacologic relief of pain during labor: systematic reviews of five methods. *Am J Obstet Gynecol* 2002; **186**(5 Suppl Nature):S131-59.

5. Chaillet N, Belaid L, Crochetiere C, et al. Nonpharmacologic approaches for pain management during labor compared with usual care: a meta-analysis. *Birth* 2014; **41**(2):122–37.

6. Cluett ER, Burns E. Immersion in water in labour and birth. *Cochrane Database Syst Rev* 2009; (2):CD000111.

7. Cluett ER, Pickering RM, Getliffe K, et al. Randomised controlled trial of laboring in water compared with standard of augmentation for management of dystocia in first stage of labour. *BMJ* 2004; **328**:314.

8. Fritschel E, Sanyal K, Threadgill H, Cervantes D. Fatal legionellosis after water birth. *Emerg Infect Dis* 2015; **21**(1):130–32.

9. American Academy of Pediatrics Committee on Fetus and Newborn and American College of Obstetricians and Gynecologists Committee on Obstetric Practice. Immersion in water during labor and delivery. *Pediatrics* 2014; **133**(4):758–61.

10. Coyle ME, Smith CA, Peat B. Cephalic version by moxibustion for breech presentation. *Cochrane Database Syst Rev* 2012; (5):CD003928.

11. Allen TK, Habib AS. P6 stimulation for the prevention of nausea and vomiting associated with cesarean delivery under neuraxial anesthesia: a systematic review of randomized controlled trials. *Anesth Analg* 2008; **107**(4):1308–12.

12. Cho SH, Lee H, Ernst E. Acupuncture for pain relief in labour: a systematic review and meta-analysis. *BJOG* 2010; **117**:907–20.

13. Skilnand E, Fossen D, Heiberg E. Acupuncture in the management of pain in labor. *Acta Obstet Gynaecol Scand* 2002; **81**:943–48.

14. Qu F, Zhou J. Electro-acupuncture in relieving labor pain. *Evid-Based Compl Alt* 2007; **4**:125–30.

15. Varelman D, Pancaro C, Cappiello EC, Camann WR. Nocebo-induced hyperalgesia during local anesthetic injection. *Anesth Analg* 2010; **110**(3):868–70.

16. Rainville P, Duncan GH, Price DD, et al. Pain affect encoded in human anterior cingulate but not somatosensory cortex. *Science* 1997; **277**:968.

17. Derry S, Straube S, Moore RA, et al. Intracutaneous or subcutaneous sterile water injection compared with blinded controls for pain management in labour. *Cochrane Database Syst Rev* 2012; (1):CD009107.

18. Mello LF, Nóbrega LF, Lemos A. Transcutaneous electrical stimulation for pain relief during labor: a systematic review and meta-analysis. *Rev Bras Fisioter* 2011; **15**(3):175–84. PubMed PMID: 21829980.

19. American College of Obstetrics and Gynecologists and Society for Maternal-Fetal Medicine. Obstetric care consensus number 1: safe prevention of the primary cesarean delivery. *Obstet Gynecol* 2014; **123**(3):693–711.

Chapter 9

Systemic Pharmacologic Analgesia

Grace McClune and David Hill

Case Study

A previously fit and healthy 65-kg nulliparous woman presented at 20 weeks' gestation with pleuritic chest pain and acute shortness of breath. Arterial blood gas measurement showed a reduced PaO_2 on room air of 8.8 kPa. White cell count was within normal limits, and C-reactive protein was mildly elevated at 12 mg/liter. Due to a clinical suspicion of pulmonary embolism, the patient was admitted to hospital for further investigation and treatment. A chest x-ray and a lung ventilation-perfusion scan were performed, and the patient was diagnosed with a pulmonary embolus. She was started on a therapeutic dose of the low-molecular-weight heparin (LMWH) enoxaparin at a dose of 1.5 mg/kg daily. After 72 hours in hospital, the patient was discharged home with ongoing anticoagulation at the same dose of enoxaparin. She was reviewed 1 week later and then every 2 weeks at a joint antenatal/hematology clinic. By 29 weeks' gestation she reported complete resolution of her respiratory symptoms. Measurement of her anti-factor Xa levels (0.93 unit/ml) indicated that the enoxaparin dose was appropriately effective.

A multidisciplinary plan was put in place for induction of labor at term (40 weeks) with the cessation of therapeutic anticoagulation 24 hours before in order to facilitate neuraxial analgesia or anesthesia if required and reduce the risk of postpartum hemorrhage.

The patient presented following spontaneous rupture of membranes at 38 weeks' gestation. On vaginal examination, her cervix was 3 cm dilated, and she was judged to be in active labor because she was experiencing moderately painful contractions lasting 30–40 seconds at a frequency of 3 in 10 minutes. She had self-administered the last dose of therapeutic enoxaparin 4 hours prior to presentation.

From an obstetric viewpoint, this patient had been advised that her prescribed dose of enoxaparin carried an increased risk of more than 500 ml blood loss after

vaginal delivery but that it was not likely to significantly increase her risk of severe postpartum hemorrhage (i.e., >1,000 ml). There was therefore an obstetric plan in place to administer an IM bolus of syntocinon 5 units with ergometrine 500 μg (Syntometrine) as active management of the third stage of labor rather than the standard of syntocinon only. This was to be followed by a syntocinon infusion at 10 units per hour for 4 hours after delivery if the time interval between the last dose of enoxaparin and delivery was less than 24 hours or if blood loss after delivery was greater than 500 ml.

The patient had been advised at antenatal anesthetic assessment that epidural analgesia would be contraindicated within 24 hours of a therapeutic dose of enoxaparin due to the increased risk of epidural hematoma. She therefore asked to speak to the duty anesthetist to discuss the advantages and disadvantages of the alternative analgesia options available. The anesthetist discussed the options of nitrous oxide and oxygen (Entonox), intermittent IM diamorphine, or a remifentanil patient-controlled analgesia (PCA) with her and she initially opted to use Entonox. However, as labor progressed, she became increasingly distressed by pain, and when vaginal examination was repeated after 4 hours and showed cervical dilation of 5 cm, she decided to escalate her analgesia use to remifentanil. The anesthetist revisited her and, after confirming her consent and midwife availability to provide one-to-one supervision, prescribed and connected a remifentanil PCA with a bolus dose of 40 μg delivered over 10 seconds with a lockout time of 2 minutes.

The patient initially found it difficult to coordinate use of the PCA with the timing of her contractions, but with coaching from her midwife, this improved, and the patient continued to use it until the time of delivery. She received one-to-one supervision from a midwife throughout with continuous oxygen saturation monitoring and 30-minute

39

Table 9.1 Contraindications to Epidural Analgesia in Labor

Maternal coagulopathy
Maternal use of LMWH within 12 hours (prophylactic) or 24 hours (therapeutic)
Localized skin infection at insertion site
Untreated maternal bacteremia
Increased intracranial pressure
Stenotic valvular lesions
Allergy to epidural analgesia agents
Spinal malformations
Preexisting neurologic deficits

observations: respiratory rate, sedation score, pain score. She experienced some nausea, for which she received ondansetron 4 mg, and some mild sedation but did not desaturate or require supplemental oxygen at any time. After laboring for 8 hours (in hospital), she delivered a healthy baby boy by spontaneous vaginal delivery. Oxytocin with ergometrine (Syntometrine) was administered IM as planned for the third stage of labor, and this was followed by a oxytocin (Syntocinon) infusion at a rate of 10 units per hour over 4 hours. Total blood loss was estimated at 850 ml.

Key Points

- Neuraxial analgesia for labor was contraindicated for this patient.
- It is the responsibility of anesthetists within the delivery area to know, understand, and be able to explain the advantages and disadvantages of systemic analgesic options available to laboring women.

Discussion

Labor pain is a virtually universal experience for childbearing women.[1] Effective pain management is therefore an important goal of intrapartum care. Epidural analgesia remains the most effective method of pain control, but it is not a universal solution.[2] For some women, such as in this case study, it is contraindicated, but many others either do not feel that their level of pain warrants this intervention or wish to avoid the risks of an invasive procedure and opt for alternative solutions to reduce pain (Table 9.1). Systemic medications in common use as labor analgesia are diverse in their mechanisms of action and display varying efficacy and side-effect profiles both for mother and for the baby.

Medications in common use can be split into four main groups: inhalational agents, nonopioid analgesics, systemic opioids administered as a bolus, and systemic opioids administered via PCA systems. The dosing, efficacy, and safety profiles, for both mother and baby, of each of these are explored next.

Inhalational Agents: Nitrous Oxide

Entonox (a 50:50 mix of nitrous oxide and oxygen) can be used alone or to supplement other methods of analgesia. A pressure-reducing valve fitted to the Entonox cylinder attaches to a breathing circuit, with a demand valve connected to a mouthpiece for the patient's use. Inhaled nitrous oxide concentrations equilibrate rapidly with arterial blood concentration, with the peak effect after initiation of Entonox for approximately 50 seconds. Women are encouraged to breathe Entonox only during contractions and room air for in-between rest periods.

The availability and use of nitrous oxide for labor analgesia across the world is very variable. In some countries such as the United Kingdom it is a popular choice for many women, but the evidence supporting its efficacy is mixed.[3] Some studies report reductions in pain scores similar to those achieved with systemic opioids,[4–6] but many report no improvement in pain scores, and up to 40 percent of mothers find its use of no benefit. Interestingly despite this, many women would choose to use nitrous oxide again for subsequent labors, suggesting that it is of some help even if not measurable with pain scores.[3,7–9]

Inhaled nitrous oxide analgesia for labor displays good safety outcomes for both mother and baby. Side effects include nausea but no increased rate of vomiting, a slight increase in the rate of maternal oxygen desaturation between contractions, and an increase in the rate of maternal drowsiness.[3,6,10,11] Nitrous oxide administration does not adversely affect uterine activity and does not cause significant neonatal respiratory depression, reduced Apgar scores, or fetal acidosis.[12,13]

Nonopioid Analgesics

Acetaminophen (paracetamol) is a widely used and effective antipyretic and analgesic medication. It is administered at a dose of 1 g (if patient weight > 50 kg) orally or intravenously every 4–6 hours, with a maximum of 4 g in 24 hours.[14,15]

Oral administration of acetaminophen in labor does not appear to offer significant analgesic benefit, but intravenous acetaminophen has been shown to be more effective than intravenous pethidine, with a duration of action of up to 2 hours.[16] Acetaminophen has many fewer maternal adverse effects than opioids and has a favorable safety profile; when used in pregnancy, it is not associated with an increased risk of fetal morbidity.[14,15,17]

Nonsteroidal anti-inflammatory drugs (NSAIDs) have an anti-inflammatory, analgesic, and antipyretic effect mediated by inhibition of prostaglandin formation. They are not in common use in labor because they do not appear to be effective as sole analgesic agents.[18] As inhibitors of cyclooxygenase, NSAIDs have the potential to prolong labor and to cause constriction of the ductus arteriosus, renal dysfunction, and hemostatic abnormalities in the fetus and neonate.[19]

Systemic Opioids (Bolus)

Opioids are the most widely used systemic analgesia in labor but exhibit variable efficacy and a wide range of side effects.[4,20] They act by binding to opioid receptors found in the central and peripheral nervous systems and the gastrointestinal tract.

In some countries, such as the United Kingdom, intermittent bolus IM injections have the advantage of being midwife prescribed and delivered and so readily available, but they may be painful, display variable drug absorption depending on the site of injection, and have an inevitable delay between time of injection and onset of action. Intermittent bolus IV injections have the advantage of quicker onset, the ability to titrate to effect, and a more predictable quality and duration of analgesia, but they require the presence of medical staff to prescribe and often administer the dose.[21]

Meperidine (pethidine) is a synthetic opioid and worldwide is the most extensively used and investigated opioid analgesic in labor. The usual dose in labor is 50–100 mg or 1 mg/kg (maximum dose 200 mg) IM (peak effect at 2 hours). Morphine is a mu receptor agonist acting primarily in the CNS. The dose of morphine for maternal analgesia is 2–5 mg IV (peak effect at 10–20 minutes) or 5–10 mg IM (peak effect at 1–2 hours). Diamorphine (heroin) is a prodrug that is converted to the active components of acetylmorphine and morphine by esterases in the liver, plasma, and CNS. Diamorphine is administered intramuscularly at a dose of 2.5–5 mg, half that of morphine (peak effect at 1–2 hours). A second dose of all these drugs can be administered after 3–4 hours. Tramadol (Ultram) can be used at doses of 50–100 mg every 4 hours and can be given orally as well as via the IM or IV route.[22]

Despite being in widespread use, published evidence suggests that less than 25 percent of women receive satisfactory pain relief from pethidine administration; morphine and tramadol have not been shown to be any more effective. Both midwives and laboring women rate diamorphine as a more effective analgesic than pethidine, but diamorphine has been associated with significantly longer labors. It has been argued that these drugs often provide sedation rather than direct analgesia.[4,23–27]

Maternal side effects of systemic opioids include nausea, vomiting, delayed gastric emptying, sedation, disorientation, pruritus, and respiratory depression. Patient susceptibility to these effects is variable and often dose dependent rather than drug dependent.[21] Pethidine and tramadol have an added disadvantage of an increased risk of seizure activity in susceptible patients such as those with preeclampsia.[28]

The fetal effects of opioids can be direct (because the low molecular weight and high lipid solubility of opioids allow for placental transfer) or indirect (via effects on the mother, for example, such as altered minute ventilation or uterine tone).[29,30] Opioids are associated with decreased beat-to-beat fetal heart rate variability, neonatal respiratory depression, and a delay in effective feeding due to the inhibition of sucking reflexes.[24,31,32] Diamorphine and tramadol produce less neonatal respiratory depression than pethidine or morphine.[25,33] Naloxone (an opioid antagonist) may be administered directly to the neonate if required.[34]

Codeine is not commonly the opioid of choice in active labor owing to poor-quality analgesia, but it is worth mentioning that its use in children and in breast-feeding mothers has recently been discouraged by the European Medicines Agency and Medicines and Healthcare Products Regulatory Agency. Although no new recommendations have as yet been made regarding its use in pregnancy, there may be a risk of neonatal respiratory depression in babies of individuals who are ultrarapid metabolizers of codeine via the enzyme CYP2D6. It would be sensible to consider this potential effect if prescribing codeine to a laboring woman.[35]

Systemic Opioids: Intravenous Patient-Controlled Analgesia

Patient-controlled analgesia (PCA) systems require prescription and often must be set up by medical staff, but they can achieve good analgesia with lower drug doses than intermittent boluses. PCA systems have the added benefit of giving patients an increased sense of control during labor. Remifentanil (Ultiva), the most commonly used opioid in PCA for labor, is an ultra-short-acting synthetic pure mu agonist. Its rapid onset and rapid metabolism by tissue and plasma esterases mean that it has a context-sensitive half-life of 3 minutes and no accumulation.[36] The efficacy of remifentanil depends on both the dose and the manner in which it is administered. The most popular regimens used in clinical practice are either 0.5 µg/kg or 40-µg boluses with a 2- to 3-minute lockout time. The onset of effect is at around 30 seconds, and peak effect occurs at 2.5 minutes. With an average uterine contraction time of 70 seconds, it therefore can be difficult initially for women to time dose delivery so as to coincide the peak drug effect with the peak of each uterine contraction, but with tutoring from midwives, women are able to learn to anticipate the next contraction and make an early, effective demand.[37–40]

Remifentanil PCA has been shown to significantly reduce pain scores of women in labor compared with baseline[41–43] and provides superior analgesia and higher patient satisfaction than bolus administration of pethidine with a comparable degree of adverse events.[44] However, the analgesia provided by remifentanil PCA is inferior to epidural analgesia.[45–49]

The potential for maternal sedation, respiratory depression, and oxygen desaturation is significant with remifentanil PCA, and there have been a number of articles published recently questioning its safety profile.[50,51] An appraisal of the evidence suggests that 32 percent of patients experience respiratory depression,[52] but this is usually transient and easily corrected with stimulation, nasal oxygen, or a reduction in dose. The rate of nausea and vomiting is difficult to distinguish as a true opioid effect because it is common in laboring women, but remifentanil PCA does not appear to cause a significantly higher rate of nausea than other opioids.[53]

Due to the high incidence of maternal sedation and desaturation, remifentanil should not be started in women who have had other opioids administered

Table 9.2 Guidelines for the Safe Administration of Remifentanil PCA

Prescription and training	• Prescribed by an anesthetist • Only nurses/midwives who have undergone a period of supervised practice and have been deemed competent may administer this infusion
Eligibility	• 36 weeks' gestation • In established labor • Informed consent
Contraindications	• Other opioid use in preceding 4 hours • Allergy to opioids • Multiple pregnancy • Preeclampsia
Supervision and monitoring	• Continuous one-to-one nursing/midwifery supervision • Continuous SaO_2 pulse oximetry established prior to first administration • 30-minute observations: respiratory rate, sedation score, pain score
Equipment	• Dedicated IV cannula • Dedicated PCA administration pump • Unidirectional antisyphon valve on administration set
Indications for contacting anesthetist	• Excessive sedation score (not responding to voice) • Respiratory rate < 8 breaths/min • SaO_2 < 90 percent despite oxygen via nasal specs

in the preceding 4 hours, and it is imperative that there is appropriate monitoring and supervision. To date, there have been four case reports describing respiratory arrest with remifentanil PCA.[53–57] While each has its own set of circumstances and potentially confounding factors, their existence cannot and should not be ignored. High standards of supervision must be maintained, with trained midwives or nurses providing constant one-to-one care with a protocol that includes continuous oxygen saturation monitoring; regular documentation of pain scores, respiratory rate, and sedation level; and use of a dedicated cannula with an antisyphon valve. As with all areas where strong parenteral opioids are administered, full resuscitation equipment must be immediately available, with supplemental oxygen and a bag-valve/mask apparatus in the room[58] (Table 9.2). Caregivers must be trained to recognize and manage the potential adverse events. Maternity departments choosing to use remifentanil should have stringent guidelines in place to ensure appropriate safeguards for women and regular audit processes to ensure compliance, and if this cannot be guaranteed at all times, then units should not offer remifentanil as an option for laboring women.[59] Remifentanil should not be viewed as a "poor woman's epidural."[60]

Like other opioids, remifentanil readily crosses the placenta but undergoes rapid metabolism and redistribution within the neonate.[59] There is no evidence that remifentanil causes any deterioration in fetal heart rate variability and Apgar scores, and cord blood gases do not show deviation from normal practice with less neonatal desaturation compared with bolus systemic opioids.[61–64]

Learning Points

- Systemic analgesic drugs have variable efficacy and side-effect profiles. None produce analgesia comparable with that of an epidural.
- Inhaled nitrous oxide provides modest analgesic effects for some women and may be used either alone or in combination with other forms of analgesia. Acetaminophen appears to be safe to use, but its place in providing analgesia in labor is not yet established.
- Intermittent boluses of systemic opioids provide moderate analgesic effects but may be associated with significant maternal and neonatal side effects. PCA with short-acting agents such as remifentanil offers women slightly more effective analgesia with a greater sense of control in labor. However, it must be provided in the setting of one-to-one midwifery care with appropriate monitoring and resources both available and in use in order to protect against the risk of respiratory depression.
- In discussing analgesia options for labour with women it is important to highlight both the risks and the benefits of the available options

References

1. Melzach R. The myth of painless childbirth. *Pain* 1984; **19**:321–27.

2. Anim-Somuah M, Smyth R, Howell C. Epidural versus non-epidural or no analgesia in labour. *Cochrane Database Syst Rev* 2005; (4):CD000331.

3. Rosen MA. Nitrous oxide for relief of labor pain: a systematic review. *Am J Obstet Gynecol* 2002; **186**: S110–26.

4. Olofsson C, Ekblom A, Ekman-Ordeberg G, Hjelm A, Irestedt L. Lack of analgesic effect of systemically administered morphine or pethidine on labour pain. *BJOG* 1996; **103**:968–72.

5. Carstoniu J, Levytam S, Norman P, et al. Nitrous oxide in early labor: safety and analgesic efficacy assessed by a double-blind, placebo-controlled study. *Anesthesiology* 1994; **80**:30–35.

6. Yentis SM. The use of Entonox for labour pain should be abandoned (Proposer). *Int J Obstet Anesth* 2001; **10**(1):25–29.

7. Clyburn P. The use of Entonox for labour pain should be abandoned (Opposer). *Int J Obstet Anesth* 2001; **10**:25–39.

8. Wong CA. Epidural and spinal analgesia/anesthesia for labor and vaginal delivery, in Chestnut DH, Polley LS, Tsen LC, Wong CA (eds.), *Chestnut's Obstetric Anesthesia: Principles and Practice*. Philadelphia, PA: Mosby Elsevier; 2009, pp. 429–92.

9. Westling F, Milsom I, Zetterstrom H, Ekstorom-Jodal B. Effects of nitrous oxide oxygen inhalation on the maternal circulation during vaginal delivery. *Acta Anaesthesiol Scand* 1992; **36**(2):175–81.

10. Lucas DN, Siemaszko O, Yentis SM. Maternal hypoxemia associated with the use of Entonox in labour. *Int J Obstet Anesth* 2000; **9**(4):270–72.

11. McAneny T, Doughty AG. Self-administration of nitrous oxide/oxygen in obstetrics. *Anaesthesia* 1963; **18**:488–97.

12. Stefani S, Hughes S, Shnider S, et al. Neonatal neurobehavioral effects of inhalation analgesia for vaginal delivery. *Anesthesiology* 1982; **56**(5): 351–55.

13. Griffin RP, Reynolds F. Maternal hypoxemia during labour and delivery: the influence of analgesia and effect on neonatal outcome. *Anaesthesia* 1995; **50**(2): 151–56.

14. Malaise O, Bruyere O, Jean-Yves R. Intravenous paracetamol: a review of efficacy and safety in therapeutic use. *Future Neurol* 2007; **2**(6):673–88.

15. Graham GG, Scott KF, Day RO. Tolerability of paracetamol. *Drug Saf* 2005; **28**(3):227–40.

16. Elbohoty AEH, Abd-Elrazek H, Abd-El-Gawad M, et al. Intravenous infusion of paracetamol versus intravenous pethidine as an intrapartum analgesic in the first stage of labor. *Int J Gynaecol Obstet* 2012; **118**(1):7–10.

17. Hyllested M, Jones S, Pedersen JL, Kehlet H. Comparative effect of paracetamol, NSAIDs or their combination in postoperative pain management: a qualitative review. *Br J Anaesth* 2002; **88**(2):199–214.

18. Othman M, Jones L, Neilson JP. Non-opioid drugs for pain management in labour (review). *Cochrane Database Syst Rev* 2012; (11):CD009223.

19. Ostensen ME. Safety of non-steroidal anti-inflammatory drugs during pregnancy and lactation. *Inflammopharmacology* 1996; **4**:31–41.

20. Elbourne D, Wiseman RA. Types of intra-muscular opioids for maternal pain relief in labour. *Cochrane Database Syst Rev* 1998; (4):CD001237.

21. Benyamin R, Trescot AM, Datta A, et al. Opioid complications and side effects. *Pain Physician* 2008; **11**: S105–20.

22. Yentis SM, Hirsch NP, Smith GP. *Anaesthesia and Intensive Care A–Z: An encyclopedia of Principles and Practice*, 3rd edn. London: Elsevier; 2004.

23. Wee, M. Analgesia in labour: inhalational and parenteral. *Anaesth Intensive Care Med* 2004; **5**(7):233–34.

24. Fortescue C, Wee M. Analgesia in labour: non-regional techniques. *Continuing Education in Anaesthesia Critical Care and Pain* 2005; **5**(1):9–13.

25. Husslein P, Kubista E, Egarter C. Obstetrical analgesia with tramadol: results of a prospective randomized comparative study with pethidine. *Z Geburtshilfe Perinatol* 1987; **191**(6):234–37.

26. Viegas OAC, Khaw B, Ratnam SS. Tramadol in labor pain in primiparous patients: a prospective comparative clinical trial. *Eur J Obstet Gynaecol Reprod Biol* 1993; **49**(3):131–35.

27. Wee MYK, Tuckey JP, Thomas PW, Burnard S. A comparison of intramuscular diamorphine and intramuscular pethidine for labour analgesia: a two-centre randomized blinded controlled trial. *BJOG* 2013; **121**(4): 447–56.

28. Thomson AM, Hillier VF. A re-evaluation of the effect of pethidine on the length of labour. *J Adv Nurs* 1994; **19**(3):448–56.

29. Bailey PL, Egan TD, Stanley TH. Intravenous opioid anesthetics, in Miller RD (ed.), *Anesthesia*, 5th edn, vol. **1**. Philadelphia, PA: Churchill Livingstone; 2000, pp. 273–376.

30. Ala-Kokko T, Vähäkangas K, Pelkonen O. Placental function and principles of drug transfer. *Acta Anaesthesiol Scand* 1993; **37**:47–49.

31. Littleford J. Effects on the fetus and newborn of maternal analgesia and anesthesia: a review. *Can J Anaesth* 2004; **51**(6):586–609.

32. Jones L, Othman JL, Dowswell T, et al. Pain management for women in labour: an overview of systematic reviews. *Cochrane Database Syst Rev* 2012; (3):CD009234

33. Ullman R, Smith LA, Burns E, Mori R, Dowswell T. Parenteral opioid for maternal pain relief in labour. *Cochrane Database Syst Rev* 2010; (9):CD007396.

34. Maguie W, Fowlie PW. Naloxone for narcotic exposed newborn infants. *Cochrane Database Syst Rev* 2002; (4): CD003483.

35. Medicines and Healthcare products Regulatory Agency (MHRA). Codeine: restricted use as analgesic in children and adolescents after European safety review, June 2013. Available at www.mhra.gov.uk/safetyinformation/drugsafetyupdate/CON287006 (accessed January 10, 2014).

36. Egan TD. Pharmacokinetics and pharmacodynamics of remifentanil: an update in the year 2000. *Curr Opin Anesthesiol* 2000; **13**(4):449–55.

37. Babenco HD, Conard PF, Gross JB. The pharmacodynamics effect of a remifentanil bolus on ventilatory control. *Anesthesiology* 2000; **92**(2): 393–98.

38. Volmanen P, Alahuhta S. Will remifentanil be a labour analgesic? *Int J Obstet Anaesth* 2004; **13**(1):1–4.

39. Dhileepan S, Stacey RG. A preliminary investigation of remifentanil as a labor analgesic. *Anesth Analg* 2001; **92**(5):1358–59.

40. Caldero-Barcia R, Poseiro JJ. Physiology of the uterine contraction. *Clin Obstet Gynecol* 1960; **3**:386–408.

41. Volikas I, Butwick A, Wilkinson C, Pleming A, Nicholson G. Maternal and neonatal side effects of remifentanil patient-controlled analgesia in labour. *Br J Anaesth* 2005; **95**(4):504–9.

42. Balki M, Kasodekar S, Dhumne S, Bernstein P, Carvalho JC. Remifentanil patient-controlled analgesia for labour: optimizing drug delivery regimens. *Can J Anaesth*, 2007; **54**(8):626–33.

43. Tveit TO, Halvorsen A, Seiler S, Rosland JH. Efficacy and side effects of intravenous remifentanil patient controlled analgesia used in a stepwise approach for labour: an observational study. *Int J Obstet Anaesth* 2013; **22**(1):19–25.

44. Schnabel A, Hahn N, Broscheit J, et al. Remifentanil for labour analgesia: a meta-analysis of randomised controlled trials. *Eur J Anaesthesiol* 2012; **29**(4):177–85.

45. Stourac P, Suchomelova H, Stodulkova M, et al. Comparison of parturient – controlled remifentanil with epidural bupivacaine and sufentanil for labour analgesia: randomised controlled trial. Biomedical Papers of the Medical Faculty of the University Palacký, Olomouc, Czech Republic, 2012.

46. Douma MR, Middledorp JM, Verwey RA, Dahan A, Stienstra R. A randomised comparison of intravenous remifentanil patient-controlled analgesia with epidural ropivicaine/sufentanil during labour. *Int J Obstet Anaesth* 2011; **20**(2):118–23.

47. Volmanen P, Sarvela J, Akural EL, et al. Intravenous remifentanil vs epidural levobupivicaine with fentanyl for pain relief in early labour: a randomised,

controlled, double-blinded study. *Acta Anaesthesiol Scand* 2008; **52**(2):249–55.

48. Marwah R, Hassan S, Carvalho JC, Balki M. Remifentanil versus fentanyl for intravenous patient-controlled labour analgesia: an observational study. *Can J Anaesth* 2012; **59**(3):246–54.

49. Stocki D, Matot I, Einav S, et al. A randomized controlled trial of the efficacy and respiratory effects of patient-controlled intravenous remifentanil analgesia and patient-controlled epidural analgesia in laboring women. *Anesth Analg* 2013; **118**(3):589–97.

50. Sneyd R. Remifentanil on the labour ward. *Anaesthesia* 2012; **67**(9):1045–46.

51. Kan RE, Hughes SC, Rosen MA, et al. Intravenous remifentanil: placental transfer, maternal and neonatal effects. *Anesthesiology* 1998; **88**(6):1467–74.

52. Hinova A, Fernando R. Systemic remifentanil for labour analgesia. *Int Anaesth Res Soc* 2009; **109**(6):1925–29.

53. Bonner JC, McClymont W. Respiratory arrest in an obstetric patient using remifentanil patient-controlled analgesia. *Anaesthesia* 2012; **67**(5):538–40.

54. Pruefer C, Bewlay A. Respiratory arrest with remifentanil patient-controlled analgesia: another case. *Anaesthesia* 2012; **67**(9):1044–45.

55. Marr R, Hyams J, Bythell V. Cardiac arrest in an obstetric patient using remifentanil patient-controlled analgesia. *Anaesthesia* 2013; **34**(2):123–24.

56. Kinney MA, Rose CH, Traynor KD, et al. Emergency bedside cesarean delivery: lessons learned in teamwork and patient safety. *BMC Res Notes* 2012; **5**:412.

57. Volmanen P, Akural EI, Raudaskoski T, Alahuhta S. Remifentanil in obstetric analgesia: a dose-finding study. *Anesth Analg* 2002; **94**(4):913–17.

58. McMackin P, Hodgkinson P, Foley P, et al. Remifentanil PCA for labour: completing the audit cycle. Abstracts of free papers presented at the Annual Congress of the AAGBI, Edinburgh. *Anaesthesia* 2011; **66**:S1.

59. Machatuta NA, Kinsella SM. Remifentanil for labour analgesia: time to draw breath? *Anaesthesia* 2013; **68**(3):231–35.

60. Kranke P, Girard T, Lavand'homme P, et al. Must we press on until a young mother dies? Remifentanil patient-controlled analgesia in labour may not be suited as a "poor man's epidural." *BMC Pregnancy and Childbirth* 2013; **13**:139.

61. Ross AK, Davis PJ, Dear GL, et al. Pharmacokinetics of remifentanil in anesthetized pediatric patients undergoing elective surgery or diagnostic procedures. *Anesth Analg* 2001; **93**(6):1393–401.

62. Thurlow JA, Laxton CH, Dick A, et al. Remifentanil by patient controlled analgesia compared with intramuscular meperidine for pain relief in labour. *Br J Anaesth* 2002; **88**(3):374–78.

63. Evron S, Glezerman M, Sadan O, Boaz M, Ezri T. Remifentanil: a novel systemic analgesic for labor pain. *Anesth Analg* 2005; **100**(1):233–38.

64. Griffin RP, Reynolds F. Maternal hypoxemia during labour and delivery: the influence of analgesia and effect on neonatal outcome. *Anaesthesia* 1995; **50**(2):151–56.

10a

Consent Considerations in Maternity: A US Perspective

Shobana Murugan

Case Study

A 21-year-old gravida 2, para 1 woman at 23 weeks' gestation with twin pregnancy presents with headaches and blurred vision. Her history is significant for an inoperable grade IV anaplastic astrocytoma with a history of two prior craniotomies for resection and a completed course of radiation therapy. Comorbidities included morbid obesity, childhood asthma, history of transient ischemic attacks, and seizure disorder.

Neurosurgery consultation deems the tumor to be in an unresectable location. Neuro-oncology is consulted and agrees that her prognosis is poor and could progress to become fatal before the fetuses reach term. Unfortunately, without surgical resection, her options are either radiation or chemotherapy. The typical chemotherapeutic agents are teratogenic in pregnancy. Radiation Oncology states that radiation is not an option because it may contribute to more edema formation and would likely hasten her death.

Given the need to begin a treatment regimen soon, the patient is offered options of termination of pregnancy versus prolongation of pregnancy. Termination would allow immediate treatment, which might prolong her life by weeks to months. She is counseled that she has the option of deferring all treatment, which would avoid exposure of the fetuses to chemotherapy, but at the cost of likely resulting in her death in a much shorter time period and potentially even during pregnancy. After multidisciplinary discussions, the patient decides to continue her pregnancy to benefit her unborn children.

Extensive discussions are also held with the patient and family regarding her code (resuscitation) status. The patient opts for full code resuscitation, and after 4 minutes to proceed with perimortem section to increase the chances of maternal resuscitation. The patient's mother is also designated as the medical power of attorney.

Key Points

- This case illustrates the approach to a terminally ill pregnant patient who has full capacity to make decisions that will affect her future treatment.
- Informed consent should include the patient as an active partner in decision making with the health providers.
- The importance of an advance directive by the patient in this situation is emphasized.
- Is a "Do Not Resuscitate" order appropriate in this situation, and if so, how can it be implemented in someone who is pregnant?
- Does the mother have the right to make a decision that may conflict with the well-being of her babies?
- If she had opted for termination of pregnancy, would that be allowed because it conflicts with fetal interests? And if she had opted for "Do Not Resuscitate" (DNR) status, could that be implemented in the setting of pregnancy?

Discussion

Consent and Capacity in Pregnancy

Informed consent ensures that maternal wishes are respected, adhered to, and executed during the birthing event and ensures active involvement of the patient in her medical treatment. In a pregnant patient, variables such as capacity to think and process informed consent during labor, time limitations especially in urgent situations, and unexpected changes of labor course can make decision making more complicated for the treatment care team.[1] The process requires a patient with capacity, disclosure of information, voluntarily decisions, and cooperation with the plan.[2]

Advance Directives in Pregnant Patients

An *advance directive* is a formal document that dictates a patient's explicit wishes regarding her future health status and treatment. A durable power of attorney is established for healthcare, and this is a person who is appointed as the patient's surrogate decision maker or healthcare proxy. This person will execute the patient's wishes when the patient is incapable of doing so.

The wishes stated in the advance directive should be respected and carried out by the healthcare providers. If the decisions made by the patient and relayed by the surrogate decision maker cause the physician or healthcare provider to experience moral distress or ethical conflict, patient care should be transferred to someone with more experience and who is more comfortable with the choices.

In this situation, the patient opted to continue pregnancy even though it was detrimental to her health status. The obstetricians offered her termination of pregnancy before fetal viability could be reached. This would have enabled her to proceed with chemotherapy and radiation therapy to prolong her life. However, after careful consideration, the mother decided to continue with her pregnancy, and plans were made to deliver the twins after 24-week viability status was achieved.

Two issues require discussion here.

1. Maternal-Fetal Conflict of Interest

If the patient had opted to terminate the pregnancy, conflict of interests between the rights of the mother and needs of the fetuses could have occurred. Most ethicists would argue that the medical provider's duty lies with the primary patient – the mother. Patient autonomy must be respected, with the mother accepting responsibility for negative outcomes based on her own choices. In reviewing the case of Melissa Rowland, charged with murdering her fetus by refusing a cesarean delivery, the authors conclude that "[t]he best protection for a fetus lies in the protection of the rights of the individual best positioned and most highly motivated to defend its interests: an informed and empowered mother."[3] In the same way, paternal desires do not trump those of the mother. Open dialogue and compromise should always be sought, but the parturient maintains decision-making power.

In this specific case, the patient had an inoperable brain tumor with a very poor prognosis. Despite the prognosis, the patient wished to remain full code. However, if the patient had opted for a DNR status, depending on her geographic location, her end-of-life wishes could be overtaken by the rights of the fetus.

The laws governing care to a pregnant mother in this situation vary by state. Given that this case occurred in Texas, current policy in the Texas Health and Safety Code 166.049 states that "[a] person may not withdraw or withhold life-sustaining treatment under this subchapter from a pregnant patient." This was discussed early on with the patient and her family. Texas is one of approximately a dozen states that have specific legislation that requires life-sustaining treatment to pregnant women overriding any advance directives. Several other states may allow women to write in their wishes with regard to pregnancy, and their instructions should be followed.

The American College of Obstetrics and Gynecology (ACOG) has drafted ethical guidelines to follow in case of maternal-fetal conflict of interest.[4] The American Medical Association (AMA) has similar guidelines. It is extremely important for hospitals to have policies in place when such an extremely rare case occurs in their institutions.

The key point is that maternal autonomy and expressed wishes in a competent state of mind should be respected and followed through. The International Federation of Gynaecology and Obstetrics (FIGO) has similar policies.[6] There should also be room for decision making by a proxy when available. Resorting to a court-ordered decision should be the last resort in such situations.

However, in developing world, the concept of patient autonomy and individual choices may not apply because the social structure and family dynamics play an important role in many countries. Most hospitals do not have set guidelines to handle ethical issues such as this. Doing what is morally right for the patient and prioritizing the patient's wishes are widely regarded as correct by providers all over the world.

2. Can DNR Orders Be Suspended during Cesarean Delivery and under Anesthesia?

If the patient had opted for DNR and needed a cesarean delivery under anesthesia, there are arguments against enforcing the DNR orders under anesthesia and surgery.[5] The anesthesiologist cannot always separate the need for resuscitation due to the primary illness versus depression of the cardiovascular or other systems due to drugs and processes used for anesthesia. Additionally, cardiopulmonary arrests in the operating room with monitors and immediate resuscitation by medical experts increase the chance of survival from arrests compared with out-of-hospital and operating room environments. The arrest occurring from therapeutic interventions in the perioperative setting maybe fully reversible, and the patient should not be denied resuscitation based on DNR orders. Hence, if the patient has consented for surgery and anesthesia because of its therapeutic benefits, previous DNR orders may require suspension according to the American Society of Anesthesiologists (ASA).

The current ASA Ethical Guidelines for the Anesthesia Care of Patients with Do-Not-Resuscitate (DNR) Orders strongly recommend having meaningful and clear discussions regarding all patients who might have active DNR orders. In the past, DNR orders were often clearly suspended during anesthesia and surgery. However, currently, the ASA adopts the opinion that doing so could possibly undermine a patient's right to self-determination. Anesthesiologists, surgeons, and nurses could possibly be held culpable for infringing on those rights.

Patients with DNR orders often have significant physiologic dysfunctions that would make them more susceptible to the depressive effects of anesthesia. This makes it highly challenging to differentiate those effects from the patient's already deteriorated baseline health status, and efforts at resuscitation may be against a patient's wishes.

Resolution of Difficult Situations by Preoperative Discussion

In this case, prior to taking the patient to the operating room for her cesarean delivery, the discussion about resuscitation was undertaken with the patient and her family again. The patient had assigned her mother as a medical power of attorney and understood under the law that she would remain full code until after the delivery. However, if something were to occur *after delivery* and would impair her brain function permanently, the patient wanted withdrawal of care. As anesthesiologists, for us, the conversation with regards to resuscitation is often a difficult subject to address given that our field highly specializes in resuscitative efforts. It therefore remains imperative for physicians who care for pregnant patients to be familiar with advance directives and the laws of the state in which they practice.

Learning Points

- Most physicians agree that a pregnant woman's informed refusal of medical intervention should prevail if she makes it with competence and capacity.
- The clinical decision to either continue pregnancy, to terminate pregnancy in a nonviable fetus, or immediate delivery of the baby to improve chances of survival outside the womb depends on the woman's right to self-determination and decisions she has made in a rational frame of mind.
- Recommendations of FIGO, ACOG, and AMA to respect pregnant women's autonomy are available and can be accessed when maternal-fetal conflicts arise and the consensus is that maternal autonomy and decision making prevail. However, advocates of the fetus's best interests would disagree. Even in a terminally ill pregnant patient, fetal versus maternal interests could conflict, and the debate continues to grow.
- A court-ordered decision should be the last resort after all other options have been exhausted.

References

1. Broaddus B, Chandrasekhar S Informed consent in obstetric anesthesia. *Anesth Analg* 2011; **112**(4): 912–15.

2. American College of Obstetricians and Gynecologists (ACOG). Informed consent (ACOG Committee Opinion No. 439). *Obstet Gynecol* 2009; **114**:401–8.

3. Berkowitz R. Should refusal to undergo a cesarean delivery be a criminal offense?. *Obstet Gynecol* 2004; **104**(6):1220–21; and Minkoff H, Paltrow L. Melissa Rowland and the rights of pregnant women. *Obstet Gynecol* 2004; **104**(6):1234–36.

4. American College of Obstetrics and Gynecology (ACOG). Maternal decision making, ethics, and the law (ACOG Committee Opinion No. 321). *Obstet Gynecol* 2005; **106**(5 Pt 1):1127–37.

5. Blinderman CD, Krakauer EL, Solomon MZ. Time to revise the approach to determining cardiopulmonary resuscitation status. *JAMA* 2012; **307**:917–18.

6. International Federation of Gynaecology and Obstetrics (FIGO). Ethical issues in obstetrics and gynaecology, FIGO Committee for the Study of Ethical Aspects of Human Reproduction and Women's Health, 2006. Available at www.FIGO.org.

Consent Considerations in Maternity: A UK Perspective

Kate McCombe

Case Study

A 30-year-old primiparous woman requests an epidural to relieve the pain of labor. Her cervix is dilated to 4 cm, and her labor is progressing well. She has no comorbidities and no complications of pregnancy. The patient's birth plan states that she does not want an epidural under any circumstances. The patient is now settled in her decision to have an epidural, but her husband is adamant that she should not have one, as stipulated in her birth plan. On questioning, the patient had refused to consider epidural anesthesia previously because of the associated risks and because she wanted a "natural birth." Consequently, neither one of the couple has researched epidural anesthesia prior to labor.

Is it appropriate for the anesthesiologist to proceed to insert an epidural in this situation?

Key Points

- The patient no longer wishes to adhere to her birth plan.
- Her birth plan was based on her perception of the risk of epidural anesthesia and a desire to minimize medical intervention during labor.
- Her partner has not changed his opinion and does not wish you to proceed.

Discussion

Consent and Capacity

When patients give their consent to a procedure, they give their doctor permission to touch them without fear of being sued for battery or assault. Despite this legal protection, a doctor might still be sued for negligence if his or her actions fall below accepted professional standards or if he or she fails to inform the patient adequately of the risks inherent in the procedure. In order for consent to be valid, a patient must have the *capacity* to decide on a particular course of action. A person is deemed to have capacity if they can

- Understand the information relevant to the decision to be made
- Retain the information in their mind
- Weigh the information in the balance as part of the decision-making process
- Communicate the decision

Capacity is not an all-or-nothing state, so a patient's ability to make a choice may depend on how complex the factors involved in the decision are. Simple choices, with minimal consequences, may be reached by those who have limited ability for complex analysis, whereas increasingly complicated decisions associated with greater risks demand ever increasing degrees of capacity. A person who has capacity has the right of absolute autonomy over his or her body and may refuse investigation or treatment even if this results in dire consequences.[1] Disagreeing with one's doctors or making seemingly illogical or foolish decisions does not necessarily reveal a lack of capacity.

In the United Kingdom, under the terms of the Mental Capacity Act (MCA) of 2005, all people aged 16 and older are presumed to have capacity unless proven otherwise. No one can give consent on behalf of another adult who lacks capacity unless that person has been entrusted with the patient's *lasting power of attorney* (LPA) in a formal legal process. If an adult lacks capacity and has not appointed an LPA, his or her doctors are obliged to make treatment decisions on that person's behalf. These decisions must be in the best interests of the patient.

For many women, labor is an extremely painful and mind-altering experience. It is understandable that the anesthesiologist in attendance might question the patient's ability to give genuinely informed consent because a woman in the grip of frequent and powerful contractions, who may also have taken strong analgesia, may have a limited ability to participate meaningfully in the decision-making process. However, in the eyes of the law and of the medical profession, a woman in labor retains capacity and therefore the absolute right to determine what happens to her body in all but the most extreme situations. This remains true even if her decisions seem irrational, are contrary to medical advice, and may lead to severe injury or death. This was tested in court in the case of *R v. Collins*.[2] In this case, the patient, S, was in her thirty-sixth week of pregnancy when she developed severe preeclampsia. She was determined to deliver naturally and refused any treatment for the preeclampsia or to undergo cesarean delivery despite the risk this posed to her own life and to that of her unborn child. The Appeal Court judge ruled that an adult of sound mind is entitled to refuse treatment and, no matter how "morally repugnant" it might seem, this principle is not altered by her pregnant state because the fetus enjoys no legal personality or personhood.

Guidance on consent from the Association of Anaesthetists of Great Britain and Ireland (AAGBI) acknowledges that a laboring woman may be subject to many factors that might compromise her capacity, including "drugs, fatigue, pain or anxiety" but that "the compromise will need to be severe to incapacitate her."[3]

Birth Plans

A *birth plan* is a record of a woman's preferred plan of care for labor and will often include references to methods of pain relief. The birth plan does not have any formal legal status but should be respected by healthcare professionals as an expression of the woman's values and wishes. If the patient were to lose capacity, her birth plan might give doctors added insight to assist them in making decisions in her best interests. Except in the most extreme of cases, however, a woman is presumed to retain capacity during labor and so is at liberty to change her mind and request an epidural at any point, even if her birth plan contains statements to the contrary.

The MCA of 2005 gave legal authority to "advance decisions" (the kind usually associated in our minds with decisions about end-of-life care), and women are at liberty to write these prior to labor. Should the woman lose capacity, an advance decision that has been witnessed and countersigned by a legal official is binding on the doctors. Patients may refuse stipulated treatments and interventions in their advance

decisions, but they may not insist on treatment. To stress the point, such an advance decision would only be activated should the woman lose capacity. While she retains capacity, she is still at liberty to change her mind about her treatment options.

Jehovah's Witnesses often make advanced decisions forbidding healthcare professionals from administering blood products. These patients are usually well informed and settled in their religious beliefs, but it is important to have an honest conversation with them about the risks of blood loss during even the most "low risk" labors and to ascertain exactly which blood products and treatments, if any, are acceptable to them. It is good practice to clarify unambiguously that they would refuse blood products even if this refusal might result in their death. It is therefore important that these women are seen by the anesthesiologist prior to delivery so that their exact wishes can be established. A list of products that can and cannot be given should be clearly documented in their notes, along with whether or not they will accept cell salvage. This documentation should be signed and dated and countersigned by the patient.

Risks of Neuraxial Anesthesia

The perception of the risk posed by epidural anesthesia is often greatly exaggerated in the minds of laboring women when, in reality, significant risks are very rare. Table 10.1 shows the risks as quoted by the Obstetric Anaesthetists' Association, and it can be found on their website. This information is widely available in labor wards around the United Kingdom, and it is useful for women to have the opportunity to read this card and ask questions of the anesthesiologist, ideally before labor starts.

Standards of Disclosure

The recent case of *Montgomery v. Lanarkshire Health Board*,[4] which was heard by the UK Supreme Court in May 2015, disambiguated prior case law and set the legal standard for disclosure of risk. The judges in this case stated that

- Consent is a process that should promote dialogue between patient and doctor.
- The information given should be tailored to each patient, and the patient should be warned of any "material risk" inherent in the procedure. The test of materiality is "whether a reasonable person in

Table 10.1 Obstetric Anaesthetists' Association Epidural Information Card for Patients

Type of risk	How often does this happen?	How common is it?
Significant drop in blood pressure	One in every 50 women	Occasional
Not working well enough to reduce labor pain, so you need to use other ways of lessening the pain	One in every 8 women	Common
Not working well enough for a cesarean section, so you need to have a general anesthetic	One in every 20 women	Sometimes
Severe headache	One in every 100 women (epidural)	Uncommon
	One in every 500 women (spinal)	
Nerve damage (numb patch on a leg or foot, or having a weak leg)	Temporary, one in every 1,000 women	Rare
Effects lasting for more than 6 months	Permanent, one in every 13,000 women	Rare
Epidural abscess (infection)	One in every 50,000 women	Very rare
Meningitis	One in every 100,000 women	Very rare
Epidural hematoma (blood clot)	One in every 170,000 women	Very rare
Accidental unconsciousness	One in every 100,000 women	Very rare
Severe injury, including being paralyzed	One in every 250,000 women	Extremely rare

Note: The information available from the published documents does not give accurate figures for all these risks. The figures shown here are estimates and may be different in different hospitals.
Source: www.labourpains.com/assets/_managed/editor/File/Info%20for%20Mothers/EIC/2008_eic_english.pdf (accessed April 2018).[5]

the patient's position would be likely to attach significance to the risk."

- Patients must be made aware of alternative treatment options, including no treatment at all.
- Doctors must not reduce risk to a series of percentages nor bombard their patients with information because this will promote confusion rather than autonomy. Instead, information must be presented in a way that the patient can understand.

Written Consent

Consent does not begin and end with the signing of a consent form but is a process that starts with the first interaction between doctor and patient. The focus of this process should be on the exchange of information to maximize the patient's ability to make an informed decision about his or her care. The consent form is merely documentary evidence that the appropriate discussions about risk have taken place. Consent does not need to be written for it to be valid, and the patient who holds out his or her arm to allow blood to be drawn gives implied consent to the procedure.

Rightly or wrongly, it is currently accepted practice in the United Kingdom that consent to general

anesthesia is broadly subsumed into the consent for surgery. As such, the majority of anesthetic departments do not have separate consent forms for general anesthesia. An epidural in labor, however, is a primary therapeutic intervention and, as such, warrants separate discussion and documentation. The Association of Anaesthetists of Great Britain and Ireland (AAGBI) advises that "for significant planned procedures, e.g. those that are invasive or which carry significant risks, it is essential for health professionals to document clearly both a patient's agreement to the intervention and the discussions which led up to that agreement. This can be done on a standard consent form, on the anesthetic record or separately in the patient's notes."[3] The AAGBI advises that each hospital will develop its own working practices and that these are followed by employees.

Disagreement among the Couple

In the Case Study, the woman's partner does not want her to have an epidural sited in accordance with her birth plan. As already discussed, the birth plan is not legally binding, and even if it were, any patient with capacity has the right to change his or her mind at any point during treatment. Moreover, the partner has no legal right to dictate which treatments his wife can or cannot receive; as a competent adult, she retains complete autonomy over her own body. Hence, unless the anesthesiologist has grave reason to suspect that this woman's capacity is compromised, he should comply with her request and site the epidural.

The legal solution to this situation is simple, but in practice, the scenario may result in conflict and difficulty. It is worth spending some time with the couple to address the fears of each, paying particular attention to the partner's anxieties. To preserve a functioning therapeutic relationship, it is worth taking the time to try to resolve the conflict to the satisfaction of both parties. Ultimately, though, the partner cannot stand in the way of the therapeutic intervention if his wife is fixed in her desire for an epidural, and in the absolute worst-case scenario, it might be necessary to remove him from labor ward to allow the procedure to go ahead. A breakdown in relations to this extent should be avoided at all costs!

While documentation should always be thorough, it is prudent to make a meticulous record of the timing and content of all discussions and procedures when conflict arises. It is advisable to ask the woman to countersign the record of these discussions and of her decision to rescind her birth plan.

Learning Points

- In principle, women in labor retain their capacity and therefore the right to make autonomous decisions.
- Birth plans are not legally binding but should be seen as an expression of the woman's desires, values, and beliefs.
- The fetus enjoys no legal personality until the moment of birth.
- The law requires us to inform patients of any risk to which they are likely to attach significance.

References

1. Re C (Adult: Refusal of Medical Treatment) (1994) 1 WLR 290.

2. St. George's Healthcare NHS Trust v. S, R v. Collins, ex parte S (1998) 44 BMLR 160 (CA).

3. Association of Anaesthetists of Great Britain and Ireland (AAGBI). Consent for Anaesthesia. London: AAGBI; 2006, Sec. 9.4

4. Montgomery v. Lanarkshire Health Board (2015) UKSC 11, (2015) All ER(D) 113 (Mar).

5. www.labourpains.com/assets/_managed/editor/File /Info%20for%20Mothers/EIC/2008_eic_english.pdf (accessed April 2018).

Accidental Dural Puncture

Sarah Armstrong and Sioned Phillips

Case Study

A fit and well primiparous woman who was in established labor at 39 weeks requested an epidural for labor analgesia. During insertion, it was noted that free-flowing clear liquid was seen from the hub of the Tuohy needle. Initially, the anesthesiologist reinserted the stylet to stop the flow of CSF and then prepared to insert an intrathecal catheter (ITC). Two milliliters of low-dose epidural mix (0.1% bupivacaine with 2 μg/ml fentanyl) was injected down the ITC and flushed with 2 ml 0.9% saline. After the procedure, the anesthesiologist explained that an accidental dural puncture (ADP) had occurred and the implications that this may have. The woman was closely monitored with regard to her cardiovascular status and the height of the block. The ITC was clearly labeled as an intrathecal catheter rather than epidural catheter, and the midwife and obstetric team caring for the patient were informed. The attending anesthesiologist reviewed the patient regularly and provided further doses as required via the catheter. The parturient subsequently delivered vaginally without any further intervention, and the ITC was removed.

On day one after delivery, the woman described a fronto-occipital throbbing headache when sitting up and standing. She had some relief of symptoms when lying flat. Based on the history and an entirely normal neurologic examination, a post–dural puncture headache (PDPH) was diagnosed. She was advised to keep hydrated, prescribed regular analgesia, and kept under observation. Her symptoms persisted, and on day two post-ADP, she had a successful epidural blood patch. The patient was discharged later that day and followed up for 1 week via telephone by the anesthesiologist.

Key Points

- After recognition of an ADP, there are two immediate options: ITC insertion via the Tuohy needle or removal of the needle and another epidural sited.
- Regardless of the subsequent management option chosen, the complication of an ADP should be explained along with the likelihood of experiencing a PDPH.
- The patient was treated with an epidural blood patch, which provided complete relief of her symptoms. She was followed up regularly and given information about potential complications.

Discussion

A *dural puncture* refers to the puncture of both the dura and the underlying arachnoid mater. It may occur with the Tuohy needle or more rarely with the epidural catheter perforating the arachnoid mater after an initial tear by the Tuohy needle. The incidence of dural puncture during epidural insertion varies in the literature and is quoted as between 0.19 and 3.6 percent.[1] A meta-analysis of the obstetric literature described a PDPH rate of up to 52 percent after an ADP from pooled data of all needle types.[2] PDPH rates may differ depending on the needle used. A study comparing 18-gauge Sprotte with 17-gauge Tuohy needles showed a lower incidence of PDPH with the 18-gauge needles (55 versus 100 percent) after recognized ADP despite no difference in ADP rate.[3] Untreated ADP, with a persistent CSF leak, can have serious consequences such as cranial nerve palsy, subdural hematoma, seizures, and chronic headache. Senior anesthesiologists with experience of ADP should be involved in the management of these patients.

Risk Factors

Several risk factors for ADP have been identified in the literature. One proposed factor for increasing the risk of PDPH is the direction of the bevel of the needle in relation to the dural fibers. It is thought that if the

Table 11.1 Comparison of Simple Tests to Differentiate CSF from Saline

	CSF	Saline
Temperature	Warm	Cool
Glucose	Present	Absent
Protein	Present	Absent
pH	<7.5	>7.5

bevel is inserted perpendicular to the dural fibers, as opposed to longitudinal, higher rates of PDPH occur. Studies have compared these two insertion techniques. In one study, a group of patients had epidurals inserted with the bevel perpendicular to the dural fibers, and in the second group, the bevel was inserted parallel to the dural fibers and then rotated once in the epidural space.[4] There was a lower incidence of PDPH after ADP in the second group (5/21 versus 14/20). However, a similar study showed no difference in the rates of PDPH,[5] and there are concerns that the rotation of the epidural needle in itself may cause ADP. Other factors considered as risks for ADP are relative inexperience of the anesthesiologist, movement of the laboring patient, and repeated epidural attempts. Using a loss-of-resistance technique to air to locate the epidural space has been discontinued by some anesthesiologists because of concerns that it is associated with a higher rate of ADP. However, a meta-analysis of prospective randomized trials showed no difference in ADP or PDPH when using loss of resistance to air compared with saline.[6]

Signs of an ADP

It is often obvious that an ADP has occurred when free-flowing CSF streams from the Tuohy needle. This is as opposed to only a few drops of saline, which may be seen when using the loss of resistance to saline technique. If there is doubt over which fluid is coming from the Tuohy needle, the characteristics shown in Table 11.1 can be used to distinguish CSF from saline. If an epidural catheter is inserted either purposefully or unintentionally after an ADP, CSF will be continuously aspirated from the catheter.

ADP may go unrecognized until either the epidural catheter is used or the parturient describes a PDPH following the procedure. Individual studies quote the incidence of unrecognized ADP at between 16 and 36 percent of all dural punctures, which equates to 0.13–0.29 percent of all epidurals performed.[7,8] A UK survey of obstetric units reported a 10.5 percent national incidence of unrecognized dural punctures.[9]

An epidural catheter cannot perforate the dura but can perforate the arachnoid mater.[10] Therefore, if no CSF is seen flowing through the Tuohy needle initially but on use of the epidural catheter a dense motor block occurs, it may indicate that the Tuohy needle was initially placed in the subdural position.

Other mechanisms for unrecognized dural puncture have been described. The Tuohy needle may tent the dura and cause a small tear. This will not allow CSF to flow back through the needle and results in the correct placement of an epidural catheter. During the second stage of labor, the increased pressure in the epidural space may lead to an extension of the original tear into the arachnoid mater and later produce a headache.[11] Another hypothesis describes the lumen of the Tuohy needle becoming occluded by either the ligamentum flavum or a blood clot, preventing the backflow of CSF[12] despite the dura being punctured. However, this would be more likely if loss of resistance to air technique is used rather than saline.

Initial Management of ADP

Immediate options after recognition of an ADP during Tuohy needle insertion are to reinsert the stylet into the Tuohy needle, remove the whole thing, and then attempt a second epidural insertion or insert an ITC through the ADP site. Neither of these options has robust evidence to favor one over the other. Despite some literature describing safe and effective analgesia with an ITC, some anesthesiologists would reattempt epidural insertion.

Second Epidural Attempt

The stylet should be reinserted into the Tuohy needle prior to removal. This will stop further CSF leakage and reduce the incidence of tissue being caught in the needle tip on withdrawal. An epidural can then be sited one space cephalad to the previous attempt. Caution should be exercised with local anesthetic dosing because some of the epidural mixture may move through the dural tear into the intrathecal space. Given this risk, all top-ups should be administered by the anesthesiologist in an incremental manner. The patient should be closely monitored, anticipating a high block or cardiovascular compromise. The midwife and obstetric team must also be aware of an ADP and risk of catheter migration.

Intrathecal Catheter

Three to four centimeters of an epidural catheter can be inserted into the intrathecal space and used to provide labor analgesia. A dose of 2 ml of a low-dose epidural mixture such as 0.1% bupivacaine with 2 µg/ml fentanyl can be given via the ITC to provide analgesia, with all top-ups being cautiously given by an anesthesiologist. After each dose, the catheter should be flushed with 2 ml of saline to compensate for the dead space in the epidural catheter and filter. A continuous infusion of a low-dose epidural mixture running at 2–3 ml/h has also been described. Intrathecal lidocaine is not advocated after studies have shown that it is associated with neurotoxicity, the risk of which may be increased with prolonged and repeated administration.[13] All intrathecal catheters should be labeled clearly, and the midwife and obstetrician looking after the patient should be informed that the woman has an intrathecal catheter in situ.

After a difficult epidural attempt that leads to an ADP, an anesthesiologist may prefer to use the ITC to provide analgesia rather than a second attempt at an epidural.

As stated earlier, a dural puncture may not be recognized until the epidural catheter is inserted, where, on aspiration, a continuous flow of CSF is noted. In this case, the epidural catheter could be left in situ and managed as an intrathecal catheter.

Along with nerve injury, there are concerns regarding infection with intrathecal catheters and the efficacy of analgesia they provide. However, a retrospective review of 761 patients who had had intrathecal catheters over an 11-year period showed that no patients developed serious infective or neurologic complications (e.g., meningitis, spinal or epidural abscess, hematoma, arachnoiditis, or cauda equine).[14] When used for labor analgesia, the failure rate for intentional ITC placement was 2.8 percent (3/108), and for ITC placed after ADP it was 6.1 percent (40/653). Notably, there was a high failure rate when ITC was used to provide surgical anesthesia for cesarean delivery (37.2 percent). Despite this, ITCs are used to provide anesthesia at cesarean section, and doses of hyperbaric bupivacaine 2.5–7.5 mg and an opiate (fentanyl 10–25 µg, morphine 25–100 µg, or sufentanil 2.5–10 µg) have been suggested.[15]

Complications after Accidental Dural Puncture

High Spinal

A high spinal may occur if an epidural catheter is inadvertently placed in the intrathecal space and not recognized as such. Marked hypotension, bradycardia, and ascending paralysis will occur if epidural doses are given via the catheter. Consciousness will be lost if a "total" or "complete" spinal occurs, where the intrathecal drugs have reached the cranium and will affect the brainstem. The management is supportive and depends on the height and degree of the block. There may be loss of consciousness and cardiorespiratory collapse with a requirement for the mother to be intubated and ventilated with cardiovascular support until the effects of the local anesthetic have regressed. The block typically will resolve after 4–6 hours. Interuterine resuscitative techniques should be employed immediately, and delivery of the baby may be required. There may be serious consequences for maternal recovery and bonding with the baby after such a significant event, and this should be anticipated.

Post–Dural Puncture Headache

The diagnosis, investigation, and management of PDPH are discussed in Chapter 42, along with the consequences of untreated PDPH. This section focuses on the prevention of PDPH after recognized ADP. Despite several techniques being described, there is no consensus as to the most effective preventative treatment.

A small randomized, controlled trial (RCT; 25 patients) looked at the use of epidural morphine in patients with ADP to reduce the incidence of PDPH.[16] Two epidural injections were given 24 hours apart of either 3 mg morphine in 10 ml saline or 10 ml saline only. The incidence of PDPH was reduced from 48 percent (12/25) to 12 percent (3/25), respectively. This produced a small relative risk (RR) reduction for headache of 0.25 (95 percent confidence interval [CI] 0.08–0.78).

A systematic review looked at other methods to avoid PDPH.[1] These included prophylactic epidural blood patch (PEBP), intrathecal catheters, and epidural or intrathecal saline. PEBP has been studied with both RCTs and non-RCTs. Initial analysis of nine trials had a RR of 0.41 (95 percent CI 0.24–0.71), which would support the hypothesis of PEBP and coagulation of blood within the epidural space patching the dural tear therefore halting any further CSF leak. Given the significant heterogeneity within the studies, further analysis was performed, which showed that when looking at the pooled results of the RCTs only, PEBP did not significantly reduce PDPH rates. Currently, there are insufficient data to advocate PEBP. ITCs may be left in situ for the duration of analgesia (i.e., removed the same day) or left in for more than 24 hours. Removing catheters on the same day has not been shown to prevent PDPH. Two studies looking at the use of ITCs for more than 24 hours suggested a decrease in the incidence of PDPH.[17,18] When a larger study was included in the analysis, the pooled results showed no statistically significant reduction in PDPH after use of ITCs (RR 0.21, 95 percent CI 0.02–2.65). Saline boluses and infusions have been described given either via the epidural catheter or ITC, but none of the studies has achieved statistical significance in results.[19–21]

A small retrospective study showed a higher chance of headache after ADP with a 17-gauge needle if the women actively pushed during the second stage compared with delivering by cesarean section.[22] This risk was disputed in a single-blinded randomized prospective trial.[23] Women were given spinal analgesia with a 22-gauge needle at the time the fetal head was seen and then randomized to two groups, one encouraged to push during the active second phase and the other discouraged. No difference in the incidence of headache was seen.

Posture and hydration therapy have been studied in an attempt to prevent PDPH. A Cochrane review in 2016 of 24 studies looked at a variety of positions (prolonged bed rest, head-down tilt, and early mobilization) and the use of supplementary hydration therapy after lumber puncture. It concluded that there was insufficient evidence to advocate routine bed rest after a dural puncture, and any benefit from the use of hydration therapy was unclear.[24]

Long-Term Complications of ADP

A case-controlled retrospective questionnaire study has looked at the long-term sequelae in 60 women who had an ADP after epidural placement.[25] Patients who had an ADP were significantly more likely to report chronic backache: 46.7 percent complained of backache for up to 1 year, and 44.8 percent had backache for between 2 and 7 years after an ADP (at the time of questioning). Seventy-three percent of women complained that the backache interfered with performance of normal daily tasks. Long-term headaches were reported, but not as frequently as backache, and 18.7 percent of women still had symptoms of headache 3–6 years after the ADP. Four women in the ADP group and two women in the control group complained of paresthesia and weakness lasting long

than 7 days. All cases of sphincter disturbance were related to urge and stress incontinence, and constipation therefore not deemed secondary to the ADP.

Learning Points

- Accidental dural puncture is a recognized complication after epidural insertion with an estimated incidence of around 1 percent.
- Unrecognized ADP may lead to serious consequences for the patient, such as a high or total spinal.
- PDPH is common after ADP.
- No treatment has been proven to be effective for preventing a PDPH.

References

1. Apfel CC, Saxena A, Cakmakkaya OS, et al. Prevention of postdural puncture headache after accidental dural puncture: a quantitative systematic review. *Br J Anaesth* 2010; **105**(3):255–63.

2. Choi PT, Galinski SE, Takeuchi L, et al. PDPH is a common complication of neuraxial blockade in parturients: a meta-analysis of obstetrical studies. *Can J Anesth* 2003; **50**(5):460–69.

3. Morely-Forster P, Singh S, Angle P, et al. The effect of epidural needle type on post dural puncture headache. *Can J Anesth* 2006; **53**(6):572–78.

4. Norris MC, Leighton BL, DeSimone CA. Needle bevel direction and headache after inadvertent dural puncture. *Anesthesiology* 1989; **70**(5):729–31.

5. Richardson MG, Wissler RN. The effects of needle bevel orientation during epidural catheter insertion in laboring parturients. *Anesth Analg* 1999; **88**(2):352–56.

6. Schier R, Guerra D, Aguilar J, et al. Epidural space identification: a meta-analysis of complications after air versus liquid as the medium for loss of resistance. *Anesth Analg* 2009; **109**(6):2012–21.

7. Davies RG, Laxton CJ, Donald FA, et al. Unrecognised dural punctures. *Int J Obstet Anesth* 2003; **12**(2):142–43.

8. Sprigge JS, Harper SJ. Accidental dural puncture and post dural puncture headache in obstetric anaesthesia: presentation and management. A 23-year survey in a district general hospital. *Anaesthesia* 2007; **63**(1):36–43.

9. Gleeson CM, Reynolds F. Accidental dural puncture rates in UK obstetric practice. *Int J Obstet Anesth* 1998; 7:242–46.

10. Hardy PAJ. Can epidural catheters penetrate dura mater? An anatomical study. *Anaesthesia* 1986; **41**(11): 1146–47.

11. Reynolds F, Speedy HM. The subdural space: the third place to go astray. *Anaesthesia* 1990; **45**(2): 120–23.

12. Cohen S, Casciano M. Unrecognised dural punctures-revisited. *Int J Obstet Anesth* 2004; **12**(13):57–58.

13. Pollock JE. Neurotoxicity of intrathecal local anaesthetics and transient neurological symptoms. *Best Pract Res Clin Anaesthesiol* 2003; **17**(3):471–84.

14. Cohn J, Moaveni D, Sznol J, Ranasinghe J. Complications of 761 short-term intrathecal macrocatheters in obstetric patients: a retrospective review of cases over a 12-year period. *Int J Obstet Anesth* 2016; **25**:30–36.

15. ValleJo MC. Regional anaesthesia/ analgesia techniques in obstetrics, in Suresh M, Shnider SM, Levinson G. (eds.), *Shnider and Levinson's Anesthesia for Obstetrics*, 5th edn. Baltimore, MD: Lippincott Williams & Wilkins; 2013, pp. 119–43.

16. Al-metwalli RR. Epidural morphine injections for prevention of post dural puncture headache. *Anaesthesia* 2008; **63**(8):847–50.

17. Ayad S, Demian Y, Narouze SN, Tetzlaff JE. Subarachnoid catheter placement after wet tap for analgesia in labor: influence on the risk of headache in obstetric patients. *Reg Anesth Pain Med* 2016; **28**(6): 512–15.

18. Cohen S, Amar D, Pantuck EJ, Singer N, Divon M. Decreased incidence of headache after accidental dural puncture in caesarean delivery patients receiving continuous postoperative intrathecal analgesia. *Acta Anaesthesiol Scand* 1994; **38**(7):716–18.

19. Brownridge P. The management of headache following accidental dural puncture in obstetric patients. *Anaesth Intensive Care* 1983; **11**(1):4–15.

20. Trivedi NS, Eddi D, Shevde K. Headache prevention following accidental dural puncture in obstetric patients. *J Clin Anesth* 1993; **5**(1):42–45.

21. Craft JB, Epstein BS, Coakley CS. Prophylaxis of dural-puncture headache with epidural saline. *Anesth Analg* 1973; **52**(2):228–31.

22. Thompson D, Halpern S, Wilson DB. Second stage pushing correlates with headache after unintentional dural puncture in parturients. *Can J Anesth* 1999; **46**(9):861–66.

23. Ravindran RS, Viegas OJ, Tasch MD, et al. Bearing down at the time of delivery and the incidence of spinal headache in parturients. *Anesth Analg* 1981;**60**(7): 524–26.

24. Arevalo-Rodriguez I, Ciapponi A, Roqué i Figuls M, Muñoz L, Bonfill Cosp X. Posture and fluids for preventing post-dural puncture headache. *Cochrane Database Syst Rev* 2016.

25. Jeskins GD, Moore P, Cooper GM, Lewis M. Long-term morbidity following dural puncture in an obstetric population. *Int J Obstet Anesth* 2001; **10**(1):17–24.

Fetal Heart Rate Monitoring for the Obstetric Anesthesiologist

Jennifer Lucero and Julian T. Parer

Case Study

A 35-year-old gravida 1, para 0 woman at 35 + 1 weeks' gestation underwent induction of labor because of concern for intrauterine growth restriction (IUGR). The fetal heart rate had a normal baseline, moderate variability, and no decelerations (a Category I cardiotocograph [CTG]). On examination, the cervix was 1 cm dilated, long, and the presenting vertex was at a high station. A transcervical Foley balloon catheter was placed for cervical preparation (labor induction).

After several hours, the transcervical catheter fell out, and when examined, the patient's cervix was found to be 4 cm dilated, 50 percent effaced (cervical thickness), –2 station (relationship of the presenting fetal part to the maternal ischial spines during delivery). Oxytocin was started, and the patient requested an epidural for pain relief. After injection of local anesthetic, the patient's blood pressure dropped from 120/80 to 85/42 mmHg, and the fetal heart tracing was noted to have late decelerations with moderate rate variability (Category IIb CTG). The patient was given 100 μg IV phenylephrine, and her blood pressure increased to 110/60 mmHg, which was consistent with her preanalgesia blood pressure. The fetal heart rate improved, with a baseline rate of 130–140 beats/min, moderate variability, and no further decelerations (Category I CTG). Low-dose oxytocin was begun.

Two hours later, the uterine contractions were every 2–3 minutes, and the fetal heart rate tracing showed variable decelerations to a nadir of 60 beats/min, with minimal variability (Category IIc CTG). The cervical examination results were 6 cm/80 percent/–1 station, and the oxytocin infusion was stopped. The variable decelerations became moderate in depth and non recurrent, and fetal heart rate variability was moderate (Category IIb CTG).

Within 2 hours, the uterine contractions were every 2–3 minutes without an oxytocin infusion, and the fetal heart rate tracing continued to have episodes of minimal variability with accelerations and occasional decelerations. A cervical examination revealed that the patient was fully dilated (10 cm) and +2 station, and the patient began expulsive efforts. Within 15 minutes, the fetal heart rate tracing began to show severe variable decelerations and minimal variability with every contraction (Category IIc CTG). After 15 minutes, the obstetrician asked the patient to stop pushing and assessed her for an operative vaginal delivery. Before placing the forceps for delivery, there was a fetal bradycardia of 60 beats/min, and the patient was urgently brought to the operating room, where the fetal heart rate recovered to 160 beats/min, with minimal variability and late decelerations (a Category III CTG). The forceps were placed on the fetal head, and with the next contraction the fetus was delivered.

The neonate weighed 2,500 g, had Apgar scores of 4 at 1 minute and 8 at 5 minutes. The umbilical cord was clamped at birth and blood collected for analysis. The umbilical cord arterial blood gases showed a pH of 7.11, PCO_2 of 64 mmHg, and a base excess of –8 mEq/liter, and the umbilical cord venous blood gases showed a pH of 7.20, PCO_2 of 55 mmHg, and a base excess –6 mEq/liter.

Key Points

- This pregnancy was complicated by intrauterine growth restriction, which is associated with uteroplacental insufficiency and may result in fetal heart rate tracing abnormalities and the development of metabolic acidosis.
- Maintaining maternal blood pressure during induction of neuraxial anesthesia is important to fetal oxygenation because placental perfusion is pressure dependent.
- Severe variable decelerations with minimal variability and late decelerations with minimal variability are both associated with fetal metabolic acidosis.

Discussion

This discussion is based primarily on guidance commonly followed in North America. Please also refer to the Appendix for clinical management based on the interpretation of electronic fetal monitoring (CTG) from the UK National Institute of Health and Care Excellence (NICE).

Electronic tracing of the fetal heart rate (FHR) was initially designed as a noninvasive measure of adequacy of fetal oxygenation and of fetal hypoxia so that timely intervention could prevent the development of fetal acidemia. The challenge has become how to interpret this multivariate technique and provide a consensus for clinicians on which to base clinical management. The ultimate goal in FHR interpretation should be not to miss the presence of acidemia, but prevention of acidemia should not result in an unduly rate of high obstetric intervention. To maintain this balance, the FHR description and interpretation should be performed in a systematic fashion using accepted guidelines.

In interpreting the FHR tracing, the baseline FHR (110–160 beats/min is the normal range) and the FHR variability (moderate, minimal, or absent) should be noted initially. Next, the presence or absence of decelerations and whether they are late or variable in nature, as well as their severity, have to be assessed. Understanding the evolution of these decelerations over time is very important in determining the level of obstetric intervention necessary.

FHR Pattern Nomenclature

The nomenclature and definitions of FHR patterns have been standardized in the United States since the first US National Institute of Child Health and Human Development (NICHD) conference in 1997[1] and were reiterated in 2008[2] (Table 12.1).

How Do FHR Patterns Relate to Fetal Acidemia?

The significance of these patterns for predicting the risk of fetal acidemia can be surmised from four principles based on empirical evidence (Table 12.2). The evidence points to the paramount importance of FHR variability, as well as the depth and type of deceleration.[3]

Spectrum (Continuum) of Acidemia

This spectrum of fetal acidemia can be determined by classifying the FHR patterns within the CTG based on the baseline rate, baseline variability and/or accelerations, the presence and recurrence of decelerations, the type and severity of decelerations, and the time course of changes in these patterns.[4–9] The NICHD[1] has classified the CTG patterns into three categories:

Category I. A FHR tracing with normal baseline rate (110–160 beats/min), moderate FHR variability, absence of late or variable decelerations, and possible presence of early decelerations

Category II. Everything not included in Categories I and III. Most authorities believe that this middle category needs to be subdivided into two further subcategories based on increasing severity of the periodic changes (IIb) and then reduction of FHR variability (IIc).

Category III. A FHR tracing with absent FHR variability, recurrent decelerations or bradycardia, or a sinusoidal pattern (Table 12.3).

Expanded Five-Tier System of Classification

In 2008, the NICHD convened an expert panel to develop categories of FHR tracings for the purposes of developing a system for interpretation and management to better evaluate and respond to concerns about fetal acidemia. The expert panel developed a three-tier system for interpretation of FHR patterns. In the development of this system, there was concern regarding the potential of heterogeneity within Category II, but at the time of the NICHD conference, there was insufficient data to further subdivide Category II with regard to the association between FHR patterns in this category and a specific risk of fetal acidemia. As such, the three-tier system resulted in heterogeneity within Category II.

As the three-tier system was adopted, studies evaluating the sensitivity and specificity of the system documented the lack of sensitivity and specificity of Category II, making it an ineffective screening tool.[7] As a result of this heterogeneity, the American College of Obstetricians and Gynecologists (ACOG) and several large medical institutions started to identify subcategories within Category II for the purposes of clinical management. ACOG published what is essentially a four-tier system in its clinical practice bulletin published in 2010.[9] Parer and Ikeda[4] further refined a color-coded five-tier system (Figure 12.1).

Table 12.1 National Institute of Child Health and Human Development Research: Electronic FHR Monitoring: Pattern Definitions

Pattern	Definition

Baseline	• The mean FHR rounded to increments of 5 beats/min during a 10-minute segment, excluding
	    · Periodic or episodic changes.
	    · Periods of marked FHR variability.
	    · Segments of baseline that differ by more than 25 beats/min.
	• The baseline must be for a minimum of 2 minutes in any 10-minute segment, or the baseline for that time period is indeterminate. In this case, one may refer to the prior 10-minute window for determination of baseline.
	• Normal FHR baseline: 110–160 beats/min
	• Tachycardia: FHR baseline > 160 beats/min
	• Bradycardia: FHR baseline < 110 beats/min

Baseline variability	• Fluctuations in the baseline FHR that are irregular in amplitude and frequency
	• Variability is visually quantitated as the amplitude of peak-to-trough in beats per minute.
	    · Absent: amplitude range undetectable
	    · Minimal: amplitude range detectable but 5 beats/min or fewer
	    · Moderate (normal): amplitude range 6–25 beats/min
	    · Marked: amplitude range > 25 beats/min

Acceleration	• A visually apparent abrupt increase (onset to peak in less than 30 seconds) in the FHR • At 32 weeks' gestation and beyond, an acceleration has a peak of 15 beats/min or more above baseline, with a duration of 15 seconds or more but less than 2 minutes from onset to return. • Before 32 weeks' gestation, an acceleration has a peak of 10 beats/min or more above baseline, with a duration of 10 seconds or more but less than 2 minutes from onset to return. • Prolonged acceleration lasts 2 minutes or more but less than 10 minutes in duration. • If an acceleration lasts 10 minutes or longer, it is a baseline change.
Early deceleration	• Visually apparent, usually symmetrical gradual decrease and return of the FHR associated with a uterine contraction • A gradual FHR decrease is defined as from the onset to the FHR nadir of 30 seconds or more. • The decrease in FHR is calculated from the onset to the nadir of the deceleration. • The nadir of the deceleration occurs at the same time as the peak of the contraction. • In most cases, the onset, nadir, and recovery of the deceleration are coincident with the beginning, peak, and ending of the contraction, respectively.
Late deceleration	• Visually apparent, usually symmetrical gradual decrease and return of the FHR associated with a uterine contraction • A gradual FHR decrease is defined as from the onset to the FHR nadir of 30 seconds or more. • The decrease in FHR is calculated from the onset to the nadir of the deceleration. • The deceleration is delayed in timing, with the nadir of the deceleration occurring after the peak of the contraction. • In most cases, the onset, nadir, and recovery of the deceleration occur after the beginning, peak, and ending of the contraction, respectively.
Variable deceleration	• Visually apparent abrupt decrease in FHR • An abrupt FHR decrease is defined as from the onset of the deceleration to the beginning of the FHR nadir of less than 30 seconds. • The decrease in FHR is calculated from the onset to the nadir of the deceleration. • The decrease in FHR is 15 beats/min or greater, lasting 15 seconds or greater and less than 2 minutes in duration. • When variable decelerations are associated with uterine contractions, their onset, depth, and duration commonly vary with successive uterine contractions.
Prolonged deceleration	• Visually apparent decrease in the FHR below the baseline • Decrease in FHR from the baseline that is 15 beats/min or more lasting 2 minutes or more but less than 10 minutes in duration • If a deceleration lasts 10 minutes or longer, it is a baseline change.
Sinusoidal pattern	• Visually apparent, smooth sine wave-like undulating pattern in FHR baseline with a cycle frequency of 3–5 per minute that persists for 20 minutes or more

Sources: Data taken from references 1 and 2.

Table 12.2 Fetal Acidemia and FHR Patterns: Associations between FHR Patterns and Newborn Acidemia

- Moderate FHR variability, even in the presence of decelerations, is associated with an absence of an umbilical arterial pH < 7.15 or Apgar score < 7 at 5 minutes in over 98 percent of cases.
- Minimal or less FHR variability with decelerations is associated with a 23 percent incidence of umbilical arterial pH < 7.15 or Apgar score < 7 at 5 minutes.
- The likelihood of fetal acidemia increases with the depth of deceleration, especially with late decelerations and with reduced FHR variability.
- Potentially hazardous fetal acidemia develops over a period of 1 hour or more in a fetus whose pattern is evolving from normal to one with decelerations and reduced FHR variability.

Source: Reference 3.

Table 12.3 Five Gradations of Fetal Acidemia Based on FHR Patterns and Their Color-Coded Equivalents Based on the Five-Tier System

I	Green	No acidemia
IIa	Blue	No central fetal acidemia (adequate oxygen)
IIb	Yellow	No central fetal acidemia, but FHR pattern suggests intermittent reductions in O_2 that may result in fetal O_2 debt.
IIc	Orange	Fetus potentially on the verge of decompensation
III	Red	Evidence of actual or impending damaging fetal asphyxia

The five-tier system identifies three subcategories within Category II based on three levels of clinical risk for acidemia. Within Category II there are (a) FHR patterns that have minimal variability and are not associated with fetal acidemia (Category IIa), (b) FHR patterns that are associated with central oxygenation that could develop into acidemia if persistent, and these are often treated with some form of intrauterine resuscitation (Category IIb), and (c) FHR patterns that are not improved with management changes and need to be delivered for concern for fetal acidemia (Category IIc). Adoption of this five-tier system in Japan has been studied in clinical management settings and has resulted in the reduction of metabolic acidemia in umbilical artery cord gases without increases in cesarean and operative delivery rates[6] (see Tables 12.4, 12.5, and 12.6).

Fetal Scalp Sampling

Fetal scalp sampling has not been widely used in North America as a way to assess fetal acidemia. Instead, physicians have relied largely on the assessment of FHR variability with the occasional use of fetal scalp stimulation. In some part, this may be because the paper speed used in the United States is different from that used in Europe. The United States uses a 3 cm/min paper speed, which allows a fuller

MODERATE (NORMAL) VARIABILITY

	No	Early	Mild VD	Mod VD	Sev VD	Mild LD	Mod LD	Sev LD	Mild PD	Mod PD	Sev PD
Tachy	B	B	B	Y	O	Y	Y	O	Y	Y	O
Normal	G	G	G	B	Y	B	Y	Y	Y	Y	O
Mild Brd	Y	Y	Y	Y	O	Y	Y	O	Y	Y	O
Mod Brd	Y	Y			O		O	O			O
Sev Brd	O	O			O			O			O

MINIMAL VARIABILITY

	No	Early	Mild VD	Mod VD	Sev VD	Mild LD	Mod LD	Sev LD	Mild PD	Mod PD	Sev PD
Tachy	B	Y	Y	O	O	O	O	R	O	O	R
Normal	B	B	Y	O	O	O	O	R	O	O	R
Mild Brd	O	O	R	R	R	R	R	R	R	R	R
Mod Brd	O	O			R		R	R			R
Sev Brd	R	R			R			R			R

ABSENT VARIABILITY

	No	Early	Mild VD	Mod VD	Sev VD	Mild LD	Mod LD	Sev LD	Mild PD	Mod PD	Sev PD
Tachy	R	R	R	R	R	R	R	R	R	R	R
Normal	O	R	R	R	R	R	R	R	R	R	R
Mild Brd	R	R	R	R	R	R	R	R	R	R	R
Mod Brd	R	R			R		R	R			R
Sev Brd	R	R			R			R			R

Sinusoidal	R
Marked Variability	Y

VD, Variable decelerations; LD, Late decelerations; PD, Prolonged decelerations; Brd, Bradycardia; Tachy, Tachycardia; G, Green; B, Blue; Y, Yellow; O, Orange; R, Red

Figure 12.1 Management color grid for fetal heart monitoring

Table 12.4 Proposed Management System Based on a Five-Tier System

Category	Color code	Conservative techniques	Operating room	Obstetrician	Anesthetist	Newborn resuscitator	Patient location
I	Green	No	–	–	–	–	–
IIa	Blue	Yes	Available	Informed	–	–	–
IIb	Yellow	Yes	Available	At bedside	Informed	Informed	–
IIc	Orange	Yes	Immediately available	At bedside	Present	Immediately available	OR
III	Red	Yes	Open	At bedside	Present	Present	OR

Table 12.5 Expanded Version of the Three- and Five-Tier Systems

Category	Definition	Risk of acidemia at time of evaluation	Risk of progression of acidemia	Management
Green (primarily Category I)	No acidemia	None	Very low	None
Blue (Category IIa)	No central acidemia	None	Low	Conservative Interventions
Yellow (Category IIb)	Intermittent hypoxia that may lead to acidemia	None	Moderate	Conservative interventions with surveillance
Orange (Category IIc)	Potential for fetal decompensation	Low	High	Conservative interventions and preparation for delivery
Red (Category III)	Possible actual or impending fetal asphyxia	High	Present	Deliver unless FHR abnormality can be immediately resolved

Source: Courtesy of Dr. Mark Tomlinson, Portland, OR, USA.

Table 12.6 Conservative Therapeutic Interventions to Improve FHR Patterns

- Position change (the full left or right lateral position)
- Hyperoxia (administer face mask oxygen to the mother)
- Correct hypotension (administer IV fluids and/or vasopressors)
- Adequate intravascular volume (administer IV fluids)
- Correct excessive contractions (reduce or stop oxytocin infusions if present)
- Avoid constant pushing
- Tocolysis
- Amnioinfusion to correct amniotic fluid deficit

analysis of FHR variability, whereas a speed of 1 cm/min is used in most European countries.[8] In addition, with fetal scalp sampling, the results obtained can only indicate the status of the fetus at that moment in time, not 10 minutes later. The provider cannot be reassured by a fetal scalp sample that indicates no fetal acidemia is present in what is an evolving FHR pattern. A meta-analysis of limited RCTs failed to show any significant beneficial effect of scalp blood sampling.[10]

Learning Points

- Interpretation of FHR tracings relies on the understanding of established nomenclature, the continuum of acidemia, and the evolution of a FHR tracing, knowing what interventions are necessary to prevent fetal acidemia.
- The presence of moderate FHR variability, even with decelerations, is 98 percent associated with absence of pH < 7.15 or an Apgar score < 7 at 5 minutes.
- Minimal or less FHR variability with decelerations has a 23 percent association with pH < 7.15 or an Apgar score < 7 at 5 minutes.

- The likelihood of acidemia increases with the depth of decelerations, especially with late decelerations, and with reduced FHR variability.
- Potentially hazardous acidemia develops over a period of 1 hour or more in a fetus whose pattern evolves from normal to one with FHR decelerations together with reduced FHR variability.
- The umbilical cord blood gases in the Case Study show a mild mixed respiratory and metabolic acidemia and are not in the range where fetal asphyxial damage would be expected.
- Evaluation of the FHR tracing should take into account the maternal and fetal clinical issues (e.g., intrauterine growth restriction, preeclampsia with severe features).
- While making interventions based on the FHR tracing, also consider the current clinical situation. For example, if the blood pressure is low, this needs to be treated urgently, knowing that placenta perfusion is pressure dependent. Such therapeutic maneuvers may have a direct impact on the FHR pattern and lead to clinical improvement.

References

1. National Institute of Child Health and Human Development (NICHD). Electronic fetal heart rate monitoring: research guidelines for interpretation. *Am J Obstet Gynecol* 1997; 177:1385–90; and *JOGN Nurs* 1997; 26:635–40.

2. Macones GA, Hankins GD, Spong CY, Hauth J, Moore T. The 2008 National Institute of Child Health and Human Development Workshop report on electronic fetal monitoring: update on definitions, interpretation, and research guidelines. *Obstet Gynecol* 2008; 112: 661–66.

3. Parer JT, King T, Flanders S, Fox M, Kilpatrick SJ. Fetal acidemia and fetal heart rate patterns: is there evidence of an association? *J Mat Fet Neo Med* 2006; 19: 289–94.

4. Parer JT, Ikeda T. A framework for standardized management of fetal heart rate patterns, *Am J Obstet Gynecol* 2007; 197:26.e1–e6.

5. Parer JT. Standardization of fetal heart rate pattern management: is international consensus possible? *Hypertens Res Pregnancy* 2014; 2:51–58.

6. Katsuragi S, Parer JT, Noda S, et al. Mechanism of reduction of newborn metabolic acidemia following application of a rule-based 5-category color-coded fetal heart rate management framework. *J Mat Fet Neo Med* 2015; 28(13):1608–13.

7. Coletta J, Murphy E, Rubeo Z. The 5-tier system of assessing fetal heart rate tracings is superior to the 3-tier system in identifying fetal academia. *Am J Obstet Gynecol* 2012; 206:226.e1–5.

8. Peleg D, Ram R, Warsof SL, et al. The effect of chart speed on fetal monitor interpretation. *J Mat Fet Neo Med* 2016; 29(10):1577–80.

9. American College of Obstetricians and Gynecologists. Management of intrapartum fetal heart rate tracings: Practice Bulletin 116. *Obstet Gynecol Nov* 2010; 116(5): 1232–40.

10. East CE, Leader LR, Sheehan P, et al. Intrapartum fetal scalp lactate sampling for fetal assessment in the presence of a non-reassuring fetal heart rate trace. *Cochrane Database Syst Rev* 2015; (5):CD006174.

Multidisciplinary Team Management

Katherine Kosman and Rebecca D. Minehart

Case Study

A fit and well nulliparous woman at 34 weeks' gestation presented to the delivery suite with her fetus in an incomplete breech position and threatened preterm labor. Soon after arrival, she felt a gush of fluid and "something between [her] legs." The labor nurse immediately examined the patient and identified a cord prolapse.

The labor nurse shouted for help, explicitly indicating a cord prolapse, and also calmly informed the patient of the seriousness of the situation. Providers from anesthesiology, obstetrics, and nursing quickly arrived. The obstetric resident was only partially successful in relieving the cord obstruction. An anesthesiology team member went to ensure that the operating room (OR) was prepared, including informing the scrub nurse and neonatal team. The patient entered the OR within 1 minute of prolapse identification. A provider identified herself as the "event manager" and proceeded to clearly announce updates and ask specific questions, such as whether the cord had a palpable pulse. The obstetric resident replied that the pulse was not strong. The event manager alerted the room of the plan for emergency cesarean delivery, and the anesthesiologists proceeded with general anesthesia. Incision was made 2 minutes after OR arrival, and an active, crying male infant was delivered with Apgar scores of 8 and 9 at 1 and 5 minutes, respectively. The patient emerged uneventfully and had an uncomplicated postoperative course. After a brief stay in the neonatal intensive care unit, the infant was discharged home with his mother.

The patient commented that despite her son's potentially devastating condition and her fears for his safety, she felt full trust and confidence in the team and that they were all working together to help her.

Key Points

- This patient experienced an obstetric crisis. If care were delayed or disorganized, this could have led to a disastrous outcome.

- Such teamwork does not usually occur spontaneously but is manifested via deliberate education and training in crisis-management principles, ideally in multidisciplinary teams using high-fidelity simulation to teach concepts and behaviors.

Discussion

The field of obstetrics poses unique challenges to effective team performance and communication. For a patient in the delivery ward, providers from multiple healthcare disciplines are involved, including anesthesiologists, obstetricians, midwives, nurses, neonatologists, and other specialists. The number and variety of staff make interdisciplinary teamwork a challenging but critical necessity. In addition, pitfalls arise from the false sense of security that obstetric patients are generally young and healthy, because they may not exhibit deterioration until the situation is late and urgent.[1]

Poor teamwork on the obstetrics ward can lead to devastating consequences. Several reports have shown that better teamwork and communication could have prevented maternal morbidity, including hysterectomies, multiple organ dysfunction, coma, shock, and intensive care admission.[2] Observations of simulated maternal cardiac arrests highlight common weaknesses in team performance, including slow problem recognition, delayed cardiopulmonary resuscitation, and poor communication.[3] Poor multidisciplinary teamwork can also have a negative impact on the fetus and neonate. Suboptimal communication, poor teamwork, and deficient team training contribute to the most common root causes for infant death in the developed world.[2] Optimal teamwork is essential in the management of high-risk delivery scenarios such as abnormal fetal heart rate and shoulder dystocia.[2] With the potential for a rapid decline in maternal and/or fetal stability, obstetric care necessities that a multidisciplinary team be able to perform immediately, work well together, and communicate effectively.[1]

Crisis-management principles were initially adopted for anesthesiology by David Gaba in the 1980s. This approach uses principles from high-reliability organizations (HROs) such as the military, aviation, and nuclear power industries. Like high-stakes patient care, HROs have the potential for catastrophic outcomes, crisis time constraints, multiple decision makers, and complex communication networks yet use principles to operate nearly error free.[1] HROs foster *collective mindfulness*, meaning that everyone in the organization is on high alert for safety threats and aware that small process failures could create devastating errors. At the core of HROs are five key concepts essential for safety[1]:

- **Sensitivity to Operations:** aims to maintain situational awareness for potential errors.
- **Reluctance to Simplify Tasks:** avoids introducing new errors from bypassing standardized steps.
- **Preoccupation with Failure:** uses "near misses" as positive opportunities to analyze process weaknesses and build improvements into the current system.
- **Deference to Expertise:** recognizes that the person with the most relevant knowledge may not be the person with the most expertise and hence a team approach is critical for sharing information.
- **Resilience:** acknowledges that systems may fail in unanticipated ways and that staff must be prepared to perform quick situational solutions.[1]

As described in *To Err is Human*, an estimated 98,000 Americans die each year as a result of medical errors.[4] Among patients admitted to a labor and delivery floor, Forster observed 110 *triggers* (events likely to indicate an actual or potential adverse event) in a prospective cohort study of 425 obstetric patients at a tertiary care academic hospital. Notably, poor teamwork and protocol violations were identified as the most important contributing issues, whereas technical proficiency and therapeutic decision making were less important.[5] Similarly, other studies reveal team communication failures as the most commonly avoidable factor.[6,7] In a survey study of more than 1,000 healthcare workers, the most common recommendation to improve patient safety was "improved communication."[8]

How can a team communicate well? Under time pressure and the high stakes of obstetric cases,

a communication style that allows quick and efficient information sharing and critical feedback is key. Whereas an advocacy style of communication declares an opinion, an inquiry style elicits information.[8] A balanced use of both advocacy and inquiry by both obstetricians and anesthesiologists may lead to better shared understanding during a crisis.[8] Effective communication tools can also include structured methods for patient handoffs and checklists for information sharing.[9]

In addition to communication, what promotes good multidisciplinary teamwork? Salas[10] proposes five key dimensions of effective teams:

- Team leadership
- Mutual performance monitoring
- Backup behavior
- Adaptability
- Team organization

Studies show that team leadership is best established by the person who has the most experience with this type of emergency and when that person clearly states that he or she is assuming the manager role, as seen in the Case Study.[2] Mutual performance monitoring allows identification of task overload, whereas backup behavior requires sufficient understanding of others' tasks to support them when needed.[9] Adaptability is similar to the HRO concept of resilience. It is possible that the system may fail in unexpected ways, and the team must be prepared to devise alternative solutions. Clear team organization may be hindered by shift changes and unfamiliarity with new team members. Introductions at the start of each shift are suggested so that staff can know team members' names, roles, and experience levels in order to efficiently allocate tasks in an emergency.[11]

In addition, an effective multidisciplinary team also includes the patient. Almost one-fifth of women cite dissatisfaction with their labor and birth experience, particularly in emergency situations or after intervention becomes necessary.[2] Therefore, it is crucial to train team members to communicate not just with each other but also with the patient and/or her supporters. As illustrated in the Case Study, the team ensured that the patient was aware of the seriousness of her situation and that she felt informed and included in her own care.

In addition to the five dimensions of effective teamwork set forth by Salas, good teams are coordinated by underlying mechanisms of *mutual trust,*

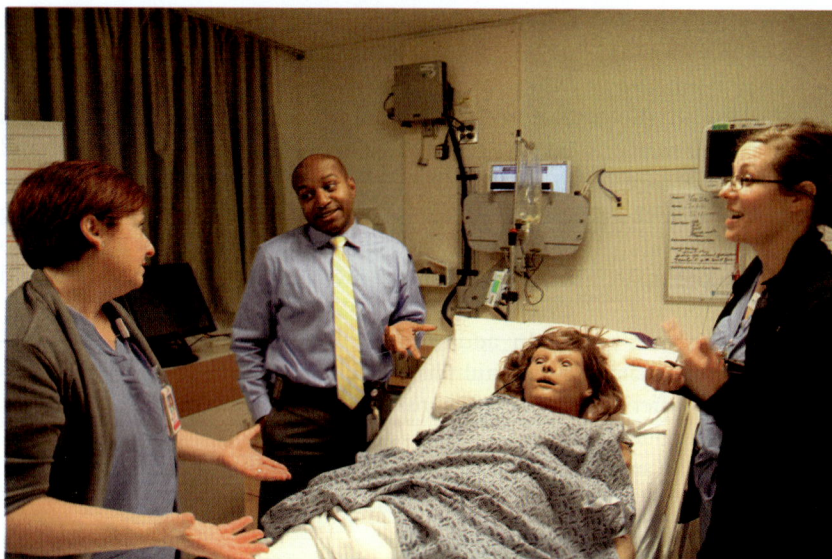

Figure 13.1 A multidisciplinary team debriefing at the simulator "bedside" after a simulated obstetric crisis

shared mental models, and *closed-loop communication*. Mutual trust forms from rapport with team members and from familiarity with each other's roles, expertise, and prior experiences.[11] A shared mental model is a critical foundation for effective teamwork. Given the compressed timeline in a crisis, it is valuable to have the same mental framework regarding patient management, medical issues, and allocation of staff and resources. It is important for staff to identify the problem early and to verbalize information loudly to the entire team so that everyone has a shared view and can provide information to support or refute that view. Closed-loop communication ensures that essential instructions are correctly interpreted and performed by identifying the recipient by name or touch and then confirming that the task has been performed. This directed communication is associated with fewer errors, less work, less noise, and better team efficiency.[2]

It is also important to be aware of factors that could have a negative impact on the success of a multidisciplinary team. The social identity theory of the *tribal phenomenon* suggests that group members of one specialty may perceive other groups' attributes as less desirable.[9] This can create tension and communication barriers when multidisciplinary teammates have different expectations about how things should be done.[9]

Additional potential psychological barriers may exist in hierarchical structures, with less senior staff reluctant to offer suggestions or challenge decisions. Weller et al.[9] set forth several interventions to overcome barriers to information sharing. Teams should be redefined as inclusive rather than specialized silos. Creating democratic teams allows each team member to feel valued and able to communicate information.

Finally, the bedrock for effective multidisciplinary teams is an organizational culture that champions patient safety. Whereas *safety culture* can be defined as the integration of safety practices into clinical activities, *safety climate* is a quantitative description of this culture. This quantitative approach uses outcome measures such as adverse events and adherence to processes or cultural measures such as attitudes toward patient safety. By asking staff to respond to statements such as "The staff works together as a well-coordinated team," questionnaires can help explore differences in perspective, such as the level of teamwork culture perceived by nurses, residents, obstetricians, and anesthesiologists in the department.[12]

In the pursuit of effective multidisciplinary team management, simulation can be a valuable modality to develop, reinforce, and research ideal crisis-management behaviors (Figure 13.1). Simulation provides an opportunity for participants to explore communication styles and to better understand other

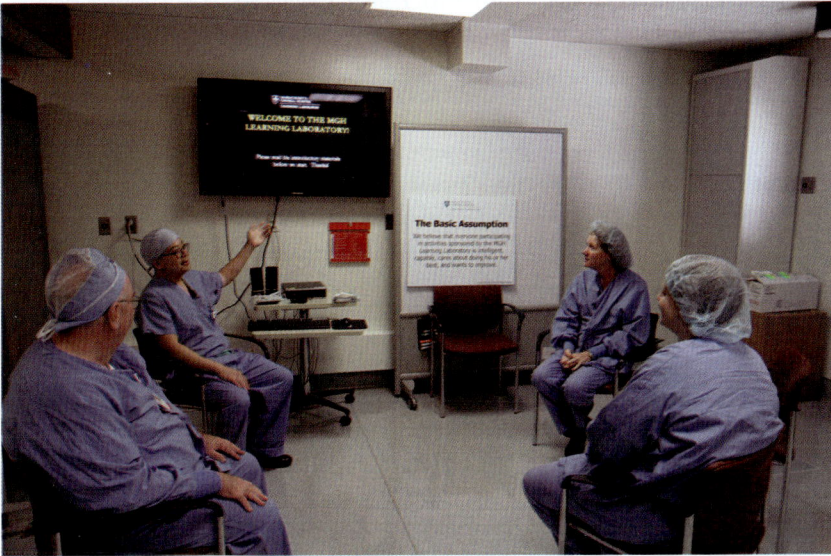

Figure 13.2 Debriefing space for a larger multidisciplinary team engaging in a simulation session. Note the attention to including all members of the group in a circle-seating arrangement and the inclusion of visual aids designed to promote a learning environment and a "safe container."

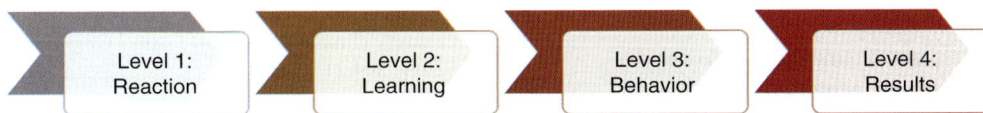

| Level 1: Reaction | Level 2: Learning | Level 3: Behavior | Level 4: Results |

Figure 13.3 Kirkpatrick's four-level training evaluation
Source: Model adapted from Fransen et al.[13,14]

roles within the team.[13] During simulation, it is important to also consider threats to positive learning environments, such as preexisting tensions. Sufficient representation by all groups is needed to effectively model a multidisciplinary case and to yield valuable discussions around multidisciplinary team processes. Good facilitation is critical for creating a supportive atmosphere and a valuable debriefing discussion[14] (Figure 13.2).

To evaluate medical team training and the effectiveness of simulation, Donald Kirkpatrick's model for training evaluation can be applied (Figure 13.3). In this four-level model, response to training is considered beginning with *reaction* and then proceeding to *learning, behavior*, and finally, *results*. Moving up this pyramid-shaped model leads to implementation of learned skills, with level 4 demonstrating results and measurable clinical outcomes. With the use of

this Kirkpatrick framework in conjunction with the Clinical Teamwork Scale (CTS; a validated tool measuring team performance in five domains) to assess obstetric team performance, the benefits of simulation and team training can be analyzed.[15–17]

Using this framework, studies have explored whether simulation improves obstetric team performance. A multidisciplinary study by Fransen et al.[15] used a training course followed 6 months later by an unanticipated clinical simulation. Compared with the group without training, the group with prior simulation more frequently used predefined obstetric procedures and overall had better teamwork performance. In addition, the simulation group had higher scores on the CTS, with clear improvement in "communication" and "decision making" domains. Similarly, in a study by Daniels et al.[18] comparing simulation versus traditional didactic instruction, both groups of multidisciplinary teams knew the correct maneuver sequence for shoulder dystocia, but the simulation-trained team consistently performed better.

Learning Points

- High-reliability organizations (HROs) have an attitude of *collective mindfulness* and five key attributes essential for safety: sensitivity to operations, reluctance to simplify tasks, preoccupation with failure, deference to expertise, and resilience.[1]
- Key dimensions of effective teams are team leadership, mutual performance monitoring, backup behavior, adaptability, and team organization.[10]
- Mutual performance monitoring and backup behavior require familiarity with team members, their level of expertise, and the tasks they can perform. Take the time to introduce yourself, to learn teammates' names, and to be aware of their level of training.[9,11]
- An effective multidisciplinary team also includes the patient.[2] Simulation is a valuable modality to learn the perspectives of multidisciplinary teammates and to try a new communication style of advocating or inquiring. Moving up Kirkpatrick's model of training leads to implementation of learned skills and improved clinical outcomes.[16]

References

1. Goffman D, Lee C, Bernstein PS. Simulation in maternal-fetal medicine: making a case for the need. *Semin Perinatol* 2013; **37**:140–42.

2. Cornthwaite K, Edwards S, Siassakos D. Reducing risk in maternity by optimizing teamwork and leadership: an evidence-based approach to save mothers and babies. *Best Pract Res Clin Obstet Gynaecol* 2013; **27**: 571–81.

3. Lipman SS, Daniels KI, Carvalho B, et al. Deficits in the provision of cardiopulmonary resuscitation during simulated obstetric crises. *Am J Obstet Gynecol* 2010; **203**(2):179.e1–5.

4. Kohn LT, Corrigan JM, Donaldson MS. *To Err Is Human: Building a Safer Health System*. Washington, DC: Institute of Medicine, National Academy of Press; 2000.

5. Forster AJ, Fung I, Caughey S, et al. Adverse events detected by clinical surveillance on an obstetrics service. *Obstet Gynecol* 2006; **108**:1073–83.

6. White AA, Picher JW, Bledsoe SH, Irwin C, Entman SS. Cause and effect analysis of closed claims in obstetrics and gynecology. *Obstet Gynecol* 2005; **105**:1031–38.

7. Joint Commission on Accreditation of Healthcare Organizations. *JCAHO Sentinel Event Alert, Issue 30: Preventing Infant Death and Injury during Delivery*. Washington, DC: The Joint Commission; 2004, pp. 1–2.

8. Minehart RD, Pian-Smith MCM, Walzer TB, et al. Speaking across the drapes: communication strategies of anesthesiologists and obstetricians during a simulated maternal crisis. *Simul Healthc* 2012; **7**:166–70.

9. Weller J, Boyd M, Cumin D. Teams, tribes and patient safety: overcoming barriers to effective teamwork in healthcare. *Postgrad Med J* 2014; **90**:149–54.

10. Salas E, Sims DE, Burke CS. Is there a "big five" in teamwork? *Small Group Res* 2005; **36**(5):555–99.

11. Siassakos D, Fox R, Bristowe K, et al. What makes maternity teams effective and safe? Lessons from a series of research on teamwork, leadership and team training. *Acta Obstet Gynaecol Scand* 2013; **92**:1239–43.

12. Pettker CM, Thung SF, Raab CA, et al. A comprehensive obstetrics patient safety program improves safety climate and culture. *Am J Obstet Gynecol* 2011; **204**:216e1–6.

13. Rudolph JW, Raemer DB, Simon R. Establishing a safe container for learning in simulation: the role of the presimulation briefing. *Simul Healthc* 2014; **9**(6): 339–49.

14. Freeth D, Ayida G, Berridge EJ, et al. Multidisciplinary Obstetric Stimulated Emergency Scenarios (MOSES): promoting patient safety in obstetrics with teamwork-focused interprofessional simulations. *J Contin Educ Health Prof* 2009; **29**(2):98–104.

15. Fransen AF, van de Ven J, Merien AER, et al. Effect of obstetric team training on team performance and medical technical skills: a randomised controlled trial. *BJOG* 2012; **119**:1387–93.

16. Kirkpatrick D. *Evaluating Training Programmes: The Four Levels*. San Francisco, CA: Berrett-Kochler; 1994.

17. Guise JM, Deering SH, Kanki BG, et al. Validation of a tool to measure and promote clinical teamwork. *Simul Healthc* 2008; **3**:217–23.

18. Daniels K, Arefeh J, Clark A, Waller S, Chueh J. Prospective randomized trial of simulation versus didactic teaching for obstetrical emergencies. *Simul Healthc* 2010; **5**(1):40–45.

Obstetric Early Warning Systems

Michael Y. K. Wee and Richard Isaacs

Case Study

A low-risk nulliparous woman at 30 weeks' gestation presented to the delivery suite at 11 P.M. complaining of abdominal pain, fever, and vaginal blood loss. Her initial observations were heart rate 125 beats/min, blood pressure 100/60 mmHg, respiratory rate 28 breaths/min, oxygen saturation 98 percent on air, and core temperature 40.1°C. After midwifery and junior obstetrician assessment, routine bloods and cultures were taken. Vaginal examination revealed "bulging" membranes, noted to be "very warm" to touch. An ultrasound scan confirmed an intrauterine death; this was considered secondary to a presumed diagnosis of chorioamnionitis.

The decision to labor was made by the senior obstetric registrar, and assisted rupture of membranes (ARM) occurred at 1:00 A.M. Heavily blood-stained liquor and a cervical dilatation of 6 cm were noted. At 3:10 A.M., spontaneous vaginal delivery of a stillborn male fetus occurred. IV antibiotics were administered an hour after ARM, and IV fluids were running at 125 ml/h.

At 3:30 A.M., the parturient's observations were heart rate 130 beats/min, blood pressure 87/60 mmHg, and temperature 38.2°C, with no recorded values for respiratory rate or oxygen saturation. At 7:30 A.M., she remained tachycardic and hypotensive. After further review following a shift changeover, her persistent tachycardia and borderline urine output prompted arterial blood gas analysis. This revealed a raised lactate level of 2.8 mmol/liter, and subsequent care was escalated to an obstetric high-dependency area, invasive blood pressure monitoring, and aggressive fluid management. This process was managed by the consultant anesthetist and obstetrician and facilitated by the senior midwife.

The parturient's physiologic status slowly improved over the day, and she subsequently made a full recovery. Blood cultures grew group B streptococcus, and placental histology later demonstrated florid chorioamnionitis. Her Modified Early Obstetric Warning Score (MEOWS) chart is shown in Figure 14.1.

Key Points

- Parturients may present with severe sepsis, where time-critical assessments, investigations, and treatments are crucial in preventing morbidity and mortality.
- The Modified Early Obstetric Warning Score (MEOWS) chart enables early identification of deterioration as well as changing trends and guides appropriate escalation in care.
- Inaccurate and incomplete recording of physiologic observations can seriously delay prompt intervention.
- Admission observations may reveal physiologic triggers such as a "red" heart rate and temperature, "yellow" systolic blood pressure, and a "yellow" respiratory rate.
- In this case, the first 8 hours displayed a distinct lack of blood pressure readings, almost no respiratory rate or oxygen saturation documentation, and a persistent tachycardia. It was not until the morning, with a changeover of staff, that she received the appropriate senior level of care.
- The importance of the early warning score chain of action and its four essential steps should be highlighted.
- The first tracks the physiologic parameters, and when they fall outside the normal ranges, a clinical response is triggered.
- An escalation policy should state whom to call, how urgently they should respond, and appropriate interventions.
- The final step analyzes the intervention effectiveness and correction of the physiologic derangement. This process is underpinned by education, training, and audit, without which the chain will fail.

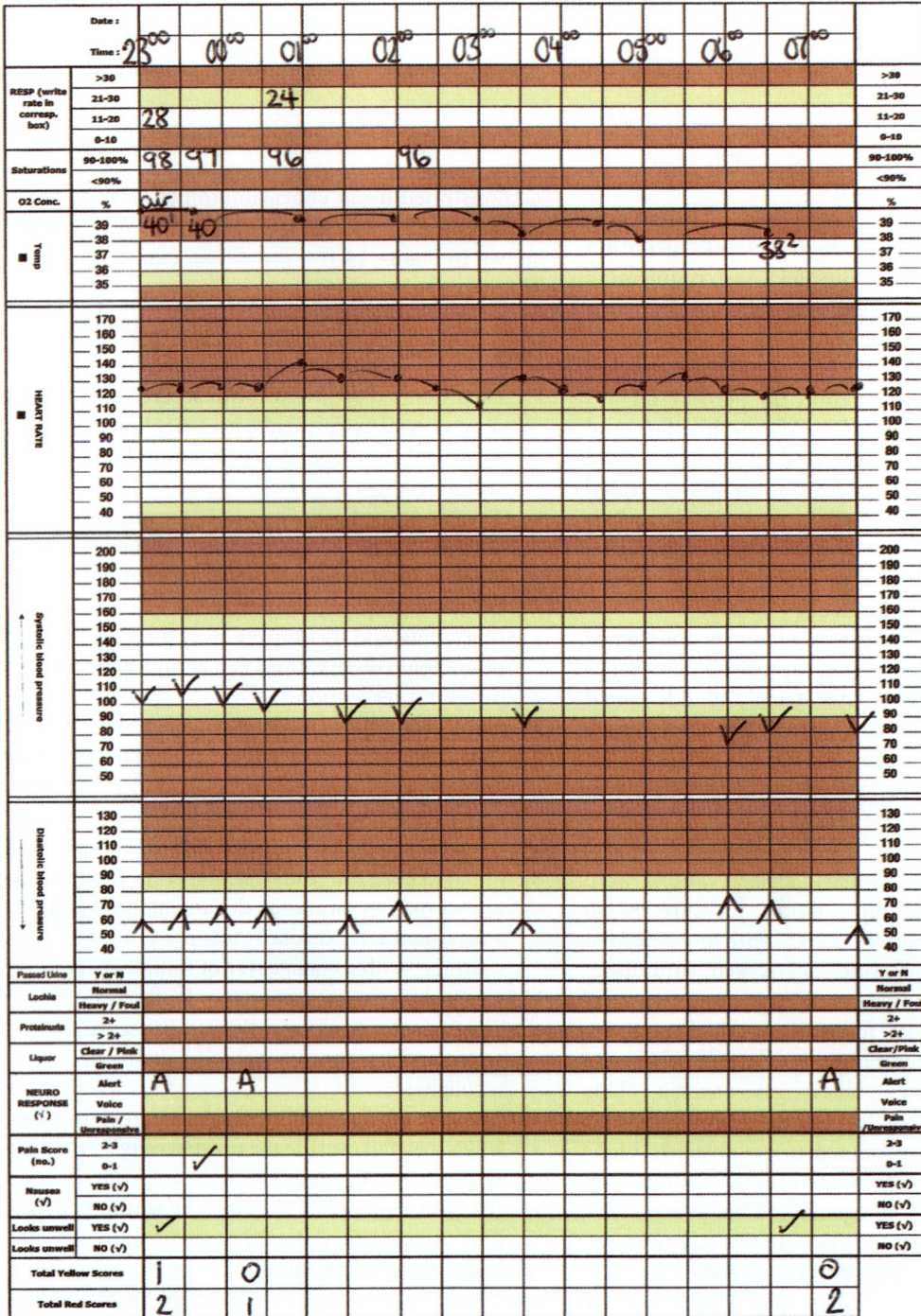

Figure 14.1 Reproduction of the parturient's MEOWS chart

Discussion

Early warning scores (EWSs) were introduced to aid detection of early deterioration in general medical patients in the belief that they may lead to a reduction in deaths, cardiac arrests, and unanticipated critical care admissions. In 2007, the National Institute of Health and Care Excellence (NICE) recommended that physiologic "track and trigger" scoring systems be used for monitoring all patients in acute care settings.[1] They identified six key physiologic parameters one or more of whose deviation from normal could generate a risk score. These vital signs were respiratory rate, oxygen saturation, heart rate, systolic blood pressure, temperature, and consciousness level.

Such track and trigger systems can be categorized as single parameter, multiple parameter, aggregate weighted, or a combination.[2] Single-parameter systems will trigger on one extreme observation value, and although they are simple to use, they do not permit risk stratification and a graded response. In multiparameter and aggregate-weighted systems, a score is obtained by adding together weighted values of abnormal vital signs. This permits charting of progress with time and/or intervention and enables classification of patients into low, medium, or high risk and their appropriate graded response.

Obstetric EWSs

Using these systems in obstetrics has proved challenging because those designed for adult medical patients may be considered unsuitable primarily because of changing physiology during pregnancy. However, the NICE recommendations apply the recording of vital signs to all acute admissions, including obstetrics. Despite lack of good evidence and validation, national organizations have recommended EWS use in obstetrics.[3–5]

The recommended MEOWS chart, based on the Stirling Royal Infirmary chart, permits a graphical display of specific calling criteria and their trigger points via a color-coding, parameter-based EWS. This is a simple visual display whereby a "red" or two "yellows" suggests that the parturient's condition is worsening, triggering escalation of clinical intervention. The MEOWS chart records six vital signs: respiratory rate, heart rate, systolic and diastolic blood pressures, oxygen saturation, and temperature. It also records secondary observations such as proteinuria, lochia, pain scores, and whether the parturient looks subjectively unwell. Values within an arbitrarily agreed "normal" range fall into white squares, "mildly abnormal" observation values into yellow squares, and "abnormal" observations into red squares.

Practicalities of EWSs

The importance of accurate and complete documentation cannot be overemphasized. As highlighted in the Case Study, the actual value for respiratory rate and oxygen saturation must be written down in the correct color-coded box. A rate of 28 breaths/min was wrongly documented in the "normal" zone, and as a consequence, this early trigger was missed. Clearly marked points connected by straight lines must be used for heart rate, blood pressure, and temperature to highlight trends. The lack of respiratory rate recordings is problematic because this is one of the most sensitive indicators of serious morbidity.[6] If MEOWS does trigger, the unit's escalation policy must be adhered to. Of concern in this case was the lack of early anesthetic/critical care involvement and early senior input toward the management of sepsis and the critically unwell patient. This is particularly pertinent in severe sepsis, where rapid patient deterioration and death can ensue. The parturient triggered on several parameters at the initial assessment but without clinical escalation, and this may have led to further deterioration without intervention. The classic stepwise deterioration (rising heart rate and falling blood pressure in sepsis) was not evident, but instead, there was the constant maintenance of a high EWS trigger score. This is not unexpected in young, fit patients, who often can maintain their functional reserve despite abnormal vital signs until eventually reaching a point of critical and rapid deterioration.

Current Problems in Practice

Clinical validation of any obstetric EWS system is necessary to demonstrate improved outcome. A study in a tertiary center reviewed 676 consecutive obstetric admissions, analyzing their completed EWS charts and notes for evidence of morbidity.[7] Two hundred parturients (30 percent) triggered and 86 parturients (13 percent) experienced morbidity according to predefined criteria. The study found that the MEOWS chart was 89 percent sensitive and

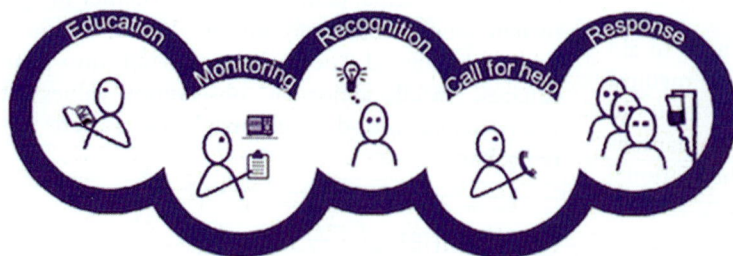

Figure 14.2 Chain of prevention
Source: Reproduced from Smith.[12]

79 percent specific, with a low positive predictive value of 39 percent. The authors concluded that the MEOWS chart is a useful bedside tool for predicting morbidity and suggested adjustment of trigger parameters to improve positive predictive value. However, there is evidence of limitations of MEOWS in women with chorioamnionitis or other serious infections during pregnancy.[8]

Recent UK surveys of lead obstetric anesthetists and heads of midwifery have revealed intriguing insights into the use of such charts in practice.[9,10] Although fewer than half the respondents use the Confidential Enquiry into Maternal and Child Health (CEMACH)–recommended chart, several use a slightly modified version. There is widespread inter-hospital variation in the type of EWS and thresholds for escalating care but good agreement between anesthetists and midwives regarding the top six physiologic parameters to be included in any obstetric EWS. There are also differing opinions as to exactly which women need an obstetric EWS.[9]

The more subjective assessments of a woman's health status by a midwife should not be overlooked. Concerns of midwives, patient partners, and relatives have been highlighted to be of importance.[10] An ethnographic study provides excellent insight into the contextual, cultural, and practical barriers to implementation of MEOWS into clinical practice.[11] Many healthcare professionals felt that MEOWS might have some benefit for high-risk women but that it was of limited value in "normal, healthy" pregnancies and deliveries. Midwives also felt that it led to a number of unnecessary interventions and limited their autonomy and judgment. Staffing pressures, lack of support for EWSs, and limited education and training are considered to be the three biggest barriers.[9]

Chain of Prevention

Recognizing patient deterioration and responding appropriately require effective multidisciplinary teamwork. The *chain of prevention* (Figure 14.2) outlines various steps that are critical in achieving a safe and effective outcome.[12] Every link needs to be equally strong or the chain will fail. Education and training ensure competence in accurate patient assessments, measurements of physiologic parameters, documentation, and the ability to escalate care appropriately. Mandatory training days and obstetric emergency courses exist to promote sound knowledge and training. The high workload pressures due to staff shortages and chart duplication may conflict with recording the maternal EWS. Recognition of abnormality is necessary before escalation. Calculation of a score, action protocols, and standardized communication tools such as the Situation, Background, Assessment, and Response (SBAR) template[13] have empowered the provider to "call for help". Finally, the "response" considers the actions taken by the individual or team summoned to provide a higher level of care. The speed of this response and supportive measures taken are vital in preventing serious morbidity, but if action is slow or inappropriate, the belief in the value of the EWS will be lost.[10]

Obstetric EWSs: The Future

The Royal College of Physicians has implemented the National Early Warning Score (NEWS) throughout the UK National Health Service for all adult inpatients.[14] This is in line with NICE recommendations.[1] However, the authors state that NEWS should not be used in pregnant women because of modified physiologic responses to acute illness. At present, there is no national or international "gold standard" obstetric EWS. Carle et al.[15] attempted to create and internally validate a clinical obstetric EWS. Similar to NEWS with a single color-coded table and risk stratification depending on total score, this aggregate-weighted system was based on physiologic parameters derived from obstetric admissions to a critical care unit. Although the clinical EWS correlated well with existing EWSs when internally tested against retrospective Intensive Care National Audit and Research Centre (ICNARC) data, caution must be exercised because mortality rather than morbidity was the main outcome measure, and the study population does not represent the normal obstetric population.

Through the formation of a national multidisciplinary group, and with the backing of all 19 maternity units, the Irish Maternity Early Warning System (IMEWS) was developed and then implemented nationally in April 2013.[16] By standardizing the system, the aim was to facilitate staff training via specific educational packages, allow instant familiarity when moving between units, and enable national audits to be conducted.

The threat of sepsis from the community and the need for a simplified EWS to trigger admission and further monitoring and treatment must be addressed. The Centre for Maternal and Child Enquiries emergent theme briefing was published because of the significance of the findings related to genital tract sepsis from group A streptococcus.[17] There were a number of deaths in healthy women with uncomplicated pregnancies and deliveries in which signs and symptoms of acute illness went unrecognized, and most of these women were from the community.[18] In the United Kingdom, the Welsh Transforming Maternity Services mini-collaborative developed a specific tool to be used by community midwives, the Community Early Warning Score (CEWS), in an attempt to improve detection of early sepsis.[19]

Regardless of future developments toward standardized and validated obstetric EWSs, the key to success undoubtedly includes all the elements of the chain of prevention. Improved training and audit for all healthcare professionals must follow through the use of specific educational packages. The importance of standardized and clear monitoring of physiologic parameters, trigger, and escalation policies cannot be overemphasized. Future research should concentrate on breaking the barriers to implementation of obstetric EWSs, consider the merits of targeting potentially vulnerable obstetric populations, and improve the positive predictive value of obstetric EWS not only in the hospital setting but also in the community.

Learning Points

- Use of physiologic parameters in EWSs can reduce morbidity and mortality, provided that every link of the chain of prevention is adhered to.
- Monitoring, triggers, and escalation of EWSs should be clear and simple to improve detection and treatment of the deteriorating parturient.
- Education, training, and audit of EWS use will improve their utility and efficacy.

References

1. National Institute for Health and Care Excellence (NICE). *Acutely Ill Patients in Hospital: Recognition of and Response to Acute Illness in Adults in Hospital (CG50).* London: NICE; 2007.

2. Department of Health and NHS Modernisation Agency. *The National Outreach Report 2003.* London: Department of Health; 2003.

3. Lewis G, ed. *Saving Mothers' Lives: Reviewing Maternal Deaths to Make Motherhood Safer 2003–2005. The Seventh Report on Confidential Enquiry into Maternal Deaths in the United Kingdom.* London: CEMACH; 2007.

4. Lewis G, ed. *Saving Mothers' Lives: Reviewing Maternal Deaths to Make Motherhood Safer: 2006–08. The Eighth Report on Confidential Enquiries into Maternal Deaths in the United Kingdom.* London: CMACE, 2011.

5. Royal College of Obstetricians and Gynaecologists. Providing equity of critical and maternity care for the critically ill pregnant or recently pregnant woman, 2011. Available at www.rcog.org.uk/en/guidelines-research-services/guidelines/providing-equity-of-critical-and-maternity-care-for-the-critically-ill-pregnant-or-recently-pregnant-woman/ (accessed June 18, 2016).

6. Fieselmann JF, Hendryx MS, Helms CM, et al. Respiratory rate predicts cardiopulmonary arrest for internal medicine patients. *J Gen Intern Med* 1993; 8:354–60.

7. Singh S, McGlennan A, England A, Simons R. A validation study of the CEMACH recommended modified early obstetric warning system (MEOWS). *Anaesthesia* 2012; 67:12–18.

8. Lappen JR, Keene M, Lore M, et al. Existing models fail to predict sepsis in an obstetric population with intrauterine infection. *Am J Obstet Gynecol* 2010; 203:573.

9. Isaacs RA, Wee MYK, Bick DE, et al. A national survey of obstetric early warning systems in the United Kingdom: five years on. *Anaesthesia* 2014; 69:687–92.

10. Bick DE, Sandall J, Furuta M, et al. A national cross-sectional survey of heads of midwifery services of uptake, benefits and barriers to use of obstetric early warning systems (EWS) by midwives. *Midwifery* 2014; **30**:1140–46.

11. Mackintosh N, Watson K, Rance S, Sandall J. Value of a Modified Early Obstetric Warning System (MEOWS) in managing maternal complications in the peripartum period: an ethnographic study. *Br Med J Quality & Safety* 2014; **23**:26–34.

12. Smith GB. In-hospital cardiac arrest: is it time for an in-hospital "chain of prevention"? *Resuscitation* 2010; **81**:1209–11.

13. Pope BB, Rodzen L, Spross G. Raising the SBAR: how better communication improves patient outcomes. *Nursing* 2008; **38**:41–4.

14. Royal College of Physicians. National Early Warning Score (NEWS): standardising the assessment of acute illness severity in the NHS. Report of a working party, RCP, London, 2012.

15. Carle C, Alexander P, Columb M, Johal J. Design and internal validation of an obstetric early warning score: secondary analysis of the Intensive Care National Audit and Research Centre Case Mix Programme database. *Anaesthesia* 2013; **68**:354–67.

16. Irish Maternity Early Warning System (IMEWS), 2013. Available at www.hse.ie/eng/about/Who/clinical/nat clinprog/obsandgynaeprogramme/imews/guideline .PDF (accessed December 10, 2014).

17. Centre for Maternal and Child Enquiries. CMACE emergent theme briefing 1: genital tract sepsis, 2010. Available at www.oaaanaes.ac.uk/assets/_managed/edi tor/File/CMACE/CMACE_sepsis_briefing_2010 .10.pdf (accessed June 18, 2015).

18. Knight M, Kenyon S, Brocklehurst P, et al., eds., on behalf of MBRRACEUK. Saving lives, improving mothers' care: lessons learned to inform future maternity care from the UK and Ireland Confidential Enquiries into Maternal Deaths and Morbidity 2009–12. National Perinatal Epidemiology Unit, University of Oxford, 2014. Available at www.npeu.ox.ac.uk/mbrrace -uk/reports (accessed June 16, 2016).

19. 1000 Lives Plus. Are you feeling well? Community bundles, 2013. Available at www.1000livesplus.wales .nhs.uk/sitesplus/documents/1011/powys_story board_ls41.pdf (accessed June 18, 2016).

Obesity in Pregnancy

Thunga Setty and Sohail Bampoe

Case Study

A high-risk nulliparous woman with a body mass index (BMI) of 45 kg/m^2 at booking, and now estimated to be 55 kg/m^2, presented to the labor ward at 39 weeks' gestation. On arrival, she was in spontaneous labor and contracting three times in 10 minutes. Vaginal examination revealed that her cervix was 3 cm dilated.

The woman had been reviewed in the antenatal clinic by an obstetric anesthesiologist, who had advised her to consider an early epidural and had warned her that epidural insertion may be technically challenging. Airway assessment demonstrated a Mallampati grade 3 jaw slide B with good mouth opening.

Based on the advice she had received, she requested an epidural for labor analgesia. A 16-gauge IV cannula was inserted on the dorsum of her left hand under ultrasound guidance. The ultrasound was then used to locate the midline, and an estimation of the depth of epidural space of 8 cm was made.

The epidural was inserted after three attempts. The epidural space was found at a depth of 8.5 cm, and 4 cm of catheter was left in the space. Patient-controlled epidural analgesia was started.

Labor pain was initially well controlled. However, as labor progressed, the patient needed further clinician boluses of the low-dose epidural mixture (0.1% bupivacaine and 2 μg/ml fentanyl) because of a unilateral block.

Before the labor epidural could be resited, a pathologic cardiotocographic (CTG) trace necessitated an emergency Category 2 cesarean delivery, and the patient was transferred to the operating room (OR).

In the OR, the patient's epidural was topped up using 20 ml 2% lidocaine and 1:200,000 epinephrine with alkalization using 2 ml 8.4% sodium bicarbonate (equivalent to 2 mmol). On testing with ethyl chloride following the epidural top-up, the patient was found to have an established block to T8 unilaterally. This was deemed unsatisfactory, requiring conversion to general anesthesia (GA).

Because the patient had an anticipated difficult airway, an airway strategy had already been devised. Plan A consisted of using a videolaryngoscope. She was placed on an Oxford Head Elevating Laryngoscopy Pillow (HELP) pillow, given antacid prophylaxis, and underwent a rapid-sequence induction with preoxygenation and cricoid pressure. On induction of anesthesia, IV propofol 3 mg/kg and rocuronium 1.2 mg/kg were administered. After a Cormack-Lehane grade 1 intubation, anesthesia was maintained with 50% nitrous oxide in oxygen and sevoflurane.

Key Points

- This high-risk patient with morbid obesity class 3 experienced inadequate pain relief in labor and subsequently required emergency cesarean delivery.
- Epidural top-up failed to establish adequate anesthesia for surgery, requiring conversation to general anesthesia.

Discussion

In recent years, the prevalence of obesity among women in the United Kingdom has increased substantially, with approximately 40 percent being overweight and 25 percent obese in 2010.[1] In women of childbearing age, the excess body weight is of concern because obese parturients experience an increased incidence of complications compared with normal-weight mothers. In addition to the maternal risks associated with excess body weight, fetal morbidity and mortality are also increased compared with pregnancies of normal-weight mothers. Furthermore, the increased use of maternity services associated with obesity in pregnancy adds significantly to healthcare costs compared with normal-weight mothers. With an ever-increasing number of obese parturients, the

Table 15.1 The WHO Classification of Obesity

	BMI	Risk of comorbidities
Underweight	<18.5	Low
Normal	18.5–24.9	Average
Overweight	25–29.9	Increased
Mild obesity: class 1	30–34.5	Moderate
Moderate obesity: class 2	35–9.9	Severe
Morbid obesity: class 3	>40	Very severe

Source: From the World Health Organization.[28]

labor ward anesthesiologist will be required to anticipate and safely assist in the prevention of peripartum complications associated with excess body weight.

Obesity can be quantified by using the body mass index (BMI). The BMI classification is currently the preferred standard by which to stratify maternal body weight (Table 15.1).

$$BMI = weight\ (kg)/height\ (m^2)$$

BMI does not consider frame size or the distribution of body fat.

Obese parturients have severely limited physiologic reserve and a higher risk of emergency surgical intervention. Hence the anesthetic risks increase greatly. Obesity and pregnancy each have multisystem effects, many of which are additive (Table 15.2).

Neuraxial Procedures in Obese Parturients

The anesthetic management of obese parturients should begin in the antenatal clinic, with obese women being offered a consultation with an obstetric anesthesiologist. Many maternity units will refer all pregnant women with a BMI greater than 40 kg/m^2 to the anesthetic high-risk clinic for assessment. As obesity in pregnancy becomes more prevalent, some units are raising the threshold for referral and are referring only women with a BMI greater than 50 kg/m^2 for assessment. During the consultation, maternal expectations should be explored, and an anesthetic management plan for labor and delivery should be discussed and agreed to. Specific risks associated with obesity in pregnancy should be identified and explained. The anesthesiologist should pay close attention to the possibility of associated cardiopulmonary pathology. Practical issues with difficult venous access, regional anesthesia, and pain relief for labor and operative procedures should be discussed.

Risk factors for fetal macrosomia and shoulder dystocia, which are increased in obese parturients, result in more painful contractions and complicated labors.[2] Although there are various modalities of pain relief, analgesia using neuraxial blockade has been shown to be the most effective.[3] The anticipated technical difficulties should not preclude the use of epidural analgesia in obese parturients. It has been shown that effective pain relief during labor can improve maternal respiratory function and attenuate sympathetically mediated cardiovascular responses.[4,5] Available evidence shows that the rate of cesarean delivery does not increase with epidural analgesia during labor,[3] although obesity increases the need for cesarean delivery. Therefore, electively placing a functional epidural catheter early in labor is advantageous to avoid any time delay because of difficult insertion, should any emergency operative intervention be required. In addition, epidural analgesia can be extended into the postoperative period, where adequate pain relief can optimize care.

Technical problems for neuraxial block include achieving appropriate positioning of the patient, identification of the midline, and a high failure rate for epidural catheter placement (up to 42 percent),[6] and multiple attempts at catheter placement are common. The sitting position often allows for easier identification of the midline and should be used routinely in obese parturients.[7]

Early placement and confirmation of optimal epidural analgesia during early labor are prudent. This allows sufficient time to manage a failed epidural block. Not only is the incidence of failed initial epidural catheter placement high in obese parturients, but the incidence of failed epidural during labor due to migration of the epidural catheter in fatty subcutaneous tissues is also high.[8–10] An appropriate length of epidural catheter should be left in the epidural space in anticipation of such migration, and an appropriate fixation device should be used.[11]

General Anesthesia in the Obese Parturient

Obese parturients need thorough preoperative assessment for difficult airway because the incidence of failed intubation is eight times higher than in

Table 15.2 Multisystem Effects of Pregnancy and Obesity

	Anatomic changes in pregnancy	Physiologic changes in pregnancy	Physiologic changes in obese parturient
Airway	↑ Risk of difficult airway and intubation Breast tissue/fat pad on back makes head positioning difficult for intubation	Mucous membranes in the airway are edematous and prone to bleeding	Limited mouth opening Limited neck movements Narrowing of pharyngeal opening due to excess adipose tissue
Respiratory		↓ Functional residual capacity (FRC) with risk of hypoxia of ~15–20% ↓ Expiratory reserve volume (ERV) and residual volume (RV) ≃ 15–20% ↓ Closing capacity Poor respiratory compliance ↑ Alveolar ventilation ↑ Pulmonary resistance due to low lung volumes Risk of atelectasis and shunt, Ventilation/Perfusion (V/Q) mismatch	Restrictive respiratory pattern due to additional weight gain on the thorax and restriction of diaphragm movement leading to impaired diaphragm function Risk of obstructive sleep apnea (OSA) with risk of pulmonary hypertension and cor pulmonale Risk of obese hypoventilation syndrome
Cardiovascular		↑ Blood volume ↑ Cardiac output of ~50% ↓ Afterload Risk of supine hypotension secondary to aortocaval compression	↑ Cardiac output proportional to degree of obesity (fat needs 2–3 ml of blood/100 g/min) Hypertension found in up to 60% of obese patients, leading to increased afterload and left ventricular hypertrophy Right ventricular hypertrophy secondary to OSA ↑ Risk of arrhythmia due to fatty deposits in myocardium Heart failure; ↑ risk with duration of obesity ↑ Risk of supine hypotension syndrome
Gastrointestinal		↑ Acid reflux ↑ Residual volume of stomach ↓ Lower esophageal sphincter tone	↑ Risk of hiatal hernia
Metabolic		↑ Oxygen demand	↑ Plasma lipids, which ↑ risk of atheroma
Renal		↑ Angiotensin-converting enzyme and renin levels ↑ Glomerular Filtration Rate (GFR) ↑ Intra-abdominal pressure can decrease renal blood flow	
Endocrine		Insulin resistance Hyperinsulinemia Impaired endothelial function	↑ Diabetes; risk increases as BMI increases
Hematology		↑ Risk of deep vein thrombosis	

Table 15.3 Effects of Obesity on Obstetric Management

- Higher chance of failure to progress[12]
- Prolonged second stage of labor[12]
- Failed induction of labor[12]
- Higher risk of instrumental delivery (~18% in BMI = 35–40 and ~34% in BMI > 40 kg/m^2)[7]
- Increased risk of failed instrumental delivery leading to cesarean delivery[13–15]
- Overall three times higher risk of cesarean delivery due to fetal macrosomia, higher risk of shoulder dystocia and/or failed cervical dilatation[13–15]
- Increased presentation as emergency cesarean delivery (~66%)[6]
- Higher risk of having a prolonged incision to delivery time[7]
- Higher risk of blood loss greater than 1,000 ml[7]
- Risk of prolonged operative time[7]
- Increased risk of wound infections, endometritis, and dehiscence[16,17]
- Increased risk of postpartum hemorrhage (30% for a moderately raised BMI and approximately 70% more frequent in morbid obesity)[7]
- Increased risk of thromboembolism[7]

nonobese patients. In the obstetric population, between 1 in 280 and 1 in 750 attempted tracheal intubations fails[6] compared with 1 in 2,230 in the general population.[8,18,19] In contrast, the incidence of difficult intubation in obese population is as high as 15.5 percent.[20] Dewan[21] found the incidence as high as 33 percent in morbidly obese parturients. A 6-year review of failed intubations in parturients in a UK region reported 36 cases of failed intubation, and it was found that the average BMI of these women was 33 kg/m^2.[20] It is evident that the incidence of difficult or failed tracheal intubation in obese parturients is very high and emphasizes optimal assessment and management of the airway.

An airway assessment should include a Mallampati classification, thyromental distance, neck extension (atlanto-occipital joint extension), and mouth opening (vertical dimension). Other features shown to be significant are short neck, receding mandible, and protruding incisors.[22] It is of interest to note that neck circumference, not BMI, is more predictive of a difficult intubation in morbidly obese patients.[23] A study has shown that a gestational weight gain of more than 15 kg is associated with a threefold increase in a suboptimal laryngoscope view compared with that in nonobese parturients of the same age.[20,24] A history of snoring, diagnosis of sleep apnea, lack of teeth, and large breasts all increase the risk of difficult intubation, and awake fiberoptic intubation should be considered in all patients with limited range of neck, head, or jaw movements, short neck, neck circumference of 15 inches and above, and Mallampati score of 3 and above.

Before induction, preoxygenation should be performed in a reversed Trendelenburg position because this extends the time to desaturation during apnea. Desaturation occurs rapidly because of the physiologic effects of a reduced functional residual capacity secondary to both adipose tissue and the gravid uterus. This is further compounded by the increases in oxygen consumption associated with both pregnancy and obesity. Consideration should be given to modifying the traditional "sniffing the morning air" intubation position to the ramped position. This position is achieved by ramping the patient's upper body until there is horizontal alignment between the external auditory meatus and the sternal notch. This can be achieved by using pillows underneath the patient's upper body and head to elevate it (Figure 15.1).

The potential for an anticipated difficult airway requires the anesthesiologist to have prior local knowledge and training in the use of aids for difficult intubation and ventilation. Safe general anesthesia will often require assistance from an experienced anesthesiologist.

Women with obesity are more likely to have obstructive sleep apnea (OSA), but the prevalence is unknown in pregnancy. Sleep disturbances and daytime fatigue are normal at the end of pregnancy, so OSA may go undiagnosed. Mhyre[25] has suggested that women with a BMI greater than 35 kg/m^2, neck circumference greater than 16 inches, symptoms of suspected airway obstruction during sleep (include frequent or loud snoring, observed pauses in breathing during sleep, or arousal with a choking sensation) should be screened by polysomnography for OSA and advised continuous positive airway pressure (CPAP) if required. If obesity hypoventilation syndrome is suspected, arterial blood gas determination is useful to screen hypoxia, hypercarbia, and acidosis, and an echocardiogram should be done to evaluate cardiac function. Referral to a cardiologist should be considered.[26,27] Caution should also be exercised in the use of long-acting opioids because of the risk of sensitivity to adverse effects, especially respiratory depression.

Perioperative issues such as transfers, beds, intravenous access, difficulty in measuring noninvasive blood pressure, arterial cannulation, and different-sized regional anesthesia equipment should be anticipated, discussed, and planned for.

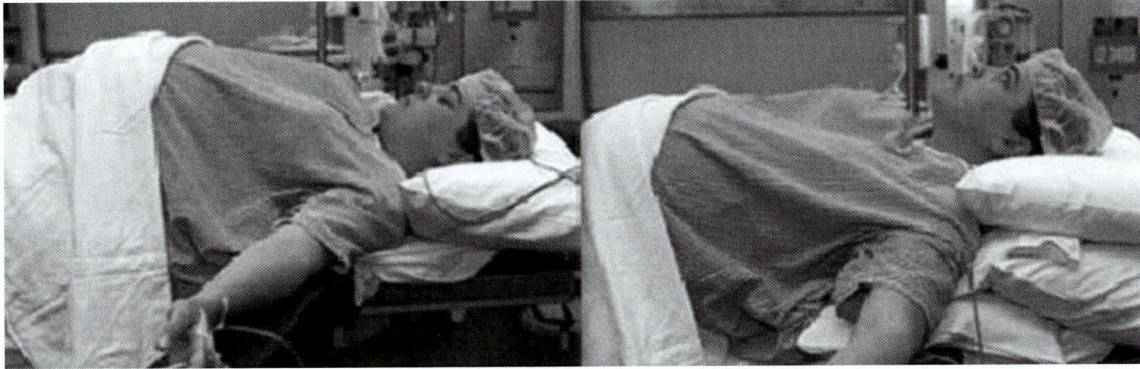

Figure 15.1 Improved airway positioning obtained using a ramping technique[29]

Learning Points

- Identification of obesity in pregnancy should result in early assessment with regard to analgesia for labor and anesthesia for cesarean delivery.
- A strategy for airway management should be devised in case of the need for general anesthesia.
- Early senior multidisciplinary discussion, including obstetricians, anesthesiologists, and the patient, should occur regarding epidural placement, as well as a plan for labor management including thromboprophylaxsis.
- The risk of potential failure/inadequacy of neuraxial blockade should be actively managed.
- Early recognition of logistical problems (e.g., requirement for appropriate equipment/monitoring) should occur.

References

1. Gupta A, Faber P. Continuing education in anaesthesia. *Crit Care Pain* 2011: **11**:143–46.

2. Hess PE, Pratt SD, Lucas TP, et al. Predictors of breakthrough pain during labor epidural analgesia. *Anesth Analg* 2001; **93**:414–18.

3. Howell CJ. Epidural versus non-epidural analgesia for pain relief in labour. *Cochrane Database Syst Rev* 2004; (4):CD000331.

4. Von Ungern-Sternberg BS, Regli A, Bucher E, Reber A, Schneider MC. The effect of epidural analgesia in labour on maternal respiratory function. *Anaesthesia* 2004; **59**: 350–53.

5. Cascio M, Pygon B, Bernett C, Ramanathan S. Labour analgesia with intrathecal fentanyl decreases maternal stress. *Can J Anaesth* 1997; **44**: 605–9.

6. Hood DD, Dewan DM. Anesthetic and obstetric outcome in morbidly obese parturients. *Anaesthesiology* 1993; **79**:1210–18.

7. Shah N, Latoo Y. Anaesthetic management of obese parturient. *Br J Med Pract* 2008; **1**:15–23.

8. Saravankumar K, Rao SG, Cooper GM. Obesity and obstetric anaesthesia. *Anaesthesia* 2006; **61**:36–48.

9. Robinson HE, O'Connell CM, Joseph KS, McLeod NL. Maternal outcomes in pregnancies complicated by obesity. *Obstet Gynecol* 2005; **106**:1357–64.

10. Vallejo MC. Anaesthetic management of the morbidly obese parturient. *Curr Opin Anaesthesiol* 2007; **20**: 175–80.

11. Odor PM, Bampoe S, Hayward J, Chis Ster I, Evans E. Intrapartum epidural fixation methods: a randomised controlled trial of three different epidural catheter securement devices. *Anaesthesia* 2016; **71**:298–305.

12. Johnson SR, Kolberg BH, Vasrner MW, Railsback LD. Maternal obesity and pregnancy. *Surg Gynecol Obstet* 1987; **164**:431–37.

13. Sebire NJ, Jolly M, Harris JP, et al. Maternal obesity and pregnancy outcome: a study of 287,213 pregnancies in London. *Int J ObesRelat Metab Disord* 2001; **25**(8):1175–82.

14. Ehrenburg HM, Mercer BM, Catalano PM. The influence of obesity and diabetes on the prevalence of macrosomia. *Am J Obstet Gynecol* 2004; **191**:964–68.

15. Weiss JL, Malone FD, Emig D, et al. Obesity, obstetric complications and caesarean delivery rate. *Am J Obstet Gynecol* 2004; **190**:1091–97.

16. Usha Kiran TS, Hemmadi S, Bethel J, Evans J. Outcome of pregnancy in a woman with an increased body mass index. *BJOG* 2005; **112**:768–72.

17. Myles TD, Gooch J, Santolaya J. Obesity as an independent risk factor for infectious morbidity in

patients who undergo caesarean delivery. *Obstet Gynecol* 2002; **100**:959–64.

18. Munnur U, de Boisblanc B, Suresh MS. Airway problems in pregnancy. *Crit Care Med* 2005; **33**(10 Suppl):259–68.

19. Schneider MC. Amaesthetic management of high-risk obstetric patients. *Acta Anaesthesiol Scand* 1997; **41**(1 Suppl. 111):163–65.

20. Juvin P, Lavaut E, Dupont H, et al. Difficult tracheal intubation is more common in obese than lean patients. *Anesth Analg* 2003; **97**:595–600.

21. D'Angelo R, Dewan DD, Chestnut DH. Obesity, in Chestnut DH (ed.), *Obstetric Anesthesia: Principles and Practice*. Philadelphia, PA: Elsevier Mosby; 2004, pp. 893–903.

22. Rocke DA, Murray WB, Rout CC, Gouws E. Relative risk analysis of factors associated with difficult intubation in obstetric anaesthesia. *Anesthesiology* 1992; **77**:67–73.

23. Bell RL, Rosenbaum SH. Postoperative considerations for patients with obesity and sleep apnea. *Anesthesiol Clin North Am* 2005; **23**:493–500.

24. Kodali BS, Chandrasekhar S, Bulich LN, Topulos GP, Datta S. Airway changes during pregnancy. *Anaesthesiology* 1997; **87**:895.

25. Mhyre J. Anaesthetic management of morbidly obese patients. *Int Anesthesiol Clin* 2007; **45**(1):51–70.

26. Vasan RS. Cardiac function and obesity. *Heart* 2003; **89**:1127–29.

27. ACOG. Obesity in pregnancy (Committee Opinion No. 315). Obstetr Gynecol 2005; **106**:671–75.

28. World Health Organization. *Obesity: Preventing and Managing the Global Epidemic* (Report on a WHO consultation, WHO Technical Report Series 894). Geneva: WHO; 2000.

29. Mace HS, Paech MJ, McDonnell NJ. Obesity and obstetric anesthesia. *Anaesth Intensive Care* 2011; **39**:559.

Complex Adult Congenital Heart Disease in Pregnancy

Daryl Dob, Zara Edwards, and Lorna Swan

Case Study

A 26-year-old woman with a single-ventricle circulation treated with the Fontan procedure wanted to become pregnant. She was advised by a multidisciplinary clinic including her adult congenital heart disease cardiology physician, the obstetrician, anesthetist, and midwife in the specialist referral center that this would be possible because she had good underlying cardiac function. She was taking warfarin anticoagulation therapy. A full anesthetic and obstetric management plan was made and put into her medical notes to communicate with the multidisciplinary team. The patient had good exercise tolerance with baseline observations of systemic arterial oxygen saturation of 94 percent on air, arterial blood pressure 110/70 mmHg, and heart rate of 90 beats/min in sinus rhythm.

She was seen again after conception and followed up regularly every 6 weeks in the joint clinic, having echocardiographic checks by her cardiology doctors and regular obstetric checks. Her normal warfarin was stopped to avoid embryopathy and substituted with a therapeutic dose of enoxaparin 40 mg SC twice a day.

She was well at 20 weeks' gestation and continued her pregnancy with no signs of cardiac decompensation. At 35 weeks' gestation, she was admitted to the specialist referral center for bed rest and more careful observation until 38 weeks, which is routine in cases such as this. At this point, delivery by induction of labor was planned. Enoxaparin anticoagulation was stopped 24 hours before induction to allow safe regional anesthesia and delivery. Because she had good cardiac function, induction of labor was planned with early low dose combined spinal epidural (CSE) analgesia. She was monitored with noninvasive blood pressure, ECG, and pulse oximetry. The baby was monitored with a cardiotocograph (CTG).

CSE anesthesia was performed with 1 ml hypobaric 0.25% bupivacaine and 25 μg fentanyl for the spinal component. Then 8-ml doses of 0.1% bupivacaine and 2 μg/ml fentanyl low-dose epidural mixture were given by patient-controlled epidural analgesia (PCEA) pump for the epidural component with a lockout time of 15 minutes. The analgesia worked well, and there was no need for any additional physician-administered rescue doses. The patient was carefully monitored throughout the day, and a decision was made not to place a radial artery catheter for invasive blood pressure monitoring because the patient was hemodynamically stable.

After a 9-hour labor that was augmented with oxytocin, the patient reached full cervical dilatation and was transferred to the operating room (OR) for an outlet forceps delivery to reduce the maternal effort of pushing. Her obstetricians were confident of a vaginal delivery.

In the OR, the epidural catheter was topped up in four divided doses of 5 ml low-dose bupivacaine 0.1% with 2 μg/ml fentanyl. The standard low-dose mixture was used for hemodynamic stability in the likelihood that delivery would be vaginal. If cesarean section were required, a higher concentration of local anesthetic (e.g., plain bupivacaine 0.5% or lidocaine 2% with epinephrine) would have been administered. An arterial line was inserted to accurately monitor blood pressure.

At delivery, there was a rapid vaginal blood loss of 500 ml. The patient felt faint, increased her heart rate to 110 beats/min, and became hypotensive with a blood pressure of 80/50 mm Hg. The blood loss was immediately replaced with 500 ml colloid solution IV, leading to an improvement in blood pressure and symptoms.

After delivery, the patient was given a low-dose oxytocin infusion (0.02 IU/ml at 36 ml/h) and restarted on a therapeutic dose of enoxaparin 40 mg twice daily SC (6 hours after epidural catheter removal). She spent 24 hours in the obstetric high-dependency unit under observation, after which time the arterial line was removed. Her warfarin was restarted. She went home after 3 days to be followed up in the multidisciplinary clinic and also at her specialist cardiac hospital. She and her baby were very well 1 year later.

Key Points

- Complex patients with congenital heart disease (CHD) such as those with a double-outlet right ventricle, large ventricular septal defect, and pulmonary atresia treated with the Fontan repair may present to a specialist referral center antenatal clinic.
- In such cases, comprehensive multidisciplinary planning and regular antenatal review may allow a smooth labor, timely regional anesthesia, and safe instrumental vaginal delivery with minimal hemodynamic compromise.

Discussion

Congenital heart disease (CHD) complicates 0.8 percent of all live births worldwide. In this century, more than 80 percent of neonates with moderate to complex CHD survive to adulthood, and over the last two decades, patients with complex congenital lesions are successfully completing pregnancies with careful planning and meticulous antenatal care. This is also true for patients with univentricular hearts and Fontan palliation. A comprehensive understanding of the individual patient's cardiac anatomy, previous operations, and current physiology is crucial to successfully managing pregnancy and childbirth.

The normal cardiac configuration can be divided into seven features[1]:

1. The atrial situs (position) – situs solitus being normal with the left atrium on the left.
2. The draining pattern of the systemic and pulmonary veins.
3. The relationship between the atria and the ventricles. In the normal heart, this is a concordant relationship (i.e., the left atrium is connected to the left ventricle and the right to the right).
4. The absence of intracardiac defects – for example, an atrial septal defect (ASD) or a ventricular septal defect (VSD).
5. The status of the atrioventricular valves. These may be atretic (absent) or hypoplastic or draining into the wrong ventricle (i.e., blood that flows through the mitral valve drains into the right ventricle, instead of the left ventricle, and blood

that flows through the tricuspid valve drains into the left ventricle, instead of the right ventricle).
6. The relationship between the ventricle and the great arteries (pulmonary and aorta). In the normal heart, there should be ventriculoarterial concordance (i.e., the ventricles are connected normally to the corresponding great arteries – left ventricle to the aorta and right ventricle to the pulmonary artery).
7. No extracardiac lesions such as patent ductus arteriosus (PDA) or coarctation of the aorta.

The patient was born with a large ventricular septal defect (VSD), a double-outlet right ventricle, and pulmonary atresia shown in Figure 16.1. This leads to mixing of oxygenated blood from the left atrium and deoxygenated blood from the right atrium in the ventricles. It also limits pulmonary blood flow due to pulmonary atresia. For this reason, the patient required bilateral Blalock-Taussig shunts as a baby. This shunt involves a conduit between the subclavian artery and the pulmonary artery. It helps to increase pulmonary blood flow – helping to improve oxygenation and growth of the pulmonary arteries. In this patient, the VSD was too large to permit a repair, which would result in a biventricular circulation, so her surgical team advised a Fontan repair with a fenestrated total cavopulmonary connection (TCPC) done in two stages. This results in anatomy with a "single ventricle," or univentricular physiology, as shown in Figure 16.2 and in the MRI scan in Figure 16.3.

The Fontan procedure separates pulmonary and systemic circulations, therefore greatly improving oxygenation. It involves a direct connection between the systemic venous return and the pulmonary artery (the total cavopulmonary connection), bypassing the right ventricle. This has the advantage that deoxygenated blood is oxygenated in the lungs and does not mix with deoxygenated systemic venous return in the single ventricle. Because the right ventricle is disconnected from the lungs, pulmonary flow must come from the remaining kinetic energy of the systemic circulation driven by the single ventricle. The two circulations are separated, and systemic oxygen saturation is high, whereas the functional single ventricle only pumps blood through the aorta.[2,3]

Early versions of the Fontan procedure involved connecting the right atrium directly to the pulmonary artery with a valved conduit. This was called the *atriopulmonary Fontan* or *classic Fontan procedure*. Unfortunately, this resulted in sluggish and inefficient

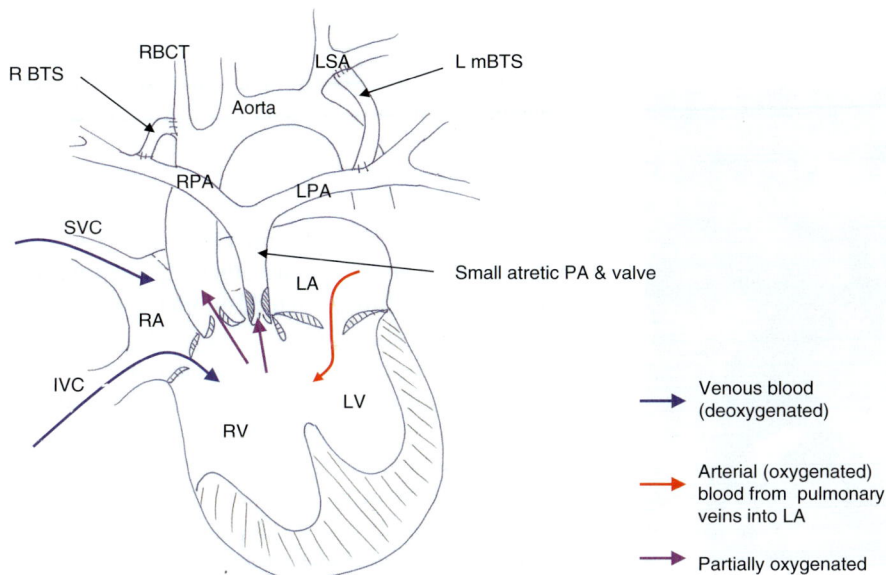

Pre-total cavopulmonary connection (lateral-tunnel Fontan) anatomy – Double outlet RV with pulmonary atresia

IVC/SVC – inferior/superior vena cava   RA/LA – right/left atrium   RV/LV – right/left ventricle

RBCT – brachiocephalic trunk   LSA – left subclavian artery   RPA/LPA – right/left pulmonary artery

R BTS – right Blalock-Taussig shunt   L mBTS – left modified Blalock-Taussig shunt

Figure 16.1 Pre-total cavopulmonary connection (lateral-tunnel Fontan) anatomy – double-outlet right ventricle with pulmonary atresia

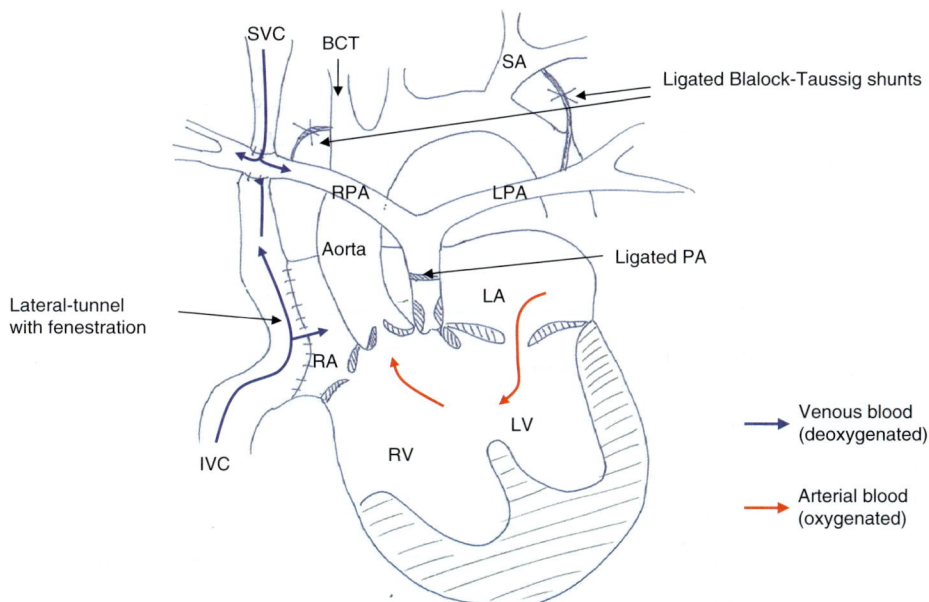

Post-total cavopulmonary connection (lateral-tunnel Fontan)

IVC – inferior vena cava   SVC – superior vena cava   RV/LV – right/left ventricle

PA - pulmonary artery   RPA – right pulmonary artery   LPA – left pulmonary artery

RA/LA – right/left arium   SA – subclavian artery   BCT – brachiocephalic trunk

Figure 16.2 After total cavopulmonary connection (lateral-tunnel Fontan)

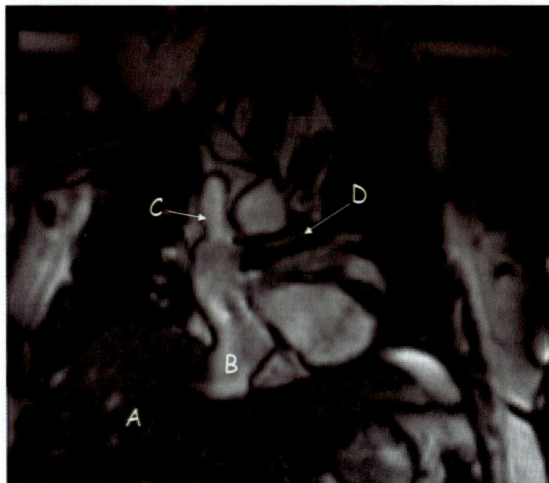

Cardiac MRI scan of a lateral tunnel Fontan

A - Liver   B - Dilated IVC entering lateral tunnel TCPC

C - SVC   D - Left pulmonary artery

Figure 16.3 Cardiac MRI scan of a lateral-tunnel Fontan

blood flow through the lungs and very high venous pressures. This caused many problems such as right atrial dilatation, pleural effusions, ascites, liver venous engorgement, cirrhosis, and protein-losing enteropathy.

A more modern version of the original Fontan operation using an extracardiac conduit (TCPC) was developed in the 1980s. The first stage of this operation is to perform a bidirectional Glenn shunt operation, otherwise known as a *hemi-Fontan procedure*. This involves transecting the superior vena cava off the right atrium and connecting it to the right pulmonary artery. In this operation, the venous blood from the upper body, head, and neck flows passively through the lungs via the right and left pulmonary arteries, (bidirectional), becoming oxygenated and returning to the left atrium. The inferior vena cava is still connected to the right atrium, so deoxygenated blood from the lower body still mixes in the single ventricle with the oxygenated blood from the lungs. The blood pumped out has an overall oxygen saturation of about 85–90 percent and allows the pulmonary blood vessels time to accommodate a higher blood flow than before. The final stage of the procedure is to complete the TCPC. This involves transecting the inferior vena cava and connecting it to the pulmonary artery. This means that oxygenated and deoxygenated blood is completely separated, and arterial oxygen

saturations reach 90–100 percent. The completely oxygenated blood is pumped out of the aorta by the single ventricle. It delivers oxygen to the body and then returns via the superior and inferior venae cavae directly to the pulmonary artery through the lungs. The connection from the inferior vena cava to the pulmonary artery is a more efficient tube (extracardiac TCPC) or tunnel (lateral-tunnel version). This prevents massive dilatation of the right atrium.

In the early period after this operation, the high venous backpressure can still be problematic. To improve this, a small hole, or *fenestration*, can be made in the tunnel. If pulmonary venous pressure rises, then deoxygenated blood can vent out of the tunnel into the atrium. This stops the venous pressure from rising too high, but at the expense of deoxygenated blood shunting through to the single ventricle. Although this slightly reduces systemic arterial saturation, it allows the pulmonary vasculature time to adjust to the increased blood flow. At a later date, it may be possible to close the fenestration, usually with a small umbrella catheter technique. Despite these measures, even a well-functioning TCPC will have high venous pressures and be subject to a great sensitivity in preload.

Labor and Delivery

Cardiac Output

In pregnancy, plasma and blood volume are increased significantly, and it is important to watch for systemic ventricular dysfunction as the cardiac output increases. It is often necessary, as in our case, to admit mothers for bed rest and observation toward the end of their pregnancy to help both maternal oxygenation and fetal growth.

Anticoagulation

In Fontan circulations, blood flow through the lungs is often slow. To prevent thrombus formation, most patients with this circulation are anticoagulated with warfarin.

Pregnancy, which is a hypercoagulable state, puts the mother with a Fontan repair at even greater risk of thromboembolic events, so continued anticoagulation is essential. One strategy is to convert from warfarin, which crosses the placenta, to subcutaneous low-molecular-weight heparin (LMWH), which does not cross the placenta. Paradoxical embolism is a particular concern if there is a fenestration or other

Table 17.2 Von Willebrand Disease Laboratory Assays

Assay	Significance
Activated partial thromboplastin time (aPTT)	Measures the integrity of the coagulation factors in the intrinsic coagulation cascade
Factor VIII activity (FVIII, FVIII:C)	Functional assay of plasma factor VIII activity
vWF antigen (vWF:Ag, VWFA)	Quantitative measurement of plasma vWF
Ristocetin cofactor activity (vWF:RCo, RISTOC)	Functional measure of plasma vWF activity
Ristocetin-induced platelet aggregation (RIPA)	Qualitatively measures vWF and platelet activity
Multimer gel electrophoresis	Measures vWF multimer structure

vWF = von Willebrand factor.

autosomal-dominant inability to release vWF from cellular stores, resulting in a quantitative decrease in circulating vWF levels. The far more uncommon homozygous autosomal-recessive type 3, comprising approximately 1 percent of patients with vWD, is characterized by nearly absent production of functional vWF, resulting in an almost complete degradation of factor VIII and a severe disease pattern closely resembling X-linked recessive hemophilia A. Type 2 vWD comprises four subtypes of qualitative vWF defects.[2] Expert hematology input is necessary during pregnancy as part of a multidisciplinary approach for delivery, including the suitability and safety of neuraxial anesthesia. Disease severity and treatment depend on the type of vWD. Establishing the diagnosis is paramount for optimal patient care. Mild cases of vWD can be difficult to diagnose and depend on patient blood type, estrogen level, inflammation, stress, and smoking. Laboratory diagnosis of vWD often involves the assays listed in Table 17.2.

Although routine screening of normal pregnant women for coagulopathy is not indicated, patients may present to the obstetric anesthesiologist for consultation regarding an isolated elevated aPTT. An elevated aPTT prompts a differential diagnosis that includes hypo- and hypercoagulable states and laboratory error or artifact. In fact, the most common cause of an isolated elevated aPTT level is an inadequate amount of blood in the collection tube. To differentiate between the presence of a hypocoagulable (e.g., vWD) and a hypercoagulable state (e.g., anti-phospholipid antibody syndrome), a mixing study is performed with normal serum. Correction of the aPTT after mixing indicates a

deficiency in the intrinsic coagulation cascade factors (e.g., factor VIII), whereas maintenance of the elevated aPTT indicates the presence of an inhibitor (e.g., lupus anticoagulant or anti-cardiolipin antibodies).

Implications of vWD in Obstetric Anesthesia

A parturient with vWD poses unique challenges to the obstetric anesthesiologist. Concerns include provision of adequate labor analgesia and management of postpartum hemorrhage (PPH). Depending on the type and severity of vWD, parturients may not be candidates for neuraxial anesthesia or analgesia without prior laboratory assessment of coagulation or receiving empirical treatment due to the risk of epidural hematoma. Devastating neurologic injury related to neuraxial analgesia or anesthesia has *not* been reported in this population. In fact, multiple case reports and case series have described the efficacy and safety of neuraxial analgesia and anesthesia in this population after undergoing proper testing and/or treatment.[3–7]

In addition, vWD elevates the risk of early and delayed PPH. Patients with type 1 vWD, who comprise the majority of patients with vWD, often have normal laboratory values for factor VIII, VWFA, RISTOC, and aPTT by the third trimester of pregnancy; neuraxial anesthesia and analgesia are considered safe under these circumstances. However, because these levels will return to baseline within 7–21 days, 20–25 percent of patients with type 1 vWD will experience delayed (mean 15.7 days) PPH.[8]

Women on estrogen-containing oral contraceptives will have an increase in vWF antigen levels, similar to the increase found in pregnancy. Making a diagnosis of vWD in a woman on combination oral contraceptives can be difficult. The patient in this case was on levonorgestrel, a second-generation synthetic progestin, which has no impact on vWF antigen levels. Therefore, the levels in this patient can be considered to be true baseline levels.

If laboratory values do not normalize by the time of delivery, treatment based on the specific type of vWD is indicated, regardless of whether neuraxial analgesia or anesthesia is desired, because of the risk of early PPH.[9] In types 1 and 2 vWD, vWF and factor VIII generally begin increasing in the mid-second trimester. However, because of type-specific and individual variability in magnitude increase, frequent monitoring of factor VIII levels in the antepartum and postpartum periods is necessary. Treatment of vWD in the peripartum period aims to achieve vWF:RCo and FVIII activity levels at or above 50 percent, which is accepted as safe for regional anesthesia and delivery. Scheduled labor induction or cesarean delivery is optimal for those requiring replacement therapy. If laboratory values have not normalized in the third trimester of pregnancy, a multidisciplinary meeting involving the obstetrics, hematology, and obstetric anesthesia services is ideally performed in the antepartum period to formulate a treatment plan for delivery. If delivery is imminent and the factor status of the patient is unknown, treatment is indicated and should not be delayed for laboratory results.

For type 1 vWD, in which there is adequate vWF production and storage but impaired release, the synthetic antidiuretic hormone analogue DDAVP (1-deamino-8-D-arginine vasopressin, desmopressin) is the preferred treatment.[10] This drug, often administered as a 0.3 µg/kg IV infusion in 50–100 ml normal saline (NS) over 30 minutes, triggers release of stored vWF from Weibel-Palade bodies of endothelial cells, resulting in a three- to fivefold increase in factor VIII and vWF levels within 30 minutes and lasting at least 8–10 hours; redosage can occur at 12- or 24-hour intervals.[11] Side effects include headache, hypertension, flushing, nausea, vomiting, hyponatremia, seizures, and uterine contractions; tachyphylaxis can be seen after 3 days of treatment.

Because type 3 vWD involves the severely impaired synthesis of vWF, DDAVP administration, which acts to release intracellular stores, is *not* an effective treatment. The use of DDAVP in type 2B vWD is generally contraindicated because a transient thrombocytopenia can occur and further aggravate bleeding risk.[12] For types 2A, 2M, and 2N vWD, the response to DDAVP is variable, and a predelivery DDAVP response test is indicated. The results of this test may guide peripartum management.

If DDAVP is contraindicated or does not normalize factor VIII levels after administration, direct replacement of factor VIII with factor VIII–vWF concentrates (Humate P, Alphanate) can be considered. In patients with type 3 vWD, who almost completely lack vWF, administration of factor VIII–vWF has been shown to elicit an immune response to the vWF antigen in some patients, resulting in neutralization of vWF activity. In these patients, factor VIII is the treatment of choice. Cryoprecipitate contains a two- to threefold higher factor VIII and ninefold

higher vWF concentration than fresh-frozen plasma (FFP),[13] although neither is used routinely if factor VIII–vWF concentrate is available. The safety, efficacy, and pharmacokinetics of recombinant vWF are currently being studied in clinical trials.[14,15]

Thrombocytopenia in Pregnancy

Thrombocytopenia is defined as the drop in platelet count from the normal range of $150–400 \times 10^9$/liter to a count lower than 150×10^9/liter. Thrombocytopenia can be seen in up to 5–10 percent of all pregnancies due to a physiologic drop in the platelet count during pregnancy. It is important to determine the etiology of thrombocytopenia so that appropriate care and management can be given to improve maternal outcomes and decrease bleeding risks. Platelet counts below 100×10^9/liter may require further evaluation by a hematologist. Thrombocytopenia is caused by a variety of physiologic and pathologic conditions and is a relative contraindication to neuraxial anesthesia.

The most likely etiology of thrombocytopenia during pregnancy is gestational thrombocytopenia, which occurs in 70 percent of cases. The other 30 percent of cases are due to other causes, which include idiopathic thrombocytopenic purpura (ITP) and other autoimmune-associated causes of thrombocytopenia such as systemic lupus erythematosus and disorders associated with microangiopathic changes and thrombocytopenia. The latter include preeclampsia/eclampsia, HELLP (hemolysis, elevated liver enzymes, low platelets) syndrome, and thrombotic thrombocytopenic purpura–hemolytic-uremic syndrome (TTP/HUS). Rare inherited platelet disorders associated with thrombocytopenia, such as May-Hegglin anomaly, may first appear during pregnancy because it may be the first time the patient has had a complete blood count (CBC) performed.

In a patient with completely normal physical findings, normal white blood cells and morphology, and normal hematocrit, the differential diagnosis is limited to gestational thrombocytopenia and ITP. It is often difficult to differentiate ITP and gestational thrombocytopenia based on physical examination and other laboratory findings. Often it is only the level to which the platelet count drops that distinguishes between ITP and gestational thrombocytopenia. In patients with gestational thrombocytopenia, the platelet count usually does not drop below 70×10^9/liter.

A past history of thrombocytopenia, either during or unassociated with pregnancy, guides evaluation and management. In gestational thrombocytopenia, the platelet count returns to normal soon after delivery without other treatment. It can recur in subsequent pregnancies. Patients with ITP will often have low platelet counts prior to pregnancy or thrombocytopenia that persists postpartum. Gestational thrombocytopenia usually presents in the third trimester. ITP can occur during any trimester and is generally the only cause of new thrombocytopenia in the first trimester. The platelet count in gestational thrombocytopenia stays in the same general range, whereas in ITP there can be an extremely rapid drop (over the course of 1–2 weeks) from low/normal (around 120×10^9/liter) to between $10 - 20 \times 10^9$/liter.

Determining the etiology of thrombocytopenia is important to minimize potential bleeding risks for mother and fetus during gestation, labor, and delivery and for placement of neuraxial techniques.[16–18] Some disorders do not require treatment, such as gestational thrombocytopenia or May-Hegglin anomaly, whereas in other disorders, such as TTP, rapid institution of appropriate therapy can be lifesaving and have a significant impact on outcome.

Thrombocytopenia is a concern in any patient because of the risk of bleeding into the epidural space with neuraxial techniques[19] and the broad heterogeneity of underlying diagnoses. Bleeding is not a feature of gestational thrombocytopenia because the platelet count does not drop low enough. Mild trauma-induced bruising and minor mucosal bleeding can occur in ITP, but moderate to severe bleeding with platelet counts greater than 30×10^9/liter is uncommon in ITP. IV immunoglobulin G (IgG; 1 g/kg) is the initial treatment of choice for pregnant patients with ITP and platelet counts lower than 10×10^9/liter. An increased platelet count can be seen within 12 hours of administration. The platelet count will continue to rise over the next few days. IV IgG is a treatment that only temporarily raises the platelet count. The duration of response to one dose of IV IgG is variable, lasting from 1–6 weeks. Further treatment should be planned, as described below. Cesarean delivery can be performed if necessary, and epidural or spinal anesthesia can be used if necessary. These treatment plans vary somewhat depending on whether labor and delivery will occur spontaneously or will be a scheduled induction of labor or elective cesarean delivery. A platelet count of 30×10^9/liter is sufficient to prevent maternal bleeding in uncomplicated delivery, but for cesarean delivery, a minimum of 50×10^9/liter is required. The platelet threshold for neuraxial anesthesia varies from institution to institution but is generally in the range of $70–75 \times 10^9$/liter. If treatment for ITP is given in preparation for delivery, the target platelet count should be roughly 100×10^9/liter because it is difficult to achieve a precise number.

Glucocorticoids are first-line therapy in patients without clinical bleeding and a platelet count above 10×10^9/liter. The response rate is 60–80 percent. It takes longer to see an increase in the platelet count with corticosteroids than with IV IgG, with an increase in platelet count often not observed until after 5–10 days of treatment. Patients with presumed gestational thrombocytopenia do not require treatment, but platelet counts need to be followed over time in case the diagnosis is, in fact, ITP. If there is no significant change over this time period, then concern for a further decrease at the time of labor and delivery is lessened. Standard labor and delivery practices can be followed, including the use of neuraxial anesthesia. A short trial of steroids or IV IgG can be undertaken late in pregnancy (usually after 35–36 weeks) for patients with borderline platelet counts around $70–80 \times 10^9$/liter in case the patient may have ITP or there might be an increase in platelet count sufficient to allow neuraxial anesthesia. Collaboration and coordination between hematologist, obstetrician, and anesthesiologist are required to ensure safe delivery.

Thrombocytopenia and anemia with evidence of hemolysis are characteristic of preeclampsia, HELLP, and TTP/HUS. Other associated physical signs and symptoms are needed to differentiate these disorders. Preeclampsia is associated with hypertension and proteinuria, HELLP is associated with right upper quadrant pain and abnormal liver function tests, and fever, neurologic changes, and renal insufficiency are associated with TTP and HUS. Preeclampsia affects 6 percent of all pregnancies and accounts for 21 percent of cases of maternal thrombocytopenia. Thrombocytopenia may be the earliest clinical feature in some patients. It is usually moderate and is present in 15 percent of preeclamptic patients. Platelet counts that are trending downward may be an indication of worsening disease and the need for delivery. The platelet count may decrease to a nadir 24–48 hours postpartum, but clinical manifestations usually resolve after delivery. There is no absolute platelet count number that precludes the placement of an epidural catheter. The decision to perform a neuraxial technique is based on bleeding history, the platelet count trend, the airway examination, and the likelihood of a cesarean delivery.

HELLP syndrome is characterized by hemolysis, elevated liver enzymes, and a low platelet count. It occurs in up to 10 percent of pregnancies complicated by preeclampsia with severe features, usually presents in the second or third trimester or the postpartum period, and may be life threatening. Of note, it may occur in parturients with no other signs of preeclampsia, and one or all of the components of the HELLP syndrome may be present. The HELLP syndrome per se is not a contraindication to neuraxial anesthesia, but thrombocytopenia or the presence of a coagulopathy may influence the decision of whether to perform a neuraxial technique. A coagulopathy is not usually present unless the platelet count is less than 100×10^9/liter. Other coagulation factors may be affected following microangiopathic platelet destruction, and therefore, prothrombin time, activated partial thromboplastin time, and fibrinogen levels should be monitored once the platelet count is less than 100×10^9/liter.

A fundamental question for the obstetric anesthesiologist is whether or not to perform neuraxial procedures in the setting of thrombocytopenia. There are few data to support the notion that neuraxial techniques should be avoided at any one absolute platelet count. An increasing number of published cases of apparently safe epidural or spinal procedures performed with counts well below 100×10^9/liter, a traditionally accepted threshold, have appeared in recent years. The etiology of the thrombocytopenia, the rate of decline, and the magnitude of the drop in platelet count guide the decision as to whether and when to place the neuraxial technique. Most anesthesiologists feel comfortable initiating neuraxial anesthesia in parturients as long as the platelet count is greater than 70×10^9/liter and there is no evidence of bleeding unless there is a compelling indication to do so at a lower platelet count based on a risk-benefit analysis. A spinal technique is theoretically less traumatic than an epidural and is preferred by some practitioners once the platelet count is less than 70×10^9/liter. However, few objective data directly support this practice. Soft, flexible catheters are preferred for an epidural technique because they have a lower incidence of venous cannulation.

Epidural hematoma is a rare complication of neuraxial anesthesia but can cause serious complications. The incidence in the obstetric patient population is estimated to be 1 in 200,000, with the risk of permanent neurologic deficits approximately 1 in 237,000. Thrombocytopenia increases the risk of epidural hematoma. There is less risk in thrombocytopenic patients with normal platelet function, such as in ITP or gestational thrombocytopenia. Patients with coagulopathies may have a higher bleeding risk and hence risk for epidural hematoma – especially when thrombocytopenia is also present. A platelet count of 70×10^9/liter with no other bleeding risks is accepted as being adequate for neuraxial anesthesia. There has been a trend over the last two decades to accept an even lower threshold for spinal anesthesia, especially in patients with gestational thrombocytopenia or ITP (between 50 and 70×10^9/liter), but institutional practices vary widely.

Point-of-care measurements of global coagulation status have been used to try to assess bleeding risk in a wide variety of surgical patients, including pregnant patients, prior to neuraxial anesthesia. Most commonly, rotational thromboelastometry (ROTEM) has been studied in pregnant patients.[20] ROTEM provides a global assessment of coagulation, including clotting factors, platelet function, and their interaction. The technique can determine the clot strength, the rate of clot formation and strengthening, and fibrinolysis.

Learning Points

- Accurate diagnosis of a coagulopathy greatly facilitates treatment.
- vWD poses a unique challenge to the obstetric anesthesiologist.
- In type 1 vWD, vWF and factor VIII levels generally rise during pregnancy.
- Thrombocytopenia often presents to the obstetric anesthesiologist. Although the most common cause is gestational thrombocytopenia, other causes such as ITP need specialist input before deciding whether a neuraxial block can be used.

References

1. von Willebrand EA. Hereditar pseudohemofili. *Finska Lakarsallskapets Handl* 1926; **67**:7–112.

2. Tosetto A, Castaman G. How I treat type 2 variant forms of von Willebrand disease. *Blood* 2015; **125**:907–14.

3. Jones BP, Bell EA, Maroof M. Epidural labor analgesia in a parturient with von Willebrand's disease type IIA and severe preeclampsia. *Anesthesiology* 1999; **90**(4):1219–20.

4. Marrache D, Mercier FJ, Boyer-Neumann C, Roger-Christoph S, Benhamou D. Epidural analgesia for parturients with type 1 von Willebrand disease. *Int J Obstet Anesth* 2007; **16**:231–35.

5. Varughese J, Cohen AJ. Experience with epidural anaesthesia in pregnant women with von Willebrand disease. *Haemophilia* 2007; **13**:730–33.

6. Chi C, Lee CA, England A, et al. Obstetric analgesia and anaesthesia in women with inherited bleeding disorders. *Thromb Haemost* 2009; **101**:1104–11.

7. Amorde RW, Patel SN, Pagel PS. Management of labor and delivery of a patient with von Willebrand disease type 2A. *Int Anesthesiol Clin* 2011; **49**:74–80.

8. Roque H, Funai E, Lockwood CJ. von Willebrand disease and pregnancy. *J Matern Fetal Med* 2000; **9**:257–66.

9. Mannucci PM. Treatment of von Willebrand's disease. *N Engl J Med* 2004; **351**:683–94.

10. Mannucci PM, Ruggeri ZM, Pareti FI, Capitanio A. 1-Deamino-8-d-arginine vasopressin: a new pharmacological approach to the management of haemophilia and von Willebrands' diseases. *Lancet* 1977; **1**(8017):869–72.

11. Mannucci PM. How I treat patients with von Willebrand disease. *Blood* 2001; **97**:1915–19.

12. Holmberg L, Nilsson IM, Borge L, Gunnarsson M, Sjorin E. Platelet aggregation induced by 1-desamino-8-d-arginine vasopressin (DDAVP) in type IIB von Willebrand's disease. *N Engl J Med* 1983; **309**:816–21.

13. Caudill JS, Nichols WL, Plumhoff EA, et al. Comparison of coagulation factor XIII content and concentration in cryoprecipitate and fresh-frozen plasma. *Transfusion* 2009; **49**:765–70.

14. Turecek PL, Schrenk G, Rottensteiner H, et al. Structure and function of a recombinant von Willebrand factor drug candidate. *Semin Thromb Hemost* 2010; **36**:510–21.

15. Mannucci PM, Kempton C, Millar C, et al. Pharmacokinetics and safety of a novel recombinant human von Willebrand factor manufactured with a plasma-free method: a prospective clinical trial. *Blood* 2013; **122**:648–57.

16. Bernstein J, Hua B, Kahana M, et al. Neuraxial anesthesia in parturients with low platelet counts. *Anesth Analg* 2016; **123**:165.

17. Lee LO, Bateman BT, Kheterpal S, et al. Risk of epidural hematoma after neuraxial techniques in thrombocytopenic parturients: a report from the Multicenter Perioperative Outcomes Group. *Anesthesiology* 2017; **126**:1053–63.

18. Scully M, Thomas M, Underwood M, et al. Thrombotic thrombocytopenic purpura and pregnancy: presentation, management, and subsequent pregnancy outcomes. *Blood* 2014; **124**:211.

19. van Veen JJ, Nokes TJ, Makris M. The risk of spinal haematoma following neuraxial anaesthesia or lumbar puncture in thrombocytopenic individuals. *Br J Haematol* 2010; **148**:15.

20. Armstrong S, Fernando R, Ashpole K, Simons R, Columb M. Assessment of coagulation in the obstetric population using ROTEM thromboelastometry. *Int J Obstet Anesth* 2011; **20**:293–98.

Respiratory Disorders in Pregnancy

Jessica Booth and Melissa Potisek

Case Study

A 27-year-old gravida 1, para 0 woman presented to labor and delivery at 35 weeks' gestation for evaluation for dyspnea. Her pregnancy had been uncomplicated, but she had a known history of mild intermittent asthma for which she required an albuterol inhaler "occasionally." She reported wheezing for 1 day that has not been responsive to her albuterol inhaler and a fever with chills that started that morning. She denied contractions and reported good fetal movement.

On physical examination, the patient had tachypnea with diffuse wheezing. Her vital signs were as follows: heart rate 125 beats/min, blood pressure 117/75 mmHg, respiratory rate 40 breaths/min, oxygen saturation 93 percent on room air, and temperature 38.0°C. Fetal heart rate tracing was Category I. An IV infusion was started, and fluids were administered. A chest x-ray was obtained and revealed "developing consolidation of the right lower lobe and evidence of mild air trapping." The patient was given three treatments of nebulized albuterol and was started on ceftriaxone and azithromycin for treatment of possible community-acquired pneumonia.

After 1 hour of observation, the patient's wheezing was slightly improved, but she continued to be tachypneic and uncomfortable. The obstetrician prescribed continued nebulized albuterol with ipratropium bromide every 20 minutes and admitted the patient to the antepartum unit for monitoring. She was stable initially but had increasing oxygen requirements to maintain her oxygen saturation at greater than 95 percent. Her work of breathing increased progressively despite continuous albuterol treatments. An arterial blood gas was remarkable for a respiratory acidosis with the following values: pH 7.29, PCO_2 49 mmHg, PO_2 80 mmHg, and bicarbonate 28 mmol/kg. Fetal heart rate tracing was Category II with occasional deep variable decelerations.

The patient was transferred to the ICU for close monitoring and possible intubation and mechanical ventilation. Systemic IV steroids were added to her treatment regimen. Under close observation, her oxygen was gradually weaned to 4 liters/min via nasal cannula. Her care was gradually de-escalated, and she was discharged 5 days later on a steroid taper with close follow-up.

She remained stable for the remainder of her pregnancy and went into spontaneous labor at 38 weeks.

Key Points

- Patients may experience exacerbation of previously mild to intermittent asthma in the setting of possible community-acquired pneumonia.
- Subsequent hypoxia and hypercarbia despite aggressive therapy may result in the transfer to a higher level of care for further management.
- Intubation and ventilation sometimes may be required.

Discussion

Acute respiratory failure (ARF) is rare during pregnancy but is one of the most common indications for ICU admission for parturients. Asthma is one of the most common comorbidities found in pregnancy and is a risk factor for pneumonia during pregnancy. Any respiratory insult during pregnancy may be more likely to lead to respiratory failure due to the normal changes in pulmonary physiology during pregnancy. Both maternal and fetal mortality rates from ARF are reported to be around 30 percent, with maternal rates being slightly higher. Optimizing oxygen delivery, maintaining euvolemia, and treating the underlying causes of lung injury are the primary goals of therapy.[1]

Respiratory Physiology during Pregnancy

During pregnancy, hyperventilation and a chronic respiratory alkalosis are normal, stimulated both by progesterone levels and by fetal CO_2 in the maternal circulation. The diaphragm is pushed cephalad by the expanding uterus, and the anteroposterior and transverse diameters of the chest widen, leading to a stable total lung capacity (TLC). While vital capacity (VC) also remains stable, there is a significant increase in tidal volume (TV). Decreases in expiratory reserve volume (ERV) and residual volume (RV) lead to a significant reduction in functional residual capacity (FRC) by approximately 21 percent below the pre-pregnancy value. Given this reduction in FRC, there is a decrease in the difference between FRC and closing capacity (CC), making it more likely that small airway closure will occur during normal TV breathing. Obesity, multiple gestation, polyhydramnios, lung disease, and supine positioning all can exacerbate this problem, leading to increased ventilation-perfusion mismatch and hypoxia. The summation of these changes leads to poor tolerance of acute or chronic lung disease during pregnancy.

A normal pregnancy arterial blood gas determination reflects the above-mentioned changes with a fall in measured $PaCO_2$ and a rise in PaO_2. Generally, the PaO_2 will be above 100 mmHg for the duration of pregnancy, and the $PaCO_2$ will be approximately 30 mmHg. This respiratory alkalosis remains relatively stable for the duration of pregnancy and is accompanied by a compensatory increase in renal excretion of bicarbonate (normal HCO_3^- 21.7 mEq/liter).[2,3]

Asthma

About 8 percent of pregnant women carry the diagnosis of asthma, making it one of the most common comorbidities encountered in pregnancy. The disease is characterized by airway inflammation with reactivity and reversible airway obstruction.[3,4] The National Asthma Expert Panel Report has defined four classes of asthma severity: intermittent, mild persistent, moderate persistent, and severe persistent. Well-controlled asthma can be defined by the following parameters: minimal or no chronic symptoms day or night, minimal or no exacerbations, no limitation of activities, maintenance of (near) normal pulmonary function, minimal use of short-acting inhaled beta$_2$-agonist, and minimal or no adverse effects from medications. Disease course during pregnancy is known to be variable, with about 23 percent of women improving during pregnancy and 30 percent experiencing a worsening in their symptoms. Improvements in symptoms during pregnancy may be caused by pro-gesterone-mediated bronchodilation and increased

Table 18.1 Pharmacologic Management of Asthma during Pregnancy Using a Stepwise Approach

	Asthma severity	Treatment
Step 1	Mild intermittent	No daily medications; short-acting inhaled beta$_2$-agonist as needed
Step 2	Mild persistent	Low-dose inhaled corticosteroids
Step 3	Moderate persistent	Low-dose inhaled corticosteroids + long-acting beta$_2$-agonist *or* medium-dose inhaled corticosteroids
Step 4	Severe persistent	High-dose inhaled corticosteroids + long-acting beta$_2$-agonist *and*, if needed, oral systemic corticosteroids

serum cortisol levels, but the exact mechanism is unknown. Worsening of symptoms may be due to increased stress, worsening of reflux symptoms, bronchitis, or medication noncompliance.[3,5]

The National Asthma Education and Prevention Program published guidelines in 2004 on the pharmacologic treatment of parturients with asthma[5] (Table 18.1). If asthma is uncontrolled, there is an increased risk of preeclampsia, intrauterine growth restriction, preterm delivery, congenital malformations, and perinatal death. For this reason, all parturients with asthma should undergo clinical evaluation and optimization of symptom control. The treatment of asthma in pregnancy should involve assessment of asthma with objective measures of pulmonary function on a monthly basis, control of factors contributing to asthma severity, patient education, and a stepwise approach to pharmacologic therapy. Should the parturient require an emergency room visit or hospitalization, therapy should be aggressive and focused on maintaining maternal O_2 saturation above 95 percent. High-dose short-acting inhaled beta$_2$-agonists, inhaled ipratropium bromide, and either oral or IV corticosteroids are a part of the inpatient treatment algorithm.[6,7]

Pneumonia

Pneumonia is the most common cause of maternal mortality due to nonobstetric infection, but overall mortality rates have fallen below 4 percent due to

95

Table 18.2 Acute versus Chronic Causes of Dyspnea during Pregnancy

Acute dyspnea during pregnancy	Chronic dyspnea during pregnancy
Exacerbation of chronic disease (e.g., asthma)	Asthma
Pneumonia	Chronic obstructive pulmonary disease (COPD)
Acute respiratory distress syndrome (ARDS)	Emphysema
Amniotic fluid embolism	Cystic fibrosis
Pulmonary embolism	Tobacco abuse
Pulmonary edema	Cardiac disease (congenital or valvular disease)
Sepsis	Ischemic heart disease
Peripartum cardiomyopathy	
Aspiration of gastric contents	

improvements in targeted antibiotic therapy and critical care strategies. Community-acquired pneumonia is characterized by hypoxia, fever, cough, shortness of breath, and pleuritic chest pain and is most commonly due to infection by *Streptococcus pneumoniae* and *Haemophilus influenzae*. Common viral pathogens include influenza A and B, varicella-zoster virus, and coronavirus.[8] Of historic importance is the H1N1 strain of 2009–10, which led to an epidemic of severe illness in pregnant women and a reported mortality rate of 5 percent among 509 pregnant women (reported by the CDC). Due to an approximately 10-fold increase in influenza-related morbidity in pregnant women versus nonpregnant women, the CDC recommends that all pregnant women be vaccinated against influenza.

Anesthetic Considerations

The management of pulmonary disease should focus on providing adequate oxygenation to the mother and thus to the fetus. Chest radiography should not be delayed due to pregnancy if pneumonia is suspected, and an abdominal shield should be used. All potential diagnoses should be considered based on the acute versus chronic presentation of the patient's dyspnea (Table 18.2). Targeted treatment with appropriate antibiotic (monotherapy with macrolides) or antiviral therapy is appropriate, although broad-spectrum antibiotics may need to be initiated while the cause

of infection is confirmed. In the case of complicated pneumonia, involvement by infectious disease, critical care, obstetrics, and neonatology is optimal. If mechanical ventilation is necessary, rapid-sequence induction and a nonparticulate antacid with subsequent elevation of the head of the bed are important. Team preparedness for possible delivery is prudent.

In the case that a patient with systemic infection goes into labor or requires delivery, risks and benefits of regional anesthesia should be weighed, including the risk of CNS infection versus the risk of lost airway if regional anesthesia is not used. While most experts agree that neuraxial anesthesia should not be performed in *untreated* bacteremic patients, patients on appropriate treatment may safely undergo a spinal anesthetic.

If general anesthesia is required in an asthmatic patient, the highest risk of bronchospasm is during intubation and extubation. Drugs with bronchodilatory effects including propofol and ketamine should be considered. IV lidocaine may assist in blunting airway reflexes. Maintenance with halogenated agents as tolerated by the mother is typically used for additional bronchodilation. Administration of IV corticosteroids and beta$_2$-agonists should be considered prior to extubation. Postpartum hemorrhage may be more common in asthmatic patients. Ergot alkaloids such as methylergonovine maleate (Methergine) and prostaglandins such as carboprost (Hemabate) are relatively contraindicated. Oxytocin is first-line treatment. However, risks and benefits should be weighed if oxytocin alone is insufficient to treat uterine atony.

Learning Points

- Normal changes in respiratory physiology lead to decreased FRC and poor maternal tolerance of respiratory disease during pregnancy.
- Asthma is a common comorbidity during pregnancy, and its course is unpredictable. Some patients improve, some remain stable, and some have worsening of symptoms.
- Pregnant women have significantly increased morbidity from pneumonia, and its treatment should be focused on early intervention and optimization of maternal and fetal oxygenation.
- A neuraxial block in the setting of systemic infection is controversial but can be appropriate if the patient is treated with antibiotics.

References

1. Tonidandel A, Booth J. Anesthetic management of the parturient with respiratory disease, in Santos AC, Epstein JN, Chaudhuri K (eds.), *Obstetric Anesthesia: Clinical Anesthesiology Guide*. New York, NY, McGraw-Hill; 2015, pp. 409–18.

2. Bernstein H. Physiologic changes in pregnancy, in Santos AC, Epstein JN, Chaudhuri K, (eds.), *Obstetric Anesthesia: Clinical Anesthesiology Guide*. New York, NY: McGraw-Hill; 2015, pp. 6–8.

3. Mehta N, Chen K, Hardy E, Powrie R. Respiratory disease in pregnancy. *Best Pract Res Clin Obstet Gynaecol* 2015; **29**(5):598–611.

4. Kwon HL Triche EW, Belanger K, Bracken MB. The epidemiology of asthma during pregnancy: prevalence, diagnosis, and symptoms. *Immunol Allergy Clin North Am* 2006; **26**(1):29–62.

5. *Quick Reference from the Working Group Report on Managing Asthma During Pregnancy: Recommendations for Pharmacologic Treatment Update*, 2004. Available at www.nhlbi.nih.gov/files/docs/astpreg_qr.pdf (accessed October 4, 2018).

6. Bain E, Pierides K, Clifton V, et al. Interventions for managing asthma in pregnancy. *Cochrane Database Syst Rev* 2014; (**10**):CD010660.

7. National Asthma Education and Prevention Program (NAEPP) Expert Panel. *Report 3: Guidelines for the Diagnosis and Treatment of Asthma: Update on Selected Topics*, 2007. Available at www.nhlbi.nih.gov/sites/default/files/media/docs/asthgdln_1.pdf (accessed October 4, 2018).

8. Brito V, Niederman MS. Pneumonia complicating pregnancy. *Clin Chest Med* 2011; **32**(1):121–32.

Liver Disorders in Pregnancy

William John Fawcett

Case Study

A 31-year-old primigravida with a twin pregnancy presented at 34 weeks with a 2-week history of malaise, nausea, and vomiting. There was no relevant past medical history, and physical examination was unremarkable. The patient was initially presumed to have a nonspecific viral infection. Later she developed abdominal pain and began to develop some of the clinical features of preeclampsia (i.e., hypertension and proteinuria) as well as mild polydipsia and polyuria. She was admitted to hospital for observation, and blood results revealed a marked rise in transaminases and urate with a thrombocytopenia. The rest of her blood results, including serum bilirubin, coagulation, and renal function, were normal.

With 24 hours, she became confused, with deterioration in her hepatic and renal function. Her clotting screen was abnormal (international normalized ratio [INR] was elevated to 1.5) and was associated with some mild jaundice and intermittent hypoglycemia. Urgent imaging of the abdomen showed ascites. Over the course of the day, the patient became encephalopathic and developed the features of worsening renal failure and disseminated intravascular coagulation (DIC).

She required a dextrose infusion to prevent hypoglycemia and fresh frozen plasma to normalize her coagulopathy before undergoing cesarean section under general anesthesia, resulting in the birth of twin males. The mother required organ support on intensive care. Although her renal function had improved by 48 hours, her liver function remained deranged for nearly a week. By day 8, she was much improved, and other than some persistently elevated transaminases, she returned to the postnatal ward. The babies required oxygen and treatment of hypoglycemia but otherwise had an uneventful course. However, they required follow-up by pediatricians with a specialist interests in genetic screening and

dietary management of fatty acid oxygenation disorders. A diagnosis of acute fatty liver of pregnancy was made

Key Points

- Acute fatty liver of pregnancy usually presents in the second trimester, often with nonspecific symptoms.
- An acute hepatitis-like picture develops, with a marked transaminase rise but with jaundice not a prominent feature.
- There is often coexisting preeclampsia and sometimes some of the features of HELLP (hemolysis, elevated liver enzymes, low platelets) syndrome.
- The condition has a significant morbidity and mortality for both mother and fetus, and liver function may continue to deteriorate into the puerperium.
- Management of these patients requires delivery of the fetus and recognition and treatment of the complications of liver failure.
- Imaging may be unremarkable, but liver biopsy showing microvesicular fatty infiltration may aid diagnosis. However, in practice, coagulopathy may preclude this.

Discussion

Liver disease in pregnancy covers a wide spectrum of clinical entities. First, women may suffer from liver disease unrelated to pregnancy or as direct result of the pregnancy, with occasionally preexisting liver disease altered by the pregnancy itself. Second, liver disease may present in several ways, including a hepatitis-like picture, jaundice, abdominal pain, malaise, encephalopathy, variceal bleeding, and sepsis, possibly complicated by other organ failures such as renal or cardiorespiratory.

Table 19.1 Changes to Liver Function in Pregnancy

Test	Prepregnancy range	Pregnancy range	Comments
Transaminases (IU/liter) (alanine and aspartate)	0–40	0–30	–
Bilirubin (μmol/liter)	0–17	3–15	–
Gamma glutamyl transferase (IU/liter)	10–50	5–40	–
Alkaline phosphatase (IU/liter)	30–130	30–130	First and second trimesters
		130–400	Third trimester (produced by placenta)
Albumin (g/liter)	35–45	28–37	Secondary to hemodilution
Bile salts (μmol/liter)	0–14	0–14	–

Table 19.2 Liver Disease Unrelated to Pregnancy

Disease	Examples	Comments
Hepatitis	Hepatitis A, B, C, or E Herpes, CMV	Hepatitis E associated with increased perinatal mortality
Gallstones		
Drug induced	Acetaminophen Methyldopa Antibiotics Antipsychotic drugs Antiretroviral drugs Proton pump inhibitors	May be idiosyncratic or toxicity related
Autoimmune disease	Autoimmune hepatitis (AIH) Primary biliary cirrhosis (PBC) Primary sclerosing cholangitis (PSC)	May be overlapping features; many patients will require ongoing treatment throughout pregnancy
Vascular events	Budd Chiari syndrome (hepatic vein thrombosis)	
Others	Nonalcoholic fatty liver disease Sepsis, cardiac failure Mushroom poisoning Wilson's disease Hemochromatosis	From *Amanita phalloides*

Another area to consider is that the normal ranges for many biochemical tests are different in pregnancy (Table 19.1), which needs to be borne in mind in their interpretation.[1]

Unrelated or Coincidental Liver Disease

Young woman may suffer with ongoing liver disease that predates the pregnancy or is acquired coincidentally with the pregnancy. Commonly, this may be due to viral hepatitis or gallstones. Hepatitis may result from hepatitis A, B, C, D, and E, seronegative hepatitis, and other infections such as chickenpox, herpes simplex, and cytomegalovirus (which are much more commonly in immunocompromised patients). Gallstones may present with abdominal pain and jaundice. Other causes include drugs and toxins such as acetaminophen, recreational drugs, drug reactions, and mushroom poisoning from *Amanita phalloides*. Vascular events such as ischemia, veno-occlusive disease, and Budd Chiari syndrome (hepatic vein thrombosis), Wilson's disease, and autoimmune diseases also may occur (Table 19.2). Finally, pregnancy in patients with alcoholic cirrhosis, while once very rare, is now becoming more common, as is pregnancy in patients after liver transplantation. Patients require consideration of the transmission of any infective agent to the fetus, and the impact of any ongoing medication is paramount.

Pregnancy itself may or may not influence coexisting liver disease; for example, immune changes may result in a reduction in hepatitis B serology, with increased liver inflammation postpartum attributed to immune reactivation. Gallstones are more likely in pregnancy because there is gallbladder stasis associated with bile with an increased cholesterol concentration and reduced chenodeoxycholic acid.

Liver Disease Specific to Pregnancy

Hyperemeis Gravidarum

This presents in the first trimester, and when it is severe, it can induce dehydration and ketosis with concomitant elevation of transaminases. It may be related to hormonal changes, gastroesophageal reflux, or infections such as *Helicobacter pylori*. Conventional management with IV fluids and occasionally parenteral nutrition reverses these changes, and there is a good prognosis for both mother and fetus.

Intrahepatic Cholestasis of Pregnancy (ICP) or Obstetric Cholestasis

This is a relatively benign condition occurring in, on average, less than 0.5 percent of pregnancies, although there is a genetic and environmental predisposition, with increased incidence in up to 1.5 percent in women of Indian or Pakistani-Asian origin and up to 5 percent in Araucanian (South American Indian) peoples. It is more common in primiparous women, particularly if they have a multiple pregnancy.

The essential clinical features seem to arise from failure of the bile salt export pump (BESP) in the hepatocytes, with a proposed mechanism in susceptible individuals of BSEP expression being repressed by high levels of estrogen.[2] Thus bile salt export is reduced, with retention of bile salts leading to the usual clinical features of pruritus and sometimes jaundice. The pruritus (without a rash) is typically palmar and plantar, occurring at night. It can be very severe, causing excoriation and sleep deprivation. Biochemical markers include elevated transaminases, gamma-glutamyl transferase, bilirubin, and particularly bile salts beyond the normal pregnancy limits. The diagnosis is essentially one of exclusion, with the clinical features resolving soon after delivery. Differential diagnosis includes other rash-free pruritic conditions such as eczema. If a rash is present, the diagnosis is more likely to be polymorphic eruption of pregnancy or pemphigoid.

While there is little risk for the mother, if severe enough to inhibit vitamin K absorption, there is an increased incidence of postpartum hemorrhage. Women are more at risk for this condition in subsequent pregnancies and may also be at risk for a predisposition to biliary tract disease later in life. The fetus is more at risk, with an increased risk of preterm delivery and passing of meconium. Treatment is aimed at resolving the biochemical abnormalities and symptoms with ursodeoxycholic acid (UDCA) and antihistamines, respectively. In severe cases, once the fetus is past 37 weeks, delivery is indicated to minimize late fetal loss and provide symptom relief.

There are many unresolved questions, such as to whether improved detection may improve survival in fetuses most at risk. In addition, although UDCA improves pruritus and liver function, any beneficial effects on the fetus (e.g., reduction in stillbirths) are still largely unknown.

Preeclampsia and Eclampsia

Hypertension in pregnancy covers a wide spectrum of pathologies. Preexisting chronic hypertension and gestational hypertension are not considered further here, Preeclampsia is new hypertension presenting after 20 weeks with significant proteinuria (i.e., >300 mg protein/24 h or urinary protein:creatinine ratio > 30 mg/mmol). Severe preeclampsia is diagnosed when the hypertension is severe and/or there are specific symptoms (such as headache, blurred vision, liver tenderness, clonus, and papilledema) and/or biochemical and/or hematologic impairment. Finally, eclampsia is seen when preeclampsia is associated with one or more convulsions.

A major abnormality of this disease is a multifactorial placental abnormality that results in the release of antiangiogenic factors that cause widespread endothelial dysfunction, including the liver. While liver involvement may be minimal, in severe preeclampsia, 10 percent of women have liver involvement with abnormal liver function tests (two- to threefold elevation in alanine and aspartate aminotransferases levels). More seriously, liver ischemia, infarction, hemorrhage, and even liver rupture may occur, although this is seen more commonly with HELLP syndrome.

HELLP Syndrome

HELLP syndrome is usually considered to be a severe variant of preeclapmpsia (although it has been described in the absence of the classic features of preeclampsia) and deserves special mention. First described in 1982, it has specific and severe abnormalities characterized by hemolysis, elevated liver enzymes, and low platelet count. It occurs in approximately 0.5 percent of all pregnancies and in over 10 percent of patients with severe preeclampsia. It is a serious complication resulting in a maternal mortality of 1 percent or more (in some studies much higher) and a perinatal mortality 30 percent or more. Generally, the rise in aminotransferases is much higher (>500 units/liter), and lactate dehydrogenase (LDH) is elevated. Moreover, the hematologic film changes are a microangioplastic hemolytic ane-mia with schistocytosis as well as thrombocytopenia. The differential diagnosis includes acute viral hepati-tis, hemolytic-uremic syndrome (HUS), thrombotic thrombocytopenic purpura (TTP), antiphospholipid syndrome, and acute fatty liver of pregnancy (AFLP). There are two classifications of HELLP (Tennessee and Mississippi), with the former indicating partial or full HELLP and the latter describing prognosis in terms of platelet count; for example, the worst prog-nosis occurs in those with a platelet count of 50×10^9/liter or less.[3]

Acute Fatty Liver of Pregnancy

This is a serious condition that affects approximately 1 in 10,000 pregnancies. It is more common in primipar-ous women, as well as in multiple pregnancies and those carrying a male fetus. It may present in the third trimester with sometimes nonspecific symptoms such as nausea and vomiting, malaise, and upper abdominal pain or with signs or complications of worsening liver function such as hypoglycemia, upper gastrointestinal hemorrhage, renal failure, pancreatitis, or sepsis. It may occasionally present with fulminant hepatic failure and encephalopathy. Until the late stages, jaundice (and pruritus) may not be a feature. A little fewer than half of patients may have preeclampsia and its associated features, but AFLP is a separate condition.

A few abnormalities may be evident from bio-chemical screening, including an early marked rise in transaminases, with only mildly raised bilirubin. Later, as hepatic function worsens, bilirubin, urea, and creatinine all may rise, as may uric acid and ammonia levels. Hematologic testing may reveal a prolonged coagulation, low platelets, and markers of DIC. The Swansea criteria[4] have been described to aid in diagnosis (Table 19.3).

The major pathologic change in this condition is maternal hepatic fat deposition, which is part of a number of conditions known as *microvesicular fat disorders*. This arises from a fetal fatty acid oxidation (FAO) disorder whereby a liver mito-chondrial enzyme, long-chain 3-hydroxyacyl-coenzyme A dehydrogenase (LCHAD), is deficient, resulting in toxic fetal metabolites (long-chain fatty acids) accumulating in the maternal liver and caus-ing injury. LCHAD deficiency results from a recessive gene, which has usually undergone mutation. The combination fetal LCHAD defi-ciency with a mother who is a carrier for the

Table 19.3 Swansea Criteria for the Diagnosis of AFLP[4]

- Vomiting
- Abdominal pain
- Polydypsia/polyuria
- Hypoglycemia
- Elevated urea
- Leukocytosis
- Ascites or bright liver on ultrasound scan
- Elevated transaminases
- Elevated ammonia
- Encephalopathy
- Elevated bilirubin
- Renal impairment
- Coagulopathy – elevated PT or aPTT
- Microvesicular steatosis on liver biopsy

condition makes her susceptible to these hepato-toxic metabolites. There is also an increased inci-dence of preeclampsia and HELLP syndrome in this genetic setting.

Delivery of the fetus is a priority, and there is an increasing risk to both mother and fetus in delaying delivery. In recent years, while early and aggressive intervention has improved outcome, there is still the potential for prolonged liver dysfunction and its asso-ciated sequelae, occasionally requiring liver trans-plantation. In addition, the baby may require monitoring and specialist dietary advice.

Differential Diagnoses

There is a degree of overlap in the timing and pre-sentation of liver disease in pregnancy. The timing of the onset of liver disease is fundamental, and whereas, of course, liver disease unrelated to pregnancy may occur at any time, hyperemesis presents in the first trimester, and both the second and third trimesters are common times for the presentation of preeclampsia, eclampsia, and ICP. The third trimester alone is the usual time for the presentation for HELLP syndrome and AFLP. Finally, and commonly overlooked, is that both eclampsia and HELLP syndrome in a significant minority of cases may not be apparent until after delivery. Common presentations include a hepatitis-like picture, jaundice, pain, and acute liver failure.

Hepatitis-Like Features

A rise in transaminases may be due to viral infection or drug and alcohol misuse. Viral and autoimmune serology is required. A rise in transaminases may herald the onset of pregnancy-specific disorders with mild elevation (two to five times normal) found in uncomplicated preeclampsia and ICP, with marked elevation seen more commonly in HELLP syndrome and AFLP. A very high level of bile salts in isolation is highly suggestive of ICP.

Jaundice

Isolated jaundice is most commonly due viral infection, but other causes include drug-induced liver disease, gallstones, and cholangitis. It is a rare presentation of the pregnancy-specific disorders. Pale stools and dark urine usually signify biliary obstruction secondary to gallstones but may also occur with hepatitis, cholangitis, and the later stages of ICP.

Upper Abdominal Pain (with or without Nausea and Vomiting)

Upper abdominal pain, with or without nausea and vomiting, has many causes: gallstones and viral hepatitis are common, but severe preeclampsia, HELLP syndrome, and AFLP may also present with these symptoms.

Anesthesia and Liver Disease

Providing anesthesia for patients with established liver disease, particularly if severe, presents a huge challenge to the anesthesiologist. If the patient has infective hepatitis, great vigilance is required to prevent inadvertent seroconversion of the theater staff. Correction of hematologic abnormalities (especially coagulation and platelets) and biochemical abnormalities (especially glucose), fluid balance (e.g., treatment of ascites or edema), invasive monitoring, the prior optimization of other affected organs (e.g.,

kidney and heart), understanding of pharmacokinetic (e.g., reduced drug binding of reduced albumin levels) and pharmacodynamics changes (e.g., alterations in receptor sensitivity), and the early recognition of complications (renal failure, sepsis, encephalopathy) should all be addressed.

Learning Points

- Liver disease may present either from preexisting liver disease or de novo.
- The symptoms and signs may be nonspecific in the early stages.
- Accurate diagnosis is critical to quantifying risk and planning appropriate timing of delivery of the fetus.
- Liver dysfunction can continue into the puerperium.

References

1. Walker I, Chappell LC, Williamson C. Abnormal liver function tests in pregnancy. *BMJ* 2013; **347**:f0655.

2. Song X, Vasilenko A, Chen Y, et al. Transcriptional dynamics of bile salt export pump during pregnancy: mechanisms and implications in intrahepatic cholestasis of pregnancy. *Hepatology* 2014; **60**:1993–2007.

3. Hammoud GM, JA Ibdah. Preeclampsia-induced Liver Dysfunction, HELLP syndrome, and acute fatty liver of pregnancy. *Clin Liver Dis* 2014; **4**:69–73.

4. Ch'ng CL, Morgan M, Hainsworth I, Kingham, JG. Prospective study of liver dysfunction in pregnancy in Southwest Wales. *Gut* 2002; **51**:876–80.

Neurologic Disorders in Pregnancy

Marie-Louise Meng and Stephanie R. Goodman

Case Study

A 32-year-old woman at 39 weeks gestation presented to the labor and delivery unit in early labor. Her past medical history was notable for rapidly progressing multiple sclerosis (MS) diagnosed 5 years ago. She required a walker and assistance with the activities of daily living. She had an MS exacerbation 1 month ago requiring high-dose steroids. Ten years ago, she had a normal spontaneous vaginal delivery (NSVD) with combined spinal epidural (CSE) analgesia, and another NSVD was anticipated. Her body mass index (BMI) was 33 kg/m^2 and her airway was Mallampati class 2.

The patient was interested in labor analgesia but was concerned that it might cause a MS exacerbation. A discussion regarding the risks and benefits of neuraxial analgesia took place, noting that the postpartum period itself carries a risk of MS exacerbation. It was explained to the patient that an epidural could be performed without the spinal portion of the procedure because some evidence suggests that spinal anesthesia may increase the risk of an exacerbation.

The patient received an epidural catheter that was dosed with bupivacaine 0.125% 10 ml and fentanyl 100 μg and patient-controlled epidural analgesia (PCEA) with an infusion of 0.0625% bupivacaine with 2 μg/ml fentanyl. The patient comfortably delivered a healthy baby. Postpartum, she was followed closely by neurology and, unfortunately, did have an exacerbation of MS 1 month after delivery.

Key Points

- Patients with MS may be concerned about neuraxial analgesia worsening their medical condition.
- Although in the past MS was thought to be a contraindication to neuraxial anesthesia, current evidence suggests that it is safe.
- Patients with MS can receive epidural analgesia for labor and delivery. Spinal anesthesia should not be

avoided based on theoretical concerns that high concentrations of intrathecal local anesthesia may affect already compromised nerve tissues.
- Due to the fact that multiple triggers are present during the peripartum period, it is impossible to identify the true cause of any MS relapse.

Discussion

Multiple Sclerosis

MS is a progressive, inflammatory, and demyelinating disease with periods of remissions and exacerbations that can be triggered by infection, stress, and increased temperature. The baseline treatment of MS is immunomodulatory disease-modifying therapies (DMTs) such as interferon, glatiramer acetate, mitoxantrone, and natalizumab, which are all avoided in pregnancy. MS relapses during pregnancy are treated with steroids, which are regarded as safe.[1] Patients with MS typically have fewer exacerbations during pregnancy, but the risk of relapse is increased in the first 3 months postpartum.[2,3]

Anesthesiologists must assess patients with MS for neurologic deficits, including muscle, respiratory, and diaphragmatic weakness, and inability to cough or handle secretions. It is prudent to document all preoperative neurologic deficits. If respiratory weakness is present, pulmonary function tests (PFTs) should be obtained. Patients with MS can have autonomic system involvement, manifesting as hemodynamic instability. Anesthesiologists should be aware of patients' recent steroid use because stress-dose steroids may be indicated.

Hyperthermia is a known trigger for MS exacerbations. Labor rooms should be kept at appropriate temperatures, and maternal fever should be treated aggressively with cooling blankets and acetaminophen.

The type of anesthesia chosen for MS patients is not thought to increase exacerbations.[3,4] The PRIMS study,[3] which was large and prospective, clearly demonstrated that epidural anesthesia did not have an effect on disability nor MS relapse rate postpartum. Spinal anesthesia has been implicated, however, in increasing the risk of exacerbation possibly due to a high concentration of local anesthetic that may be neurotoxic when placed near already demyelinated CNS tissue.[4] In patients with MS presenting for cesarean delivery, spinal anesthesia can be easily replaced with epidural anesthesia. Still, the safe use of spinal anesthesia has been reported.[5]

A survey of 592 obstetric anesthesiologists in the United Kingdom revealed that 84 percent would use spinal anesthesia for elective cesarean delivery, and 90 percent would use spinal anesthesia for emergency cesarean delivery. This survey, unfortunately, was not designed to report clinical outcomes.[6] Lu et al.[7] examined the use of obstetric neuraxial anesthesia in patients with MS compared with the general population and did not find a difference in disability in patients with or without epidural or spinal anesthesia.

Choosing the appropriate anesthetic technique for a patient with MS is challenging because there are no randomized, controlled trials to guide management. Some anesthesiologists may prefer to avoid neuraxial anesthesia altogether and use general anesthesia for patients with MS, but this is only applicable to surgical procedures. For labor pain, an epidural certainly provides better pain relief than systemic medication. Therefore, if time permits, a thorough discussion with the patient about the risks and benefits of the different types of analgesia and anesthesia is recommended, and it is prudent to ensure that the patient understands that the risk of MS relapse exists regardless of the type of anesthesia used.

If general anesthesia is chosen for a patient with MS, caution must be taken when using neuromuscular blocking drugs. As with patients with any chronic motor weakness, patients with MS can have increased numbers of extrajunctional acetylcholine receptors secondary to denervation or disuse. Hence succinylcholine use may cause hyperkalemia from increased muscle release of potassium. Additionally, the increased acetylcholine receptors can decrease the sensitivity to nondepolarizing neuromuscular blocking drugs.[8]

Myasthenia Gravis

Myasthenia gravis (MG) is an autoimmune disorder in which autoantibodies are formed against the postsynaptic nicotinic acetylcholine receptor (nAChR) at the neuromuscular junction. A decreased number of nAChRs results in skeletal muscle weakness. The muscle groups usually affected are the ocular, bulbar, and proximal limb muscles. MG is progressive with relapses and periods of remission. The course of MG is unpredictable during pregnancy. Stress, pain, infection, fever, surgery, inflammation, and hypothyroidism are associated with MG relapses or crises and can occur with pregnancy and labor.[9,10] Myasthenic crisis is the extreme weakness of bulbar or respiratory muscles resulting in airway obstruction or respiratory failure and the need for mechanical ventilation.

Medical treatment of MG involves anticholinesterases and steroids. Patients refractory to medication often require plasmapheresis and may require thymectomy. Anticholinesterases, most commonly pyridostigmine, must be continued throughout pregnancy and on the day of delivery to prevent MG relapses.[9,10]

Cholinergic crisis, usually due to excess anticholinesterase medication, may be seen rarely in pregnancy due to pharmacokinetic changes. The symptoms are salivation, sweating, miosis, diarrhea, vomiting, lacrimation, bradycardia, bronchospasm, muscle weakness, and respiratory failure.[9,10] Anesthesiologists must be aware that myasthenic and cholinergic crisis can both present with muscle weakness and respiratory compromise, and immediate respiratory support and treatment are usually needed.

Preanesthetic evaluation of patients with MG should include a full assessment of symptoms, location, and weakness. Medication doses and frequency should be known, and anticholinesterases should be continued on the day of delivery and administered intravenously if oral absorption is questionable. Patients with respiratory compromise should have PFTs to assess the baseline degree of weakness and to predict the need for postoperative mechanical ventilation, should general anesthesia be needed. All patients should be counseled that mechanical ventilation and intensive care might be indicated if a myasthenic crisis develops.

Vaginal delivery is preferred in patients with MG because surgery itself is a risk factor for MG crisis. Neuraxial anesthesia (epidural, spinal, and CSE) has been safely used in patients with MG both for labor analgesia and for surgical anesthesia. Labor epidurals are preferred to avoid the respiratory depressive effects of systemic opioids and should be initiated early in labor to prevent pain and fatigue, which may precipitate a MG crisis. Anesthesiologists should closely monitor MG patients with labor epidurals for respiratory or bulbar compromise. Spread of labor analgesia should be limited to T10 to prevent any respiratory muscle weakness.[1,11]

The lowest effective concentration of local anesthetic should be used for labor analgesia infusions to minimize motor block. Patients with MG may have weakness of the pelvic and abdominal muscles and may require an assisted second stage of labor with forceps or vacuum. Ester local anesthetics should be avoided because anticholinesterases impair their degradation. If a cesarean delivery is indicated, neuraxial anesthesia is preferred to avoid prolonged mechanical ventilation following general anesthesia, but the T4 block needed may cause unsustainable respiratory compromise in MG patients with severe bulbar and respiratory symptoms at baseline.[12]

If general anesthesia is needed for cesarean delivery, neuromuscular antagonists should be avoided or used with caution. With a decreased number of nAChRs, the patient with MG is less sensitive to succinylcholine because the presence of receptors is necessary for the action of the drug, but a higher dose of succinylcholine can cause a prolonged block due to anticholinesterase activity or phase II block. Conversely, MG patients are more sensitive to nondepolarizing neuromuscular antagonists because fewer nAChRs results in a greater percentage of antagonized receptors per dose.

Medications that can exacerbate respiratory depression such as opioids and sedatives should be avoided. Certain antibiotics such as aminoglycosides can worsen muscle weakness. Magnesium is contraindicated in patients with MG because it inhibits the release of acetylcholine at the neuromuscular junction and decreases the postsynaptic response to ACh. Patients with MG who need seizure prophylaxis may receive phenobarbital instead.[9,10]

Maternal anti-nAChR antibodies can cross the placenta, resulting in neonatal MG. Poor tone and weak cry in the newborn are suggestive of this. Neonatal MG may require immediate respiratory support.[9,10,12]

Epilepsy

Epilepsy is a disorder of recurrent, nonprovoked seizures. It is estimated that the prevalence in pregnancy is 0.3–0.5 percent. While patients with epilepsy are at risk for poor neonatal outcomes such as intrauterine fetal demise (IUFD) and low birth weight, they usually have uncomplicated pregnancies and deliveries. Fetal compromise can be caused by antiepileptic drugs (AEDs) and by the hypoxia, blunt trauma, and acidosis associated with seizures.[1,13]

AEDs are known to be teratogenic. Older medications such as valproate, phenobarbital, and phenytoin are more teratogenic than newer agents such as carbamazepine, levetiracetam, and lamotrigine.[14] It is recommended that patients continue AEDs while pregnant. Ideally, patients should be switched to the less teratogenic AEDs prior to pregnancy, and AEDs should be used in the lowest dose possible. Monotherapy is preferable when possible.[11,13] AED levels should be monitored monthly because the physiologic changes of pregnancy (decreased protein binding, increased volume of distribution, greater drug clearance) can result in lower effective drug concentrations. Increased levels of estrogen during pregnancy, stress, and poor sleep can decrease the seizure threshold. AEDs should be continued during labor and delivery because acute withdrawal from AEDs can cause seizures.[15] When patients present in labor, AEDs should be switched to IV formulations because oral absorption can be diminished.

If a seizure occurs, the airway should be supported, the patient placed in the left lateral decubitus position, and IV medications given to stop the seizure. Benzodiazepines are the first-line treatment, but barbiturates and propofol may also be used. It is critical to pharmacologically stop the seizure because prolonged seizure activity in a parturient can cause uterine contractions, placental abruption, fetal intracranial hemorrhage, and fetal acidosis. More commonly, during a seizure, the fetus can become hypoxic and develop bradycardia.[14] If bradycardia persists, or if the mother's condition deteriorates despite appropriate treatment, a cesarean delivery may be appropriate. It is important to note that diazepam can cause loss of baseline fetal heart rate variability, which may lead to an unnecessary urgent cesarean delivery.

There is no need to avoid regional anesthesia (spinal, epidural, CSE) or general anesthesia in patients with epilepsy. However, it may be worth avoiding certain agents that are known to lower the seizure threshold and precipitate epileptiform activity such as etomidate, ketamine, meperidine, and sevoflurane. Epileptiform activity has been reported with higher concentrations (MAC > 1.5) of sevoflurane, so it is recommended to use lower concentrations and to coadminister a benzodiazepine when using it in epileptic patients.[16] Additionally, AEDs can alter the metabolism of commonly used anesthetic medications; for example, phenytoin induces hepatic microsomal enzymes, resulting in faster breakdown of neuromuscular antagonists and opioids.

All patients who experience seizures around the time of delivery must also be evaluated for eclampsia and other causes of seizures such as cerebrovascular lesions and metabolic abnormalities.

Learning Points

- Neuraxial anesthesia can be provided safely for patients with MS.
- Epidural anesthesia does not increase the risk of a postpartum MS exacerbation.
- Vaginal delivery under neuraxial analgesia is preferred for patients with MG to minimize pain, fatigue, and the risk of perioperative myasthenic crisis.
- Myasthenic crisis and cholinergic crisis can both present with muscle weakness and respiratory compromise.
- Anesthesiologists must be cautious using neuromuscular antagonists in MG patients because the decreased number of receptors results in sensitivity to nondepolarizing neuromuscular blockers and a resistance to depolarizing succinylcholine.
- AEDs should be continued during labor and delivery because withdrawal can result in seizures.
- If a pregnant patient has a seizure, the airway should be supported and benzodiazepines given to stop the seizure.

References

1. Hopkins AN, Alshaeri T, Akst SA, Berger JS. Neurologic disease with pregnancy and considerations for the obstetric anesthesiologist. *Semin Perinatol* 2014; **38**(6): 359–69.
2. Confavreux C, Hutchinson M, Hours MM, Cortinovis-Tourniaire P, Moreau T. Rate of pregnancy-related relapse in multiple sclerosis. Pregnancy in Multiple Sclerosis Group. *N Engl J Med* 1998; **339**(5):285–91.
3. Vukusic S, Hutchinson M, Hours M, et al. Pregnancy and multiple sclerosis (the PRIMS study): clinical predictors of post-partum relapse. *Brain* 2004; **127**(Pt 6):1353–60.
4. Bamford C, Sibley W, Laguna J. Anesthesia in multiple sclerosis. *Can J Neurol Sci* 1978; **5**(1):41–44.
5. Berger JM, Ontell R. Intrathecal morphine in conjunction with a combined spinal and general anesthetic in a patient with multiple sclerosis. *Anesthesiology* 1987; **66**(3):400–2.
6. Drake E, Drake M, Bird J, Russell R. Obstetric regional blocks for women with multiple sclerosis: a survey of UK experience. *Int J Obstet Anesth* 2006; **15**(2):115–23.
7. Lu E, Zhao Y, Dahlgren L, et al. Obstetrical epidural and spinal anesthesia in multiple sclerosis. *J Neurol* 2013; **260**(10):2620–28.
8. Naguib M, Flood P, McArdle JJ, Brenner HR. Advances in neurobiology of the neuromuscular junction: implications for the anesthesiologist. *Anesthesiology* 2002; **96**(1):202–31.
9. Ferrero S, Esposito F, Biamonti M, Bentivoglio G, Ragni N. Myasthenia gravis during pregnancy. *Exp Rev Neurotherapeut* 2008; **8**(6):979–88.
10. Kalidindi M, Ganpot S, Tahmesebi F, et al. Myasthenia gravis and pregnancy. *J Obstet Gynaecol* 2007; **27** (1):30–32.
11. Kuczkowski KM. Labor analgesia for the parturient with neurological disease: what does an obstetrician need to know? *Arch Gynecol Obstet* 2006; **274**(1):41–46.
12. Almeida C, Coutinho E, Moreira D, Santos E, Aguiar J. Myasthenia gravis and pregnancy: anaesthetic management – a series of cases. *Eur J Anaesthesiol* 2010; **27**(11):985–90.
13. Crawford P. Best practice guidelines for the management of women with epilepsy. *Epilepsia* 2005; **46**(Suppl 9):117–24.
14. Hill DS, Wlodarczyk BJ, Palacios AM, Finnell RH. Teratogenic effects of antiepileptic drugs. *Exp Rev Neurotherapeut* 2010; **10**(6):943–59.
15. Krishnamurthy KB. Managing epilepsy during pregnancy: assessing risk and optimizing care. *Curr Treat Options Neurol* 2012; **14**(4):348–55.
16. Voss LJ, Sleigh JW, Barnard JP, Kirsch HE. The howling cortex: seizures and general anesthetic drugs. *Anesth Analg* 2008; **107**(5):1689–703.

Abnormal Placentation

Elena Olearo, Pervez Sultan and Anna David

Case Study

A 35-year-old gravida 3, para 2 woman (two previous cesarean deliveries) was admitted at 35 weeks' gestation for steroid therapy administered for fetal lung maturation. Placenta accreta was suspected at the 32-week scan due to loss of regularity of the "retroplacental clear zone" and increased vascularity of the uterine serosa–bladder wall interface. The scan also revealed placenta previa. MRI was performed at 33 weeks' gestation, confirming a complete placenta previa with the placenta thinning the myometrium of the uterine anterior wall, highly suspicious for placenta accreta. The patient was scheduled for cesarean delivery with likely hysterectomy at 36 weeks' gestation. After the diagnosis, the patient underwent multidisciplinary counseling involving obstetricians, anesthesiologists, radiologists, and urologists. Prior to surgery, uterine artery angiography and catheterization were performed. The patient was transferred to the OR for cesarean delivery. During surgery, a protruding shiny-surface placenta was visualized in the lower uterine segment, cranial to the bladder, and 15 minutes following skin incision, a live-born infant was delivered. Both occlusion balloon catheters were inflated, and hysterectomy was performed with careful dissection of the planes to preserve the bladder. The estimated blood loss was 3,150 ml. The patient received 3 units of packed red blood cells, 3 units of fresh frozen plasma, and 1 unit of cryoprecipitate. She required overnight admission to the ICU and was discharged home 7 days following delivery.

Key Points

- Placental attachment disorders (PADs) are life threatening diseases associated with significant morbidity and a maternal mortality rate of 7 percent.
- The most common risk factors are placenta previa, previous cesarean delivery (particularly if repeated), and increased maternal age.

- Obstetric ultrasound remains the primary tool for diagnosis, and MRI may be additionally helpful, but controversy still exists surrounding the most accurate technique because both modalities have high false-negative and false-positive rates for diagnosis.
- The antenatal accuracy in the diagnosis of PAD should be improved to optimize peripartum maternal and neonatal outcomes.
- Whenever PAD is suspected, careful planning and close communication are essential among anesthesiologists, obstetricians, interventional radiologists, hematologists, blood bank, and specialized surgical teams.

Discussion

Definitions

Placenta previa exists when the placenta is inserted wholly or partly into the lower segment of the uterus, partially or completely covering the internal cervical os. In cases of placenta previa, there should be a high index of suspicion for placenta accreta. Placental attachment disorders (PADs) encompass a spectrum of conditions characterized by abnormal adherence of the placenta to the uterine wall, with invasion of the placental villi through the decidua. Depending on the depth of invasion, it can be divided into three categories (accreta, increta, and percreta). PAD is commonly associated with placenta previa[1,2] (Figures 21.1 and 21.2).

Epidemiology, Risk Factors, Pathophysiology

Over the last 30 years, the incidence of PAD has increased 10-fold. In developed countries, reported rates range from 1 in 530 to 1 in 2,500 deliveries.[3] The most common risk factors for PAD are placenta previa, previous cesarean delivery (particularly if repeated), and increasing maternal age. Less frequent

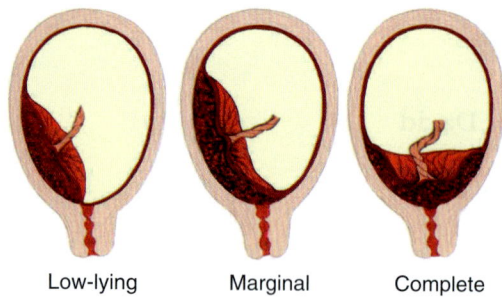

Low-lying   Marginal   Complete

Figure 21.1 Placenta previa

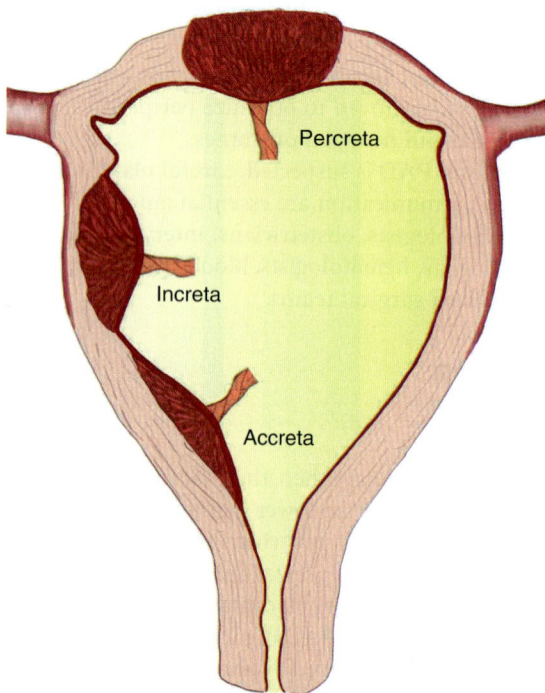

Percreta

Increta

Accreta

Figure 21.2 Placenta accreta (chorionic villi attach to the myometrium rather than being restricted within the decidua basalis), increta (chorionic villi invade into the myometrium), and percreta (chorionic villi invade through the myometrium)

risk factors include: multiparity, previous curettage, Asherman syndrome (acquired intrauterine adhesions/scarring or synechiae), and endometrial ablation. Two possible mechanisms of PAD formation have been proposed: abnormal decidualization or pathologic invasiveness of the trophoblast. The former has been considered in cases of alteration of the uterine wall, such as previous surgery, scars, and pelvic radiation,[4,5] whereas the latter may be

explained by changes in the activity of growth and angiogenesis- and invasion-related factors within the trophoblast.[6] Clinically, the most significant feature of placenta accreta is the abundant uteroplacental neo-vascularization, which can lead to life-threatening hemorrhage.[7] Patients with PAD are often asymptomatic, but it can present with antepartum hemorrhage. If associated with placenta previa, it is a life-threatening disease and represents the second leading cause of peripartum hemorrhage, with a maternal mortality rate of 7 percent and significant morbidity due to blood loss, local organ damage, requirement for urgent hysterectomy (33–50 percent), and postoperative complications.[8]

Diagnosis

The Royal College of Obstetricians and Gynaecologists (RCOG) recommend that all pregnant women should be scanned at 20 weeks' gestation to evaluate placental localization. If PAD is suspected, imaging should be performed at around 32 weeks' gestation to clarify the diagnosis and allow planning for third-trimester management, including further imaging and delivery.[2] Women with a "low-lying placenta" (diagnosed before 28 weeks) or a placenta previa (diagnosed after 28 weeks) that is overlying a uterine scar should be reevaluated in the third trimester, with attention paid to the potential presence of PAD.[9]

The main diagnostic tools are

- Two-dimensional (2D) gray-scale and color Doppler ultrasound
- Three-dimensional (3D) power Doppler ultrasound
- MRI[10]

According to Shih et al.,[11] in order to achieve the diagnosis of PAD, at least one of a number of criteria using 2D gray-scale or color Doppler ultrasound criteria should be present (Table 21.1). Three-dimensional power Doppler ultrasound can be performed as a complementary technique, as described in Table 21.1.

The techniques listed in the table were found to achieve a sensitivity of 92–100 percent, a specificity of 68–85 percent, and a positive predictive value of 76–88 percent.[2,11] MRI is no better than ultrasound, although it may be superior at detecting the depth of trophoblast invasion.[12] Dwyer et al.[13] showed comparable sensitivity between ultrasound and MRI. The main MRI features of placenta accreta include uterine bulging, heterogeneous signal intensity within

Table 21.1 Ultrasound Features of PAD

2D gray-scale or color Doppler criteria	3D ultrasound
Complete loss or an irregular retroplacental sonolucent zone (Figure 21.3)	Intraplacental hypervascularity
Thinning or disruption of the hyperechoic uterine serosa–bladder interface	Inseparable cotyledonal, intervillous circulations
Focal exophytic masses invading the urinary bladder and abnormal placental lacunae	Tortuous vascularity with "chaotic branching"
Diffuse or focal lacunar flow pattern (Figure 21.4)	
Sonolucent vascular lakes with turbulent flow	
Hypervascularity of the uterine serosa–bladder interface with abnormal blood vessels linking the placenta to the bladder (Figure 21.5)	
Markedly dilated vessels over the peripheral subplacental region	

the placenta, and dark intraplacental bands on T2-weighted imaging.[14] Many authors have recommended MRI for women in whom ultrasound findings are inconclusive.[15] The "gold standard" for diagnosis remains pathology examination after hysterectomy characterized by the absence of decidua at the placental attachment site with the chorionic villi invading deeply into the myometrium. Intraoperative diagnosis of PAD can be made when the placenta is adherent to the uterine wall with difficulty at removal and excessive hemorrhage even with minimal placental separation.[16]

Planning for Delivery

If PAD is suspected, a detailed plan for follow-up, timing for delivery, multidisciplinary discussion, and patient consent is required. The discussion with the patient should include possible maternal complications, neonatal morbidity, and interventions such as interventional radiology, cell salvage during surgery, leaving the placenta in situ, and hysterectomy.[2] The recommended gestational age for elective cesarean delivery is usually by 36–37 weeks of gestation, before labor is likely to occur, so as to avoid emergency delivery of a woman in labor who may already be compromised by hemorrhage. Administration of maternal steroids is recommended to mature the fetal lungs and prevent transient tachypnea of the newborn, which is more likely following elective cesarean delivery before 37 weeks. Women should be encouraged to take oral iron to boost their iron stores and optimize their hemoglobin level.

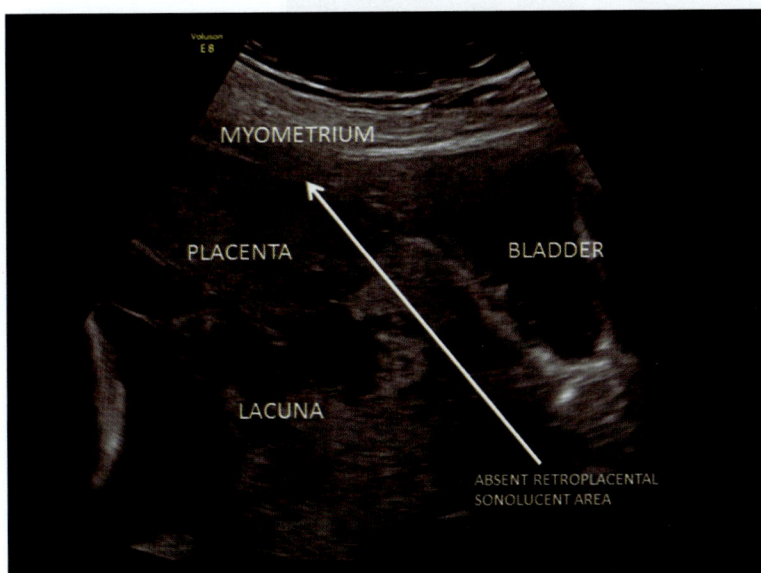

Figure 21.3 Loss and irregularity of retroplacental sonolucent zone

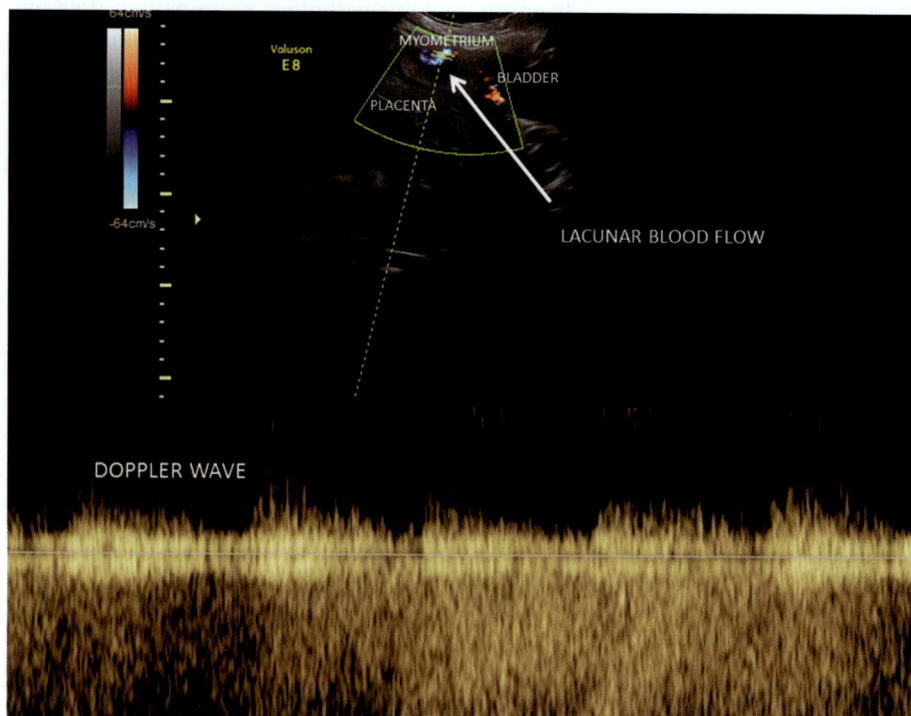

Figure 21.4 Focal lacunar flow pattern

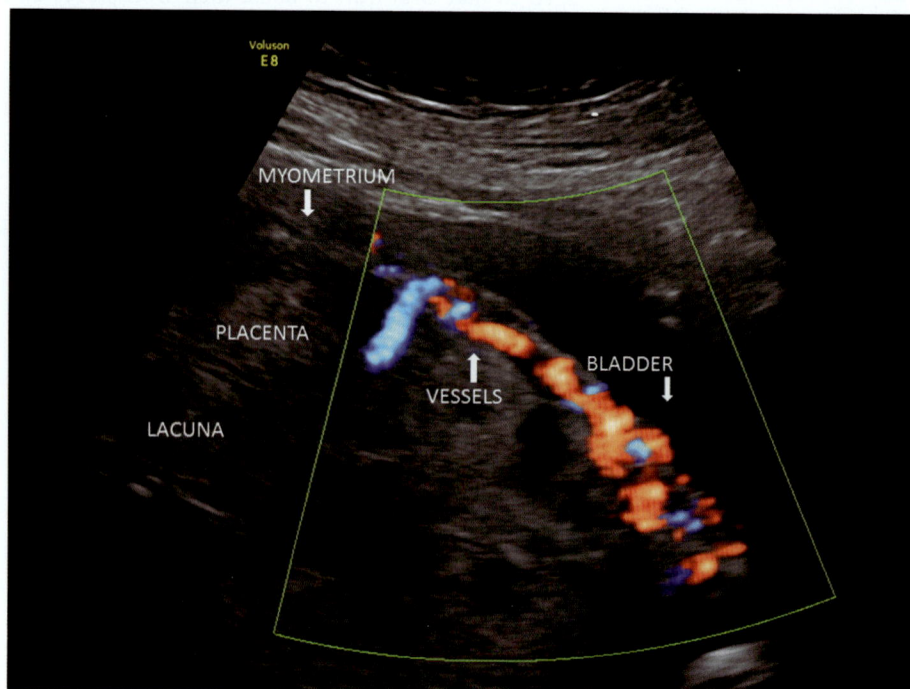

Figure 21.5 Hypervascularity of the uterine serosa–bladder interface with abnormal blood vessels linking the placenta to the bladder

Careful discussion in the case of women who refuse blood products is paramount, including documentation of which products they might consider accepting. A signed and witnessed advance decision document listing the blood products and autologous procedures that are or are not acceptable to them should be filed and a copy retained by the patient during pregnancy. There is usually no objection to intraoperative cell salvage, apheresis, hemodialysis, cardiac bypass, or normovolemic hemodilution, provided that the equipment is primed with nonblood fluids. Recombinant products, such as erythropoiesis-stimulating agents (e.g., RHuEpo) and granulocyte colony-stimulating factors (e.g., G-CSF or GM-CSF) are acceptable, as are pharmacologic agents such as IV iron or tranexamic acid. Guidelines for the use of recombinant factor VII (rFVIIa) in massive obstetric hemorrhage have been developed, although current evidence to date for use of rFVIIa in postpartum hemorrhage is limited to case reports and case series with one nonrandomized study.[17]

Management at Delivery

The traditional surgical approach to management has been cesarean hysterectomy; however, in recent years, more conservative management strategies have been employed to minimize the surgical morbidity and to preserve the woman's fertility. A *conservative approach* is defined as leaving the placenta in situ at the time of cesarean delivery, with no traction or forced manual removal, allowing instead reabsorption or expulsion to occur later. Another technique consists of resecting the invaded area of the myometrium together with the placenta and performing the uterine reconstruction as a one-step procedure.[18] These options involve accurate assessment of hemodynamic conditions, prophylactic antibiotics, and repeated screening for signs of endometritis and sepsis. Methotrexate has been considered for the retained placenta.[19,20] In the presence of suspected PAD, the senior obstetrician performing surgery can consider opening the uterus at a site distant from the placental attachment and delivering the baby without disturbing the placenta to avoid bleeding. Conservative management of PAD when the woman is already bleeding is unlikely to be successful and risks wasting valuable time.

Interventional Radiology and Urologic Management

Uterine artery embolization in cases of uncontrolled and massive postpartum hemorrhage can be lifesaving.[21] Joint angiography ORs exist and have been used with success in obstetric hemorrhage.[22,23] However, more commonly, interventional radiologists are called to perform procedures in the labor ward or cesarean delivery OR when PAD and overwhelming hemorrhage occur. Different approaches have been described, including balloon occlusion alone, a combination of balloon occlusion and embolization, and prophylactic catheter placement and pre-hysterectomy embolization.[24] If a woman is suspected to have PAD, interventional radiology should be considered, particularly if she refuses donor blood products.[2] Prophylactic placement of uterine artery balloons before cesarean delivery has the potential to reduce blood loss in women with suspected placenta accreta, but insertion requires high-quality fluoroscopy and technical skill. There is a small risk of uterine artery spasm causing fetal compromise requiring prompt delivery, and some experts advocate only performing this procedure in a joint angiography OR.[25] Because of the absence of data from large randomized, controlled trials, controversy still exists regarding the safety and efficacy for endovascular interventions used to prevent hemorrhage in cases of PAD. Complications after placement of the balloon catheters have been reported, and there is a variable rate of failure.[26]

Considering the risk of bladder invasion and bladder or ureteral injuries during hysterectomy, a senior urologist should be involved in the perioperative management. Cystoscopy and bilateral ureteric stent placement need to be discussed for each case. Eller et al.[27] attempted ureteric stent placement in 44 percent of cases of PAD, and they proposed the technique as helpful in reducing the risk of ureter injury. However, further evaluation is required before considering routine ureteric stents for all women with PAD involving the bladder.

Anesthetic Management

An antenatal anesthesia consultation should be planned for between 24 and 28 weeks' gestation if the diagnosis is known by then and certainly by 32 weeks to allow for contingency planning in the event of preterm or out-of-hours delivery. During this meeting, the following topics should be discussed with the patient: invasive monitoring, transfusion, cell salvage, requirement for ICU admission, and regional anesthesia or general anesthesia (or a combination of techniques). Dissemination of a multidisciplinary plan to all maternity healthcare staff is recommended. The number of blood products (packed red cells, fresh frozen plasma, platelets, and cryoprecipitate) requested varies according to the anticipated severity of the case.[28,29]

The anesthetic management of PAD poses a dilemma for the anesthesiologist.[30] While a catheter-based neuraxial technique can provide successful surgical anesthesia without exposing the woman to the risks of general anesthesia, planned general anesthesia may be preferable in patients with anticipated difficult airways. This patient population has an increased risk of requiring invasive ventilation following massive hemorrhage.[31] Dealing with a difficult airway in conjunction with hemodynamic instability and massive transfusion may increase airway soft tissue edema. Therefore, when either a difficult airway or a major bleeding risk is identified, elective general anesthesia from the outset may be the most appropriate technique to avoid emergency conversions in difficult conditions.

Lilker et al.[29] described the use of a catheter-based neuraxial technique for surgical anesthesia in 17 patients undergoing cesarean delivery for placenta accreta. However, five patients (29 percent) required perioperative conversion to general anesthesia for major perioperative obstetric hemorrhage (>2 liter blood loss). Despite this, there is currently insufficient evidence to recommend general anesthesia over neuraxial anesthesia in the context of placental abnormalities.[32]

Further work is necessary to compare peri- and postoperative anesthetic outcomes according to the type of suspected abnormal placentation (accreta/increta/percreta) and the respective planned anesthetic modality (general versus neuraxial anesthesia).

Learning Points

- High-risk patients for PAD should be reevaluated in the third trimester (ideally 32 weeks) with attention to the potential presence of PAD.
- All the available techniques (gray-scale and color 2D Doppler ultrasound, 3D power Doppler ultrasound, and MRI) should be used to achieve the best accuracy in antenatal diagnosis.
- Planning delivery should include optimizing maternal hemoglobin with iron medications, maternal steroids to mature the fetal lungs, confirming the acceptance of blood products and cell salvage with the patient, and

disseminating a clear plan for delivery to healthcare staff.
- The patient should be counseled for cesarean hysterectomy, but conservative management could be considered in some cases.
- Interventional radiology is a useful tool in the management of postpartum hemorrhage, but its role and the best technique in the prevention of hemorrhage in PAD need further evaluation.
- Anesthetic plans must be tailored accorded to the patient's medical, surgical, and anesthetic history. Planned general anesthesia may be advisable in patients with potentially difficult airways due to the uncertainty of potential hemorrhage.

References

1. Khong TY. The pathology of placenta accreta, a worldwide epidemic. *BMJ* 2008; **61**:1243–46.

2. Royal College of Obstetrics and Gynaecologysts. Placenta praevia, placenta praevia accreta and vasa praevia: diagnosis and management, Green-Top Guideline No. 27, January 2011. Available at www.rcog.org.uk/globalassets/documents/guidclines/gtg_27.pdf.

3. Hull AD, Resnik R. Placenta accreta and postpartum hemorrhage. *Clin Obstet Gynecol* 2010; **53**:228–36.

4. Usta IM, Hobeika EM, Musa AA, et al. Placenta previa-accreta: risk factors and complications. *Am J Obstet Gynecol* 2005; **193**:1045–49.

5. Norwitz ER, Stern HM, Grier H, Lee-Parritz A. Placenta percreta and uterine rupture associated with prior whole body radiation therapy. *Obstet Gynecol* 2001; **98**:929–31.

6. Tseng JJ, MM Chou. Differential expression of growth-, angiogenesis- and invasion-related factors in the development of placenta accreta. *Taiwanese J Obstet Gynecol* 2006; **45**:100–6.

7. Shih JC, Cheng WF, Shyu M, et al. Power Doppler evidence of placenta accreta appearing in the first trimester. *Ultrasound Obstet Gynecol* 2002; **19**:623–25.

8. Comstock CH, Bronsteen RA. The antenatal diagnosis of placenta accreta. BJOG 2014; **121**:171–82.

9. Belfort MA. Placenta accreta. *Am J Obstet Gynecol* 2010; **203**:430–39.

10. Cali G, Giambanco L, Puccio G, Forlani F. Morbidly adherent placenta: evaluation of ultrasound diagnostic criteria and differentiation of placenta accrete from percreta. *Ultrasound Obstet Gynecol* 2013; **41**:406–12.

11. Shih JC, Palacios Jaraquemada JM, Su YN, et al. Role of three-dimensional power Doppler in the antenatal

diagnosis of placenta accreta: comparison with gray-scale and color Doppler techniques. *Ultrasound Obstet Gynecol* 2009; **33**:193–203.

12. Masselli G, Brunelli R, Casciani E, et al. Magnetic resonance imaging in the evaluation of placental adhesive disorders: correlation with color Doppler ultrasound. *Eur Radiol* 2008; **18**:1292–99.

13. Dwyer BK,Belogolovkin V, Tran L, et al. Prenatal diagnosis of placenta accreta: sonography or magnetic resonance imaging? *J Ultrasound Med* 2008; **27**: 1275–81.

14. Lax A, Prince MR, Mennitt KW, et al. The value of specific MRI features in the evaluation of suspected placental invasion. *Magn Reson Imaging* 2007; **25**:87–93.

15. Palacios Jaraquemada JM, Bruno CH. Magnetic resonance imaging in 300 cases of placenta accreta: surgical correlation of new findings. *Acta Obstet Gynaecol Scand* 2005; **84**:716–24.

16. Maher MA, Abdelaziz A, Bazeed MF. Diagnostic accuracy of ultrasound and MRI in the prenatal diagnosis of placenta accreta. *Acta Obstet Gynaecol Scand* 2013; **92**:1017–22.

17. Welsh A, McLintock C, Gatt S, et al. Guidelines for the use of recombinant activated factor VII in massive obstetric haemorrhage. *Aust NZ J Obstet Gynaecol* 2008; **48**:12–16.

18. Palacios-Jaraquemada JM. Diagnosis and management of placenta accreta. *Best Pract Res Clin Obstet Gynecol* 2008; **22**:1133–48.

19. Tan SG, Jabling TW, Wallace EM, et al Surgical management of placenta accreta: a 10-year experience. *Acta Obstet Gynaecol Scand* 2013; **92**:445–50.

20. Kayem G, Davy C, Gogginet F, et al. Conservative versus extirpative management cases of placenta accrete. *Obstet Gynecol* 2004; **104**:531–36.

21. O'Rourke N, McElrath T, Baum R, et al. Caesarean delivery in the interventional radiology suite: a novel approach to obstetric hemostasis. *Anesth Analg* 2007; **104**:1193–94.

22. Kodali BS. Blodless trilogy? Anesthesia, obstetrics and interventional radiology for caesarean delivery. *Int J Obstet Anesth* 2010; **19**:131–32.

23. Uchiyama D, Koganemaru M, Abe T, Hori D, Hayabuchi N. Arterial catheterization and embolization for management of emergent or anticipated massive obstetrical hemorrhage. *Radiat Med* 2008; **26**:188–97.

24. Sadashivaiah J, Wilson R. Role of prophylactic uterine artery balloon catheters in the management of women with suspected placenta accreta. *Int J Obstet Anesth* 2011; **20**:282–87.

25. Izbizky G, Mellar C, Grasso M, et al. Feasibility and safety of prophylactic uterine artery catheterization and embolization in the management of placenta accreta. *J Vasc Intervent Radiol* 2015; **26**(2):162–69.

26. Thon S, Mclintic A, Wagner Y. Prophylactic endovascular placement of internal iliac occlusion balloon catheters in parturients with placenta accreta: a retrospective case series. *Int J Obstet Anesth* 2011; **20**:64–70.

27. Eller AG, Porter TF, Soisson O, Silver RM. Optimal management strategies for placenta accreta. *BJOG* 2009; **116**:648–54.

28. Snegovskikha D, Clebone A, Norwitz E. Anesthetic management of patients with placenta accreta and resuscitation strategies for associated massive hemorrhage.*Curr Opin Anesthesiol* 2011; **24**:274–81.

29. Lilker SJ, Meyer RA, Downey KN, Macarthur AJ. Anesthetic considerations for placenta accreta. *Int J Obstet Anesth* 2011; **20**:288–92.

30. Gallos G, Redai I, Smiley RM. The role of the anesthesiologist in management of obstetric hemorrhage. *Semin Perinatol* 2009; **33**:116–23.

31. Sentilhes L, Goffinet F, Kayem G. Management of placenta accreta. *Acta Obstet Gynaecol Scand* 2013; **92**: 1125–34.

32. Kayem G, Keita H. Management of placenta previa and accreta. *J Gynecol Obstet Biol Reprod* 2014; **43**: 1142–60.

Role of Transthoracic Echocardiography in Hypertensive Disorders of Pregnancy

Alicia T. Dennis

Case Study

A 36-year-old nulliparous woman who was previously healthy presented at 38 weeks' gestation to the delivery suite. She was contracting twice in 10 minutes. On examination, she was hypertensive (170/90 mmHg) with 3+ proteinuria, her cervix was dilated 4 cm, and cardiotocography (CTG) of the fetus was reassuring. The midwife altered the multidisciplinary team (duty obstetrician and anesthetist). An IV cannula was inserted, and blood was taken for a full blood examination (hemoglobin, platelet count, and blood film), liver function tests, and determination of urea, creatinine, and electrolyte levels. Then 1,000 ml of 0.9% saline was started, and 20 mg IV labetalol was administered to reduce the blood pressure to 150/90 mmHg. Shortly after this, the patient requested pain relief. After checking the results of the blood tests (platelet count $110,000 \times 10^9$/liter), an uncomplicated lumbar epidural was inserted, and effective analgesia was achieved with patient-controlled epidural analgesia using 0.2% ropivacaine with 2 μg/ml fentanyl, a 5-ml bolus every 15 minutes as required.

Two hours later, the patient developed a severe headache and hyperreflexia with blood pressure 180/100 mmHg. Infusions of magnesium sulfate, for seizure prophylaxis, and hydralazine, for blood pressure control, were started. There was no change in cervical dilatation, so augmentation of labor was undertaken with an oxytocin infusion. A nonreassuring CTG combined with limited labor progress led to the decision to deliver by cesarean delivery. Surgery was uncomplicated, and a healthy baby girl was born after an effective epidural top-up dose of 15 ml 2% lidocaine with 1:100,000 epinephrine and 100 μg fentanyl. IV fluid was limited to 500 ml intraoperatively, and the magnesium sulfate and hydralazine infusions continued during surgery. At the end of surgery, the epidural catheter was removed, and the patient was started on regular acetaminophen and oral slow- and intermittent-release opioid analgesia. A low-dose, high-concentration oxytocin infusion (40 units oxytocin in 40 ml 0.9% saline over 4 hours) was started to maintain uterine contractions, and the patient was returned to the delivery suite for close clinical monitoring and continuing magnesium sulfate and hydralazine infusions.

Eighteen hours later, a medical emergency team (MET) call was made when the patient developed critically high blood pressure (190/110 mmHg) followed rapidly by shortness of breath (respiratory rate of 26 breaths/min with lung crackles on auscultation) with reduced oxygen saturation (90 percent on room air). These clinical findings were consistent with pulmonary edema indicating heart failure. In order to determine whether this was reduced ejection fraction heart failure or preserved ejection fraction heart failure, bedside transthoracic echocardiography was performed. This investigation revealed a nondilated left ventricle (left ventricle end-diastolic diameter of 5.1 cm – normal nonpregnant female reference range 3.8–5.2 cm), normal fractional shortening of 38 percent (preserved ejection fraction), mitral valve E/septal e' ratio of 15 (normal nonpregnant reference value ≤ 8) consistent with diastolic dysfunction and a moderate pericardial effusion. These findings indicated that the patient had preserved ejection fraction heart failure. A bolus dose of hydralazine and furosemide was administered, and continuous positive airway pressure (CPAP) noninvasive ventilation was started. Over the next 15 minutes, her blood pressure decreased to 160/90 mmHg, respiratory rate decreased to 20 breaths/min, and oxygen saturation increased to 96 percent. Over the next hour, urine output increased to 150 ml, and the patient was weaned from noninvasive ventilation. After 24 hours, the magnesium sulfate and hydralazine infusions were ceased, and her blood pressure remained between 130 and 140/80 and 90 mmHg with no cerebral symptoms or signs.

The remainder of her hospital stay was uncomplicated, and she was discharged home on day 5. A follow-up transthoracic echocardiogram at 6 weeks, when she was normotensive, demonstrated normal cardiac structure and function with normal diastolic function evidenced by a mitral valve E/e' ratio of 7. She was advised to undergo yearly cardiovascular system follow-up with her general practitioner.

Key Points

- This patient developed severe intrapartum preeclampsia and underwent an emergency cesarean delivery. This was recognized early, and the multidisciplinary team was alerted.
- Management of severe preeclampsia involved biochemical investigations to determine the derangement in organ systems, close clinical monitoring, a magnesium sulfate infusion for seizure prophylaxis, and a hydralazine infusion for blood pressure control.
- After excluding contraindications, epidural analgesia was started that could be extended to anesthesia for cesarean delivery.
- Postoperatively, the patient developed pulmonary edema in the presence of hypertension. Bedside transthoracic echocardiography demonstrated preserved ejection fraction heart failure. Treatment involved reduction of blood pressure with hydralazine and redistribution of fluid away from the lungs using noninvasive positive end-expiratory pressure ventilation and a diuretic.

Discussion

Cardiovascular disease is a leading cause of maternal mortality worldwide.[1-3] Preeclampsia is a cardiovascular condition of pregnancy and is one of the hypertensive disorders of pregnancy. It is defined as new-onset repeatedly high blood pressure ($\geq$140 mmHg systolic and/or $\geq$90 mmHg diastolic) developing after 20 weeks' gestation and associated with another organ system involvement. It is not necessary to have proteinuria although this is a common manifestation of organ dysfunction in preeclampsia.[4-6]

Preeclampsia is frequently subclassified into mild and severe, with severe preeclampsia often defined as critically high blood pressure ($\geq$160/110 mmHg) associated with significant derangement of organ function

(e.g., 3+ proteinuria, liver enzymes twice the upper limit of normal, platelet count < 100,000/ml, headache, seizures, pulmonary edema).[7]

Anesthetists are frequently involved in the multidisciplinary management of women with severe preeclampsia because these women often require analgesia for labor, anesthesia for surgery (cesarean delivery), critical care management of hypertension, management of hemorrhage including antepartum hemorrhage, and management of life-threatening complications such as eclampsia, pulmonary edema, renal failure, or hepatic failure.[8] In addition, anesthetists need to consider other causes of hypertension when managing a woman with new-onset hypertension in pregnancy, especially when the presentation is atypical. The recent MBRRACE-UK perinatal mortality surveillance report on maternal deaths in the United Kingdom reported two deaths due to pheochromocytoma in women whose hypertension was inadequately investigated and managed.[1]

Coordinated management of a woman with severe preeclampsia is important because both stabilization of the condition and risk-reduction strategies to prevent complications need to occur simultaneously[8-11] (Table 22.1).

Echocardiography, especially transthroaicic echocardiography (TTE), is an important diagnostic and management tool in women with severe hypertension and complications related to hypertension such as acute pulmonary edema, aortic dissection, and myocardial ischemia, and international guidelines recommend its use in these situations.[12-16] In pregnancy, favorable characteristics such as anterior and lateral displacement of the heart, the requirement to lie in the left lateral position to avoid aortocaval compression, the noninvasive safe nature of ultrasound, and its high accuracy and validity mean that it is ideal for use in women with obstetric critical illness.[17,18]

Acute pulmonary edema is a dangerous complication of preeclampsia, and the reasons for its development are often multifactorial.[19] Transthoracic echocardiography can be performed at the point in patient care, often at the bedside, in the situation of breathlessness, desaturation, and hypertension, in order to determine the hemodynamic mechanism for pulmonary edema (Figures 22.1 and 22.2).

In the case of pulmonary edema occurring in a hypertensive person, the nature of the cardiac failure may be preserved ejection fraction heart failure or reduced ejection fraction heart failure. Without

Table 22.1 Key Strategies When Managing a Woman with Severe Preeclampsia

Key management strategy	General considerations
Multidisciplinary team involvement	Obstetrician, anesthetist, midwife, neonatologist, obstetric physician
Close monitoring	Maternal monitoring and fetal monitoring; activation of emergency response when observations become abnormal
Management of hypertension	Reduce blood pressure to safe levels (140–150/90–100 mmHg)
Prevention of neurologic complications	Magnesium sulfate bolus and infusion
Restrictive fluid therapy	Minimal IV fluid administration – low volume, high concentration oxytocin infusion if required
Analgesia	Neuraxial analgesia is safe, provided that there are no contraindications (thrombocytopenia)
Anesthesia	Neuraxial anesthesia is safe (assuming no contraindications); if general anesthesia is required, ablate the response to tracheal intubation using most familiar technique
High-acuity postpartum care	Monitor of complications and deterioration
Postpartum follow-up	Further investigations of hypertension and its resolution are required; lifelong regular review for early detection of cardiovascular system complications such as hypertension

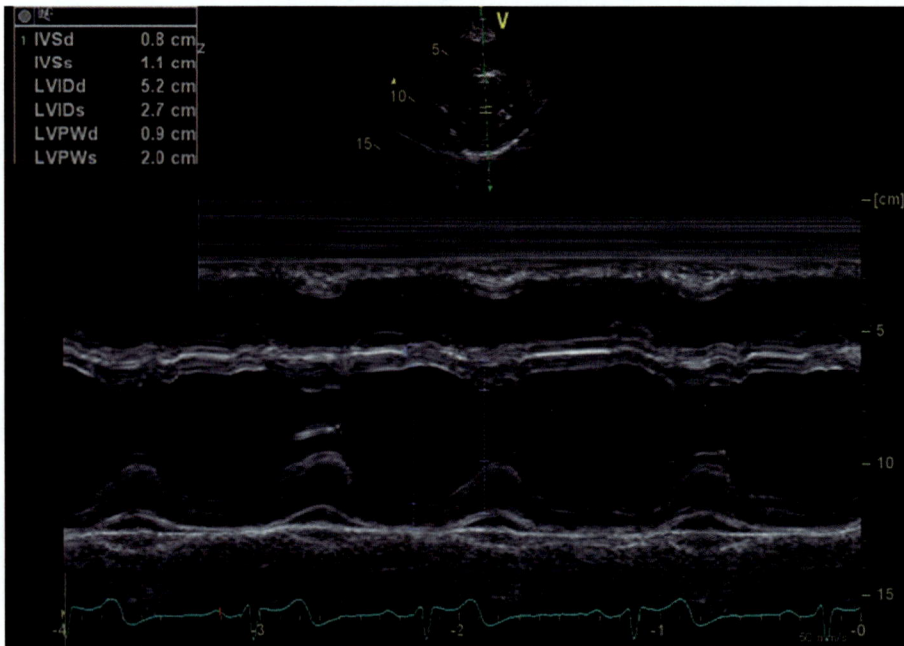

Figure 22.1 M-mode from the parasternal short-axis view demonstrating preserved fractional shortening and a nondilated left ventricle
Note: Fractional shortening = (LVIDd – LVIDs)/LVIDd ×100 = (5.2 – 2.)/5.2 × 100 = 48%, where IVSd = interventricular septal diameter during diastole; IVSs = interventricular septal diameter during systole; LVIDd = left ventricular internal diameter during diastole; LVIDs = left ventricular internal diameter during systole; LVPWd = left ventricular posterior wall diameter during diastole; and LVPWs = left ventricular posterior wall diameter during systole; written informed consent obtained to reproduce image

echocardiography, it is almost impossible to determine the difference between these two conditions because it cannot be determined from clinical examination and basic investigations alone.

Reduced ejection fraction heart failure is characterized by reduced ejection fraction or fractional shortening of less than 28 percent, often a dilated ventricle diagnosed when the left ventricular end-diastolic

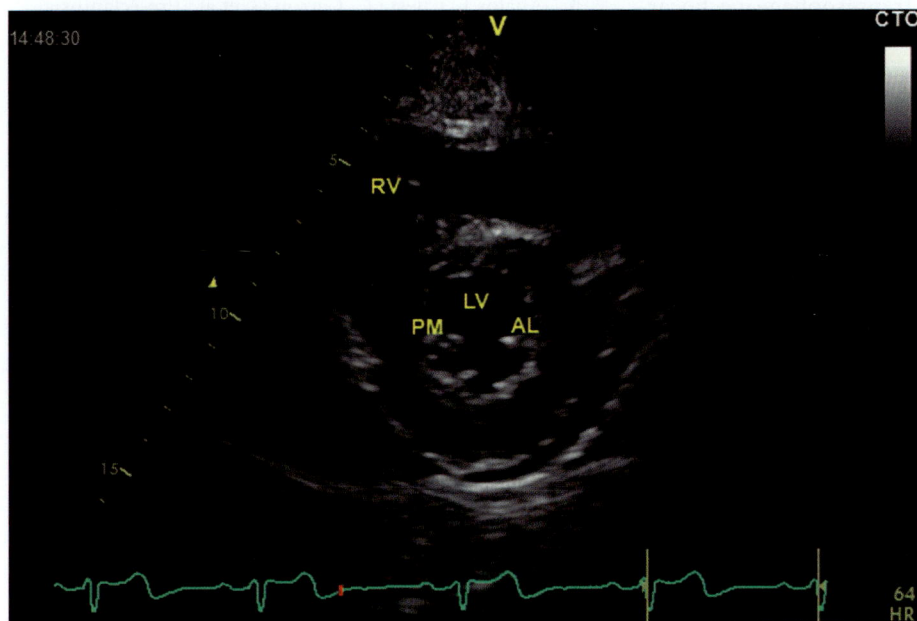

Figure 22.2 Still 2D image obtained from the parasternal short-axis view at end systole

Note: Written informed consent obtained to reproduce image.
Abbreviations: RV = right ventricle; LV = left ventricle; PM = posteromedial papillary muscle; and AL = anterolateral papillary muscle.

diameter is greater than 5.3 cm and normal or only mildly impaired diastolic function characterized by a mitral valve E/septal e' of less than 10.

Preserved ejection fraction heart failure is characterized by preserved ejection fraction or fractional shortening greater than 28 percent, usually a nondilated left ventricle and evidence of diastolic dysfunction with a mitral valve E/septal e' of greater than 10, often greater than 15. It is important to note that in the situation of preserved ejection fraction heart failure, 2D video images of the left ventricle as are obtained from the parasternal long- or short-axis view will be falsely reassuring because they will demonstrate good contractility and fractional shortening. Clinicians need to be aware that mistaking these images as normal may lead to serious diagnostic errors. It is only through assessment of diastolic function including the use of Doppler echocardiography that the reason for the heart failure will become apparent. The situation of preserved ejection fraction heart failure in women with hypertension is the reason for the inclusion of assessment of diastolic function and the use of Doppler echocardiography in an abbreviated echocardiographic examination technique in pregnant women.[18]

Once the diagnosis of either preserved ejection fraction heart failure or reduced ejection fraction heart failure is made, appropriate interventions can be started. In the situation of reduced ejection fraction heart failure, where severe hypertension has been corrected, if reduced ejection fraction heart failure is still present, inotropic agents need to be considered.

Women who survive hypertension in pregnancy complicated by acute pulmonary edema represent a group that has experienced a maternal near miss and thus is at risk of ongoing complications. Therefore, these women require close clinical monitoring after birth and specialist follow-up to determine the reasons for heart failure and to assess for resolution of the problem and lifelong screening once they have recovered so as to minimize their risks of developing uncontrolled cardiovascular disease.

Severe preeclampsia is a serious condition of pregnancy that, without adequate multidisciplinary management, including the appropriate use of echocardiography when complications occur, leads to maternal death and disability. With increasing awareness of the clinical utility of transthoracic echocardiography in critically ill pregnant women, especially those with life-threatening complications of preeclampsia, goal-directed transesophageal echocardiography (TTE) may start to be taught at more grassroots levels. This may include the teaching of echocardiography in medical schools and during basic and advanced specialty training programs that train doctors to manage critically ill adults such as anesthesia, critical care, and emergency medicine.

Learning Points

- Preeclampsia is a life-threatening hypertensive disorder of pregnancy.
- Key aspects of management include
  - A multidisciplinary team approach;
  - Reduction of high blood pressure to safe levels;
  - Prevention of eclampsia with magnesium sulfate;
  - Restrictive fluid therapy;
  - Close clinical maternal, fetal, and biochemical monitoring;
  - High-acuity care in the postpartum period; and
  - Lifelong follow-up for detection of cardiovascular disease.
- Transthoracic echocardiography (TTE) is an important diagnostic tool when a woman presents with acute pulmonary edema because it enables the differentiation of preserved ejection fraction heart failure from reduced ejection fraction heart failure.
- Echocardiography also enables the cardiac structure and function to be determined in women with severe preeclampsia and provides a baseline for serial studies and monitoring of the resolution of the condition.

References

1. Knight M, Kenyon S, Brocklehurst P, et al. *Saving Lives, Improving Mothers' Care: Lessons Learned to Inform Future Maternity Care from the UK and Ireland Confidential Enquiries into Maternal Deaths and Morbidity 2009–12*. Oxford: National Perinatal Epidemiology Unit, University of Oxford; 2104.

2. Johnson S, Bonello MR, Li Z, et al. *Maternal Deaths in Australia 2006–2010* (Maternal Deaths Series No. 4, Cat. No. PER 61). Canberra: Australian Institute of Health and Welfare (AIHW); 2014. Available at www.aihw.gov.au/publication-detail/?id=60129548319 (accessed December 27, 2014).

3. Abalos E, Cuesta C, Carroli G, et al., Pre-eclampsia, eclampsia and adverse maternal and perinatal outcomes: a secondary analysis of the World Health Organization Multicountry Survey on Maternal and Newborn Health. *BJOG* 2014; **121**(Suppl 1):14–24.

4. Magee AG, Pels A, Helewa M, et al., Diagnosis, evaluation and management of the hypertensive disorders of pregnancy. *Pregnancy Hypertens* 2014; **4**(2):105–45.

5. American College of Obstetricians and Gynecologists, Task Force on Hypertension in Pregnancy. Hypertension in pregnancy: report of the American College of Obstetricians and Gynecologists' Task Force on Hypertension in Pregnancy. *Obstet Gynecol* 2013; **122**(5):1122–31.

6. National Collaborating Centre for Women's and Children's Health. *2011 Hypertension in Pregnancy: The Management of Hypertensive Disorders during Pregnancy*. Washington, DC: National Institute for Health and Clinical Excellence; August 2010, modified 2011. Available at www.nice.org.uk/nicemedia/live/13098/50418/50418.pdf (accessed December 27, 2014).

7. Tranquilli AL, Brown MA, Zeeman G G, et al., The definition of severe and early-onset preeclampsia: statement from the International Society for the Study of Hypertension in Pregnancy (ISSHP). *Pregnancy Hypertens* 2013; **3**(1):44–47.

8. Dennis AT. Management of pre-eclampsia: issues for anaesthetists. *Anaesthesia* 2012; **67**(9):1009–20.

9. Duley L, Meher S, Jones L. Drugs for treatment of very high blood pressure during pregnancy. *Cochrane Database Syst Rev* 2013; (7):CD001449.

10. Duley L, Henderson-Smart D. Magnesium sulphate versus diazepam for eclampsia. *Cochrane Database Syst Rev* 2010; (**12**):CD000127.

11. Thornton CE, von Dadelszen P, Makris A, et al. Acute pulmonary edema as a complication of hypertension during pregnancy. *Hypertens Pregnancy* 2011; **30**(2):169–79

12. Douglas PS, Garcia MJ, Haines DE, et al. Appropriate use criteria for echocardiography. *J Am Soc Echocardiogr* 2011; **24**(3):229–67.

13. Erbel R, Aboyans V, Boileau C, et al. European Society of Cardiology guidelines on the diagnosis and treatment of aortic diseases: document covering acute and chronic aortic diseases of the thoracic and abdominal aorta of the adult. The Task Force for the Diagnosis and Treatment of Aortic Diseases of the European Society of Cardiology (ESC). *Eur Heart J* 2014; **35**(41):2873–926.

14. O'Gara PT, Kushner FG, Ascheim DD, et al. ACCF/AHA guideline for the management of ST-elevation

myocardial infarction: executive summary. A report of the American College of Cardiology Foundation/ American Heart Association Task Force on Practice Guidelines. *Circulation* 2013; **127**(4):529–55.

15. McMurray JJ, Adamopoulos S, Anker SD, et al. European Society of Cardiology guidelines for the diagnosis and treatment of acute and chronic heart failure 2012. The Task Force for the Diagnosis and Treatment of Acute and Chronic Heart Failure 2012 of the European Society of Cardiology. Developed in collaboration with the Heart Failure Association (HFA) of the ESC. *Eur J Heart Failure* 2012; **14**(8): 803–69.

16. Regitz-Zagrosek V, Lundqvist CB, Borghi C, et al. European Society of Cardiology guidelines on the management of cardiovascular diseases during pregnancy: the Task Force on the Management of Cardiovascular Diseases during Pregnancy of the European Society of Cardiology (ESC). *Eur Heart J* 2011; **32**(24):3147–97.

17. Armstrong S, Fernando R, Columb M. Minimally- and non-invasive assessment of maternal cardiac output: go with the flow! *Int J Obstet Anesth* 2011; **20**(4): 330–40.

18. Dennis AT. Transthoracic echocardiography in obstetric anaesthesia and obstetric critical illness. *Int J Obstet Anesth* 2011; **20**:160–68.

19. Dennis AT, Solnordal CB. Acute pulmonary oedema in pregnant women. *Anaesthesia* 2012; **67**(6):646–59.

Elective Cesarean Delivery

Sarah Armstrong

Case Study

A 36-year-old fit and well multiparous women presented in her third pregnancy. She had a history of two previous cesarean deliveries. The first was an elective delivery at term for breech presentation and the second following an unsuccessful trial of labor after cesarean delivery (TOLAC) in which the fetus had become distressed, requiring an emergency delivery. Following discussion with the obstetric team, a plan was made to deliver her third baby electively by cesarean.

She attended routine midwivery and obstetric appointments and was seen in the preoperative anesthetic clinic at 38 weeks' gestation. Routine blood sample were taken at this appointment, and a prescription was given for ranitidine and metoclopramide to be taken the evening before and morning of surgery. The patient was admitted to the labor ward at 39 weeks, having been NPO for food since the previous evening with clear fluids until 2 hours preoperatively.

The patient was transferred to the OR. All monitoring was placed in situ. A large-bore cannula was placed and 1 liter of Hartmann's solution started. A combined spinal-epidural was placed using a needle-through-needle technique, and 2.5 ml heavy bupivacaine 0.5% with 400 µg diamorphine was administered. A phenylephrine infusion was started. After 10 minutes, a good block was established bilaterally up to T4 to cold and light touch with a Bromage motor score grade 4. Surgery was started, resulting in a live-born baby girl. Postoperatively, multimodal analgesia was prescribed, and the patient went on to make an uncomplicated recovery.

Key Points

- The mode of anesthesia chosen for cesarean delivery will be guided by the indication for the surgery.

- In all cases, there should be adequate preoperative assessment and discussion of appropriate anesthetic technique.
- Regional anesthesia has significant advantages over general anesthesia for cesarean delivery but may result in hemodynamic instability, which should be anticipated.
- Multimodal postoperative analgesia should be used.

Discussion

The incidence of cesarean delivery is increasing, with 1.3 million (32.8 percent of all births) performed in the United States alone in 2012, a rate that has remained largely unchanged for several years.[1] Almost half of cesarean deliveries are planned. Elective cesarean delivery may be undertaken for many reasons, which are listed in Table 23.1.

It is imperative from an anesthetic viewpoint that these women are properly assessed prior to surgery so that the appropriate mode of anesthesia and analgesia may be discussed. This is ideally performed in a dedicated preoperative clinic in order to avoid any undue surprises on the date of delivery. The anesthetic assessment should be dictated by the patient's history, and in many healthy pregnancies will be straightforward. It should include at the very least an assessment of the airway, cardiovascular and respiratory status, and a discussion of the proposed anesthetic plan with the opportunity for the patient to ask questions and give informed consent.

Preoperative

Preoperative Investigations

For a healthy parturient undergoing a routine cesarean delivery with an otherwise uncomplicated pregnancy, there is currently no evidence for any specific

Table 23.1 Possible Indications for Elective Cesarean Delivery

Maternal indications	Fetal indications
• Decreased placental blood flow	• Breech or unfavorable lie
• Placental abnormalities:	• Fetal size > 4.5 kg
• Partial or complete placenta previa	• Intrauterine growth retardation
• Morbidly adherent placenta	• Fetal abnormalities (e.g., congenital heart disease) requiring planned delivery
• Active maternal infection (e.g., HIV)	• Multiple pregnancy
• Chronic maternal disease worsened by labor (e.g., maternal heart disease)	
• Demonstrated cephalopelvic disproportion	
• Increased risk of uterine rupture:	
• Previous classical cesarean delivery	
• Multiple previous cesarean deliveries	
• High maternal body mass index	
• Maternal request	

laboratory tests. Although it has been commonplace for a full blood count including platelet count, group and save, and clotting screen to be performed, the evidence suggests that this is not justified. The National Institute for Health and Care Excellence (NICE) guidance for cesarean delivery recommends that pregnant women should be offered a hemoglobin assessment to identify anemia. Blood loss of more than 1,000 ml is infrequent in cesarean delivery (it occurs in 4–8 percent), but it is a potentially serious complication.[2] The guidance also recommends that healthy women with uncomplicated pregnancies should not be routinely offered group and save or clotting screen prior to cesarean delivery.

If the patient's history warrants a platelet count in order to perform neuraxial blockade, then there must be consensus on the lower level of platelet count that is acceptable. The British Committee for Standards in Haematology has published guidance suggesting platelet counts that are safe for delivery: 50×10^9/Liter for vaginal delivery and 80×10^9/Liter for cesarean delivery and neuraxial anesthesia.[3] This is discordant with the recommendations from the American College for Hematology, which suggests any level above 50×10^9/Liter, regardless of mode of delivery.[4] There is a single

report in the literature of an epidural hematoma occurring in a pregnant woman in the presence of thrombocytopenia (71×10^9/Liter).[5] The debate surrounding the "safe" level of thrombocytopenia for neuraxial blockade is unlikely to be investigated by a clinical trial and therefore for the foreseeable future will be guided by expert consensus opinion.

Aspiration Prophylaxis

Parturients are at increased risk of aspiration of gastric contents for several reasons when compared with the nonpregnant population. First, progesterone causes relaxation of the musculature at the gastroesophageal junction and delayed gastric emptying. Second, the gravid uterus causes increased intra-abdominal pressure, tending to force the stomach contents upward. In addition, a paper by Mendelson described respiratory failure secondary to aspiration pneumonitis in pregnant women. It has been a cornerstone of anesthetic practice to prevent this.[6]

Prior to elective cesarean delivery, standard adult fasting guidelines should be adhered to.[7] Women waiting for planned surgery should not be subjected to long periods of starvation and/or fluid deprivation and should be encouraged to drink clear fluids up until 2 hours preoperatively. Women presenting for elective cesarean delivery will usually be assessed preoperatively in clinic, at which time antacid prophylaxis will be prescribed for both the evening before and the morning of surgery. A recent Cochrane review looked at interventions to reduce the risk of aspiration pneumonitis at cesarean delivery.[8] The report suggested that although the available studies were of poor quality, current evidence supported the combination of H_2-receptor antagonists and antacids as being more effective than either one alone or no prophylaxis. They concluded that neither proton pump inhibitors nor the prokinetic metoclopramide were effective. Despite this evidence, metoclopramide is currently routinely prescribed preoperatively for cesarean delivery in many units.

Intraoperative Anesthesia Antibiotic Administration

Women undergoing cesarean delivery are up to 20 times more likely to have a postpartum infection than those who have had a vaginal delivery. Until recently, all antibiotics were given after umbilical cord clamping to prevent neonatal exposure and potentially mask the signs of sepsis. Current recommendations are for

Table 23.2 Advantages of Regional Anesthesia over General Anesthesia for Cesarean Delivery

- Avoid potential for failed intubation
- Reduce risk of maternal aspiration
- Avoid pressor response to intubation (particularly in pre-eclampsia)
- Reduce perioperative blood loss
- Avoid volatile anesthetics
- Reduce perioperative venous bleeding from pelvic venous plexi
- Reduce maternal surgical stress response
- Allow maternal participation in the birth process
- Facilitate maternal bonding and breastfeeding
- Improve postoperative recovery:
    - Improved analgesia
    - Faster mobility
    - Potentially reduced pulmonary and thromboembolic complications

Table 23.3 Bromage Motor Scale

Grade	Criteria	Degree of block
1	Free movement of legs and feet	Nil (0%)
2	Just able to flex knees with free movement of feet	Partial (33%)
3	Unable to flex knees but with free movement of feet	Almost complete (66%)
4	Unable to move legs or feet	Complete (100%)

preincisional antibiotics, and a Cochrane review reported that celphalosporins are equivalent to penicillins in preventing immediate postcesarean infections.[2,9]

Neuraxial Techniques for Cesarean Delivery

The incidence of general anesthesia for cesarean delivery has dropped dramatically over the past few decades. The safety benefits of regional anesthesia over general anesthesia in pregnant patients are well documented and are summarized in Table 23.2.[10] In the United Kingdom, regional anesthesia is used for 94.9 percent of elective and 86.7 percent of emergency cesarean deliveries.[11] The choice of anesthesia ultimately rests with the competent mother. Information for mothers is available in a variety of formats, especially via the Obstetric Anaesthetist's Association website, which should help them make an informed choice in conjunction with discussion with the anesthetic team.

Spinal Anesthesia

Single-shot spinal anesthesia is probably still the most common neuraxial technique used for elective cesarean delivery. This may well be the result of the more widespread use of pencil-point spinal needles, which have lead to a reduction in post–dural puncture headache to less than 1 percent. Spinal anesthesia has become preferred in most situations over epidural anesthesia due to the shorter onset time, improved patient comfort, superior quality of surgical anesthesia, and fewer complications.[12] It is associated with less fetal exposure due to the least amount of absorption of local anesthetic into the maternal circulation.

The technique is usually performed at the level of L3 or below because in 20 percent of patients the conus medullaris has been shown to extend below the level of the body of L1, in addition to the finding that anesthetists more commonly underestimate the level of insertion.[13]

In the United Kingdom, the most commonly used intrathecal local anesthetic is bupivacaine 0.5% in dextrose 80 mg/ml ("heavy" or hyperbaric bupivacaine). The dose chosen to produce a reliable block may depend on patient height, but evidence for this is lacking. Patient positioning and the size of the gravid uterus may have more influence. A recent Cochrane review compared the use of isobaric and hyperbaric bupivacaine in cesarean delivery and concluded that the use of hyperbaric bupivacaine appeared to be associated with less likelihood of conversion to general anesthesia and that the time to reach sensory block to T4 was shorter. There was no difference in the need for supplemental analgesics and no other significant differences between the two local anesthetics.[14]

Combined Spinal-Epidural Anesthesia

Many units have adopted combined spinal-epidural (CSE) anesthesia as their primary approach for elective cesarean delivery. The technique may be performed at either two separate interspaces (usually the more cranial for the spinal component and the space below for the epidural component) or may be performed at a single interspace, often using a needle-through-needle approach using commercially available locking kits. This technique has the advantage of rapid onset of the spinal portion combined with the ability to maintain anesthesia via the epidural component and is a useful technique if the duration of surgery is longer than anticipated. Several studies have demonstrated the superiority of CSE anesthesia over conventional epidurals for cesarean delivery in terms of reliability of analgesia and muscle relaxation.

Another advantage of CSE anesthesia is the ability to use a lower initial dose in the spinal, which can be increased via the epidural component. This may be advantageous in some cardiac conditions, in pree-clampsia, and where a labor epidural has failed and there is concern that a normal-dose spinal may lead to an unacceptably high block. CSE techniques, of course, mean a risk of complications relating to both epidural and spinal anesthesia, including accidental dural puncture and possible increased risk of neural damage. Interestingly, CSE has been compared to spinals in terms of sensory block height. Although some preliminary work suggested the sensory block height may differ between CSE and spinals (using equivalent intrathecal doses) for elective cesarean delivery[15], this has not been confirmed in subsequent studies.[16,17]

General Anesthesia

Possible indications for general anesthesia for an elective cesarean delivery include contraindications to regional anesthesia or maternal request. General anesthesia for cesarean delivery is associated with higher mortality than neuraxial blockade, as demonstrated by complications arising from general anesthesia documented in the Confidential Enquiries into Maternal Deaths.[18] Airway difficulties are encountered more commonly than in the nonobstetric population. This is due to a combination of anatomical and physiological changes that occur during pregnancy, including upper airway edema (which may be exacerbated by preeclampsia), breast enlargement, and excessive weight gain.[19] The presence of the gravid uterus reduces functional residual capacity, which, combined with increased overall oxygen requirements, may accelerate the onset of desaturation during apnea.[20] Pulmonary aspiration is one of the main concerns of general anesthesia in obstetric patients, and guidelines should be strictly adhered to for the administration of antacid prophylaxis, particularly if a general anesthetic is planned. The use of a rapid-sequence induction to reduce the incidence of pulmonary aspiration has remained largely unchanged for the past six decades, traditionally with thiopentone and suxamethonium (1.5 mg/kg) but more recently using propofol and rocuronium (up to 1.2 mg/kg of body weight) with the availability of sugammadex to specifically reverse rocuronium-induced neuromuscular blockade. There has been increased interest in the use of videolaryngoscopes and second-generation supraglottic airway devices (such as the LMA Proseal™), which have been used successfully in obstetric patients undergoing general anesthesia.[21] Indeed, these devices were recommended for use in the 2015 joint Obstetric Anaesthetists' Association/Difficult Airway Society guidelines for the management of difficult and failed intubation in obstetrics.[20]

Accidental awareness under general anesthesia (AAGA) in obstetrics is another concern. It has long since been believed that the incidence of AAGA is higher in obstetrics than in nonpregnant patients, and this has been shown in several epidemiological studies.[22,23] It is thought that concerns about the deleterious effects of anesthetic drugs on the fetus (both directly and via the impact of maternal hemodynamics), the potential to increase maternal blood loss through decreased uterine tone, and the decreasing use nationally (in the United Kingdom) of thiopentone and of general anesthesia globally in obstetrics may have lead to an increase in cases of awareness. In the Fifth National Audit Project of the Royal College of Anaesthetists and Association of Anaesthetists of Great Britain and Ireland (AAGBI), obstetric general anesthesia was associated with a 10-fold overrepresentation of awareness cases when compared with other surgical specialities.[24] Monitoring of pregnant patients should be carried out according to standard AAGBI guidelines. Anesthesia is generally maintained with inhalational agents using end-tidal agent monitoring to titrate the anesthetic depth. The NAP5 study showed that the use of specific depth of anesthesia monitors (e.g., bispectral index [BIS] monitoring) during obstetric anesthesia was sparse (particularly in the United Kingdom), and it was suggested that this might reflect either the lack of confidence that these monitors provide clinically useful information or the perceived impracticality (because of slow response time) of using such monitors in obstetrics.[23,24]

Postoperative Analgesia

Effective postoperative analgesia is vital to hasten the recovery of the mother, facilitate her ability to bond with and breastfeed her child, and to allow early mobilization to reduce complications. Approaches can be divided into opioid-based techniques using intrathecal, epidural, or systemic routes with or without the use of adjuvant agents, wound infiltration, and nerve blocks and the use of oral analgesics such as acetaminophen and nonsteroidal anti-inflammatory drugs (NSAIDs). The use of a combination of these techniques is now well established in clinical practice.

Neuraxial Opioids

Neuraxial opioids have been shown in multiple studies of cesarean delivery to reduce the dose of local anesthetic required and to improve intraoperative and postoperative analgesia.[25,26] In the United Kingdom, the two most commonly used opioids intraoperatively are fentanyl and diamorphine. Fentanyl is highly lipid soluble and therefore has a rapid uptake into the lipid-rich dorsal horn. Consequently, it has a rapid onset but short duration of action, and so is excellent for intraoperative analgesia but limited in use for postoperative analgesia.[27] Morphine is lipid insoluble with a long onset of action, which means that it is not suitable for intraoperative analgesia but is effective for postoperative analgesia extending into the second postoperative day.[28] Diamorphine has intermediate solubility compared with fentanyl or morphine, meaning that it is present in both hydrophobic and hydrophilic tissue components. Diamorphine undergoes metabolism within spinal cord tissue, generating active compounds (6-acetyl morphine and morphine) that increase the analgesic effects. These metabolites are less lipid soluble than the parent drug, which limits their backdiffusion into the CSF. This property means that diamorphine can be used for both intraoperative and postoperative pain relief, where available.[29] Optimal doses of neuraxial opioids have been relatively difficult to define because multiple studies have suggested that with increasing doses, analgesia improves, as does the incidence of side effects (e.g., nausea, vomiting, pruritus, delayed gastric emptying, sedation, and respiratory depression).[30–32] In addition to intrathecal opioids, the epidural route can be used for long-acting opioid analgesia, and newer formulations of epidural opioids such as extended-release epidural morphine (morphine encapsulated in multivesicular lipid particles) have been used successfully in obstetric anesthesia, showing postoperative analgesia extending into the second postoperative day with no significant side effects.[33]

Nonneuraxial Regional Techniques

In the transversus abdominis plane (TAP), block local anesthetic is introduced into the plane between the fascia of the transversus abdominis muscle and the internal oblique muscle. It has a high margin of safety and is technically simple to perform, especially under ultrasound guidance, but despite this, TAP blocks remain overwhelmingly underused in both obstetric and nonobstetric populations. A number of studies over the years have looked at the efficacy of TAP blocks after cesarean delivery, and their utility remains controversial. Abdallah et al.[34] performed a systematic review and meta-analysis looking at five trials with 312 patients undergoing TAP block for cesarean delivery and concluded that TAP block provides superior analgesia to placebo and can reduce the first 24-hour morphine consumption in the setting of a multimodal analgesic regimen that excludes spinal morphine. There has also been interest in the literature for looking at wound infiltration using both local anesthetic and nonsteroidal analgesics. A Cochrane review in 2009 concluded that local anesthetic infiltration and abdominal nerve blocks as adjuncts to regional and general anesthesia are of benefit by reducing opioid consumption and that NSAIDs as an adjuvant in the local anesthetic mixture may confer additional pain relief.[35]

Opioid Systemic Analgesia

When neuraxial opioids have been used, studies have shown that IV opioid analgesia is usually not necessary postoperatively. However, if no neuraxial opioids have been given, such as in general anesthesia, systemic opioids may be required. IV Patient Controlled Analgesia (PCA) has been compared with IM administration of opioids, with most studies concluding that the IV PCA route is preferable, resulting in better analgesia, earlier ambulation, less sedation, and greater patient satisfaction regardless of which opioid is used.[36,37]

Nonopioid Systemic Analgesia

NSAIDs (including acetaminophen) are now widely established as a basic analgesic in the management of severe postoperative pain. In postcesarean delivery, they have been shown to potentiate opioid effect, decrease opioid consumption, and reduce side effects. Munishankar et al.[38,39] compared oral acetaminophen, diclofenac, and the combination for pain relief after cesarean in a double-blind randomized, controlled trial of acetaminophen. Patients given the combination of diclofenac and acetaminophen required 38 percent less morphine than patients given acetaminophen alone. Morphine use in patients given diclofenac alone was not significantly different from morphine use in the other two groups. Codeine phosphate has been implicated in the toxicity and death of neonates when codeine is administered to lactating mothers, particularly those who are "ultrafast metabolisers" of the drug, and as a result, codeine phosphate has been withdrawn from use in many maternity units.

Enhanced Recovery in Obstetrics

Enhanced Recovery (ER), also known as Perioperative Surgical Home (PSH), is a perioperative care pathway with the aim of improving patient outcomes and enabling earlier discharge from hospital, which has been applied successfully across multiple surgical specialities.[40] Benefits include a reduction in morbidity, reduced length of stay, and earlier return to normal activities.[40] Allowing woman to go home the day after an elective cesarean delivery is in keeping with the NICE guidance, which states that "women who are recovering well, are apyrexial and do not have complications following cesarean delivery should be offered early discharge (after 24 h) from hospital and follow-up at home, because this is not associated with more infant or maternal readmissions."[2] Aspects of ER programs in obstetrics include a reduction in the stress response to surgery, good perioperative nutrition with fluids (including carbohydrate drinks) up until 2 hours before surgery, rapid mobilization postoperatively with early removal of the urinary catheter, and postoperative pain relief that does not rely on strong opioids.[41] Increasingly, obstetric units are undertaking ER programs, and a survey of UK practice in 2013 showed that 96 percent of responding units supported the ER concept. Although only 10 units (6 percent) at the time of the survey had or were implementing ER pathways, many aspects of the routine care of parturients undergoing elective cesarean delivery were found to be consistent with fast-track surgery, with more than 70 percent of units minimizing interruption in oral intake and mobilizing parturients within 12 hours.[42] This suggests that ER pathways are a viable proposition for many units, but more rigorous research is required to examine whether the programs are safe and effective for women and their babies.[41]

Learning Points

- Patients presenting for elective cesarean delivery should be routinely assessed as for any other anesthetic.
- Women should be thoroughly assessed preoperatively to ensure that correct investigations are performed, that appropriate premedication is prescribed, and that they are given information regarding their anesthetic and recovery so that they understand what to expect.
- The mainstay of anesthesia for cesarean delivery continues to be regional anesthesia with the use of neuraxial opioids with management of expected hypotension.
- Postoperative analgesia for cesarean delivery should be based on a multimodal analgesic regimen to facilitate maternal and infant bonding and maternal recovery.
- Enhanced recovery pathways in obstetrics may improve recovery times and outcomes for parturients as part of an integrated multidisciplinary care pathway.

References

1. Hamilton BE, Martin JA, Ventura SJ. Births: preliminary data for 2012. *Natl Vital Stat Rep* 2013; **62**(3):1–20.

2. National Institute for Health and Care Excellence. Clinical guideline 132: Caesarean section, 2015. Available at www.nice.org.uk/guidance/cg132 (accessed July 11, 2016).

3. Provan D, Stasi R, Newland AC, et al. International consensus report on the investigation and management of primary immune thrombocytopenia. *Blood* 2010; **115**(2):168–86.

4. George JN, Woolf SH, Raskob GE, et al. Idiopathic thrombocytopenic purpura: a practice guideline developed by explicit methods for the American Society of Hematology. *Blood* 1996; **88**(1):3–40.

5. Yuen TST, Kua JSW, Tan IKS. Spinal haematoma following epidural anaesthesia in a patient with eclampsia. *Anaesthesia* 1999; **54**(4):350–54.

6. Mendelson CL. The aspiration of stomach contents into the lungs during obstetric anesthesia. *Am J Obstet Gynecol* 1946; **52**:191–205.

7. Association of Anaesthetists of Great Britain and Ireland (AAGBI). *Preoperative Assessment and Patient Preparation: The Role of the Anaesthetist*. London: AAGBI; 2011.

8. Paranjothy S, Griffiths JD, Broughton HK, et al. Interventions at caesarean section for reducing the risk of aspiration pneumonitis. *Cochrane Database Syst Rev* 2014; (2):CD004943.

9. Gyte GMI, Dou L, Vazquez JC. Different classes of antibiotics given to women routinely for preventing infection at caesarean section. *Cochrane Database Syst Rev* 2014; (11):CD008726.

10. Hawkins JL, Koonin LM, Palmer SK, Gibbs CP. Anesthesia-related deaths during obstetric delivery in the United States, 1979–1990. *Anesthesiology* 1997; **86** (2):277–84.

11. Jenkins JG, Khan MM. Anaesthesia for caesarean section: a survey in a UK region from 1992 to 2002. *Anaesthesia* 2003; **58**(11):1114–18.

12. Riley ET, Cohen SE, Macario A, Desai JB, Ratner EF. Spinal versus epidural anesthesia for cesarean section: a comparison of time efficiency, costs, charges, and complications. *Anesth Analg* 1995; **80**(4):709–12.

13. Broadbent CR, Maxwell WB, Ferrie R, et al. Ability of anaesthetists to identify a marked lumbar interspace. *Anaesthesia* 2000; **55**(11):1122–26.

14. Sia AT, Tan KH, Sng BL, et al. Use of hyperbaric versus isobaric bupivacaine for spinal anaesthesia for cesarean section. *Cochrane Database Syst Rev* 2013; (5): CD005143.

15. Ithnin F, Lim Y, Sia AT, Ocampo CE. Combined spinal epidural causes higher level of block than equivalent single-shot spinal anesthesia in elective cesarean patients. *Anesth Analg* 2006; **102**(2):577–80.

16. Horstman DJ, Riley ET, Carvalho B. A randomized trial of maximum cephalad sensory blockade with single-shot spinal compared with combined spinal-epidural techniques for cesarean delivery. *Anesth Analg* 2009; **108**(1):240–45.

17. Tang Y-Y, Zhou J, Ren X-H, Lin X-M. Comparison of spinal block levels between laboring and nonlaboring parturients using combined spinal epidural technique with intrathecal plain bupivacaine. *Anesthesiol Res Pract* 2012; **2012**:187132.

18. McClure JH, Cooper GM, Clutton-Brock TH, Centre for Maternal and Child Enquiries. Saving mothers' lives: reviewing maternal deaths to make motherhood safer: 2006–8: A review. *Br J Anaesth* 2011; **107**(2): 127–32.

19. O'Connor R, Thorburn J. Acute pharyngolaryngeal oedema in a pre-eclamptic parturient with systemic lupus erythematosus and a recent renal transplant. *Int J Obstet Anesth* 1993; **2**(1):53–55.

20. Mushambi MC, Kinsella SM, Popat M, et al. Obstetric Anaesthetists' Association and Difficult Airway Society guidelines for the management of difficult and failed tracheal intubation in obstetrics. *Anaesthesia* 2015; **70** (11):1286–306.

21. Munnur U, de Boisblanc B, Suresh MS. Airway problems in pregnancy. *Crit Care Med* 2005; **33**(Suppl 10):S259–68.

22. Errando CL, Sigl JC, Robles M, et al. Awareness with recall during general anaesthesia: a prospective observational evaluation of 4001 patients. *Br J Anaesth* 2008; **101**(2):178–85.

23. Paech MJ, Scott KL, Clavisi O, Chua S, McDonnell N, ANZCA Trials Group. A prospective study of awareness and recall associated with general anaesthesia for cesarean section. *Int J Obstet Anesth* 2008; **17**(4):298–303.

24. Pandit JJ, Andrade J, Bogod DG, et al. Fifth National Audit Project (NAP5) on accidental awareness during general anaesthesia: summary of main findings and risk factors. *Br J Anaesth* 2014; **113**(4): 549–59.

25. Dahlgren G, Hultstrand C, Jakobsson J, et al. Intrathecal sufentanil, fentanyl, or placebo added to bupivacaine for cesarean section. *Anesth Analg* 1997; **85**(6):1288–93.

26. Shende D, Cooper GM, Bowden MI. The influence of intrathecal fentanyl on the characteristics of subarachnoid block for caesarean section. *Anaesthesia* 1998; **53**(7):706–10.

27. Belzarena SD. Clinical effects of intrathecally administered fentanyl in patients undergoing cesarean section. *Anesth Analg* 1992; **74**(5):653–57.

28. Dahl JB, Jeppesen IS, Jørgensen H, Wetterslev J, Møiniche S. Intraoperative and postoperative analgesic efficacy and adverse effects of intrathecal opioids in patients undergoing cesarean section with spinal anesthesia: a qualitative and quantitative systematic review of randomized controlled trials. *Anesthesiology* 1999; **91**(6):1919–27.

29. Hallworth SP, Fernando R, Bell R, Parry MG, Lim GH. Comparison of intrathecal and epidural diamorphine for elective caesarean section using a combined spinal-epidural technique. *Br J Anaesth* 1999; **82**(2): 228–32.

30. Skilton RW, Kinsella SM, Smith A, Thomas TA. Dose response study of subarachnoid diamorphine for analgesia after elective caesarean section. *Int J Obstet Anesth* 1999; **8**(4):231–35.

31. Stacey R, Jones R, Kar G, Poon A. High-dose intrathecal diamorphine for analgesia after caesarean section. *Anaesthesia* 2001; **56**(1):54–60.

32. Hunt CO, Naulty JS, Bader AM, et al. Perioperative analgesia with subarachnoid fentanyl-bupivacaine for cesarean delivery. *Anesthesiology* 1989; **71**(4):535–40.

33. Carvalho B, Riley E, Cohen SE, et al. Single-dose, sustained-release epidural morphine in the management of postoperative pain after elective cesarean delivery: results of a multicenter randomized controlled study. *Anesth Analg* 2005; **100**(4):1150–58.

34. Abdallah FW, Halpern SH, Margarido CB. Transversus abdominis plane block for postoperative analgesia after caesarean delivery performed under spinal anaesthesia? A systematic review and meta-analysis. *Br J Anaesth* 2012; **109**(5):679–87.

35. Bamigboye AA, Hofmeyr GJ. Local anaesthetic wound infiltration and abdominal nerves block during

caesarean section for postoperative pain relief. *Cochrane Database Syst Rev* 2009; (3):CD006954.

36. Ballantyne JC, Carr DB, Chalmers TC, et al. Postoperative patient-controlled analgesia: meta-analyses of initial randomized control trials. *J Clin Anesth* 1993; **5**(3):182–93.

37. Hudcova J, McNicol ED, Quah CS, Lau J, Carr DB. Patient controlled opioid analgesia versus conventional opioid analgesia for postoperative pain. *Cochrane Database Syst Rev* 2006; (4):CD003348.

38. Willmann S, Edginton AN, Coboeken K, Ahr G, Lippert J. Risk to the breast-fed neonate from codeine treatment to the mother: a quantitative mechanistic modeling study. *Clin Pharmacol Ther* 2009; **86**(6): 634–43.

39. Koren G, Cairns J, Chitayat D, Gaedigk A, Leeder SJ. Pharmacogenetics of morphine poisoning in a breastfed neonate of a codeine-prescribed mother. *Lancet* 2006; **368**(9536):704.

40. Niranjan N, Bolton T, Berry C. Enhanced recovery after surgery-current trends in perioperative care. *Update in Anaesthesia* 2010; **26**(1):18–23.

41. Wrench IJ, Allison A, Galimberti A, Radley S, Wilson MJ. Introduction of enhanced recovery for elective caesarean section enabling next day discharge: a tertiary centre experience. *Int J Obstet Anesth* 2015; **24**(2):124–30.

42. Aluri S, Wrench IJ. Enhanced recovery from obstetric surgery: a UK survey of practice. *Int J Obstet Anesth* 2014; **23**(2):157–60.

Emergency Delivery for Fetal Distress

Ruth E. Murphy and Stephen Michael Kinsella

Case Study

A term nulliparous woman presented at 3–4 cm dilated in labor with irregular contractions. An epidural was established with 16 ml 0.1% bupivacaine and fentanyl 2 µg/ml in two equal divided doses and maintained using patient-controlled epidural analgesia (PCEA) of 8-ml boluses of the same low-dose mixture available every 15 minutes as required. Labor progress was slow, and an oxytocin infusion was started. On reexamination, the patient's cervix was found to be 6 cm dilated. The cardiotocograph (CTG) became nonreassuring, demonstrating late decelerations for 15 minutes occurring with over 50 percent of contractions. A decision was made to perform a fetal scalp blood sample, but while sampling in the supine position a prolonged deceleration to 65 beats/min occurred. The obstetrician ordered a Category I emergency cesarean delivery (immediate threat to life of woman or fetus) with a maximum intended decision-delivery interval of 30 minutes.

While in the labor room, intrauterine resuscitation was instituted (syntocinon infusion stopped, left lateral position adopted, 0.25 mg terbutaline injected subcutaneously [a tocolytic beta-agonist], oxygen by mask, and rapid IV infusion of 1 liter crystalloid solution). The fetal bradycardia recovered partially to 110 beats/min with these measures. The anesthetist arrived in the delivery room and rapidly assessed the epidural to determine the suitability and safety of an epidural top-up to provide surgical anesthesia. Analgesia during contractions had been complete, and the last PCEA bolus was administered 35 minutes previously. Then 20 ml of a top-up mixture containing 17 ml 2% lidocaine with 1 ml 1:10,000 epinephrine and 2 ml 8.4% preservative-free sodium bicarbonate was prepared in the room by the anesthetist. After a negative aspiration test, a fractionated epidural top-up was given. A 3-ml test dose was given with a check for signs of spinal placement after 30 seconds, and then a further 3-ml test dose was given, observing for signs of IV placement after 30 seconds. The remaining 14 ml then was given over 90 seconds in the labor room. By this time, the patient was ready for transfer, and the anesthetist accompanied her to the OR. The epidural block was checked using ethyl chloride spray, and complete loss of cold sensation was found between T4 (nipples) and S5 (perianal). The anesthetist gave the all-clear to start surgery, an emergency cesarean delivery was performed, and the neonate was delivered safely. Three milligrams of diamorphine was administered via the epidural catheter at the end of the operation for postoperative analgesia, and the epidural was then removed before discharge from the OR.

Key Points

- An abnormal CTG that requires early delivery is often preceded by nonreassuring changes, allowing advanced preparations for surgery.
- Intrauterine resuscitation measures will often lead to partial or complete recovery of fetal heart decelerations or bradycardia.
- Good function of the epidural block for labor analgesia is an indicator that surgical anesthesia for operative delivery is likely to be successful.
- Epidural top-up for surgery should include fractionation of the drug dose and assessment for misplacement.
- If the epidural catheter is topped up in the delivery room, the anesthetist should accompany the patient during transfer to the OR.

Discussion

Although the primary aim of epidural analgesia is to provide relief from painful uterine contractions, the secondary purpose is to provide surgical anesthesia should this be necessary for cesarean delivery,

- Stop oxytocin infusion if it is being used

- Position in full left / right lateral position (guided by FHR trace)

- Tocolysis with terbutaline 0.25mg subcutaneously

- Oxygen using reservoir mask and high flow

- Fluid intravenous infusion e.g. Hartmann's solution 1000 ml

- Ephedrine if low maternal blood pressure

Figure 24.1 An example intrauterine fetal resuscitation guideline (FHR, fetal heart rate)

operative vaginal delivery, or postpartum procedures. As surgery becomes more likely, the obstetric anesthetist should make a judgment as to whether the labor epidural will work to provide anesthesia for surgery; if he or she is not confident about the function of the epidural, then he or she should consider whether it should be resited if time allows or accept that an alternative method of anesthesia will have to be used.

Initial Assessment of Epidural Function

The assessment of whether an epidural is likely to give effective analgesia for the duration of labor and anesthesia for surgery should be made early and continued during labor. Quick onset of analgesia, bilateral cutaneous sensory changes between the midthoracic and sacral dermatomes, and bilateral autonomic motor block evidenced through increased foot temperature are all desirable features. Very frequent epidural top-ups may be indicators that the epidural is functioning poorly, with two provisos. The first is that women who are anxious or wish to have no sensation at all may self-administer frequent PCEA boluses; this will be demonstrated by low pain scores and no breakthrough pain. The second is that obstructed labor (dystocia) is more painful than normal labor, and therefore, breakthrough pain may occur even with a good epidural.[1,2] This is a difficult situation to clarify; sometimes this is only shown when an oxytocin infusion is switched off at the point of an obstetric decision to attempt operative delivery, when the epidural function immediately becomes normal.

Good communication with the attending midwife/obstetric nurse is important to monitor the effectiveness of analgesia and to identify any problems early. If an epidural is functioning poorly, the anesthetist should have a low threshold for resiting, unless straightforward vaginal delivery is imminent.

Urgency and Intrauterine Fetal Resuscitation

The four-category urgency classification for cesarean delivery is well established in the United Kingdom.[3] Category I is defined as immediate threat to life of woman or fetus. The use of these categories is a useful start to communication by the obstetrician to the rest of the team, but he or she should also communicate important details of the case, such as presence and severity of maternal and fetal compromise, and any response to resuscitation (see below) to the anesthetist. This will help the anesthetist to make an appropriate decision on the type of anesthetic to be used.

Most cases of Category I cesarean delivery for fetal bradycardia are likely to be associated with a transient cause, and therefore, the use of intrauterine resuscitation allows the best chance of reversing the process, allowing extra time to review the surgery and anesthesia[4,5] (Figure 24.1). For high-risk women, it may be necessary for junior anesthetic staff to await the assistance of a senior anesthetist. Even if the process is irreversible and immediate general anesthesia is required, administration of oxygen and IV fluid prepares for this eventuality.

Clear communication between obstetrician and anesthetist must be maintained; a Category I situation can be downgraded to Category II when the fetal condition is reassessed (and improves) in the OR and vice versa (when the fetal status worsens).

Assessment of the Epidural Block before Surgery

It is rare that the anesthetist cannot consider the possibility of providing regional anesthesia for operative delivery. It is undeniable that starting an epidural top-up in the delivery room allows the maximum length of time for the block to develop, although there is debate over the safety of this practice.[6,7]

Safety assessment (15 sec)
- Is the epidural in? i.e. not leaking
- Is it spinal? Has there been excessive motor block, recurrent hypotension.
- Is it intravenous? Has there been poor block, need for frequent top-ups, symptoms of local anaesthetic toxicity.

Perform aspiration test

Test dose (90 sec)
- Give 3 mL; wait 30 sec; assess change in block (e.g. any global subjective change, cold sensation at S1, ankle dorsiflexion) indicating spinal placement.
- Give 3 mL; wait 60 sec, assess symptoms (strange taste, tinnitus, sedation) indicating intravenous placement.

Main dose (90 sec)
- Give remainder while observing for any changes as above.
- Stay with woman and maintain communication. Monitor pulse and BP. Be prepared to deal with high block.

Figure 24.2 Safety assessment and rapid epidural top-up for Category I cesarean delivery

The concerns relate to the potential for a high/total spinal or IV misplacement and the lack of monitoring during transfer.[6,7]

The chance that an epidural catheter is misplaced is greatest when first inserted and decreases after initial establishment of block and assessment. Although it is sometimes assumed that correct epidural placement is guaranteed by continued function during labor, a recent report shows that this is incorrect; in one case, an epidural that provided satisfactory analgesia during labor was found, on review by the anesthetist, to be in the spinal space, and surgical anesthesia was provided using 2.5 mg bupivacaine. In a second case, 75 mg bupivacaine administered after a negative aspiration test was followed by total spinal and cardiorespiratory arrest.[8]

A national survey of Obstetric Anaesthetists' Association members found that almost two-thirds did not use a test dose when topping up an epidural for emergency cesarean delivery.[9] However, in contrast, we recommend a systematic approach to evaluating the patient and rapid but fractionated administration of the epidural top-up solution with attention to adverse changes indicating misplacement (Figure 24.2).[10] An initial assessment should be performed to ensure that the epidural catheter is sited correctly, seeking signs that the epidural is working excessively (possible spinal placement) or inadequately (possible IV placement). If indicated, the insertion site should be assessed for signs of leakage. The epidural catheter should be aspirated to check for free flow of CSF or blood. At this stage, the anesthetist may decide that topping up the epidural is likely to be ineffective or dangerous and should plan on performing general or spinal anesthesia (Figure 24.3).

Rapid Epidural Top-Up

Typical top-up mixtures used in our institution include 20 ml 2% lidocaine with 1 ml 1:10,000 epinephrine and 2 ml 8.4% sodium bicarbonate or 0.5% levobupivacaine. A meta-analysis including 779 patients suggests that a lidocaine with epinephrine 1:200,000 mixture provides the fastest onset of surgical block.[11] One milliliter of sodium bicarbonate 8.4% per 10 ml of lidocaine may be added to increase the speed of onset.[12] The addition of fentanyl to the top-up mixture may decrease the onset time,[11] but if it is not readily available, then the top-up should be given without waiting.

A spinal test dose of 3 ml of the chosen epidural top-up mixture should be given, with an assessment after 30 seconds for early block changes. A further 3 ml should be given to complete an IV test dose, seeking systemic signs or symptoms after 30 seconds. The remaining top-up dose then should be given over 90 seconds while still observing for the above-mentioned changes, allowing for potential epidural vein-to-brain circulation to occur before completion

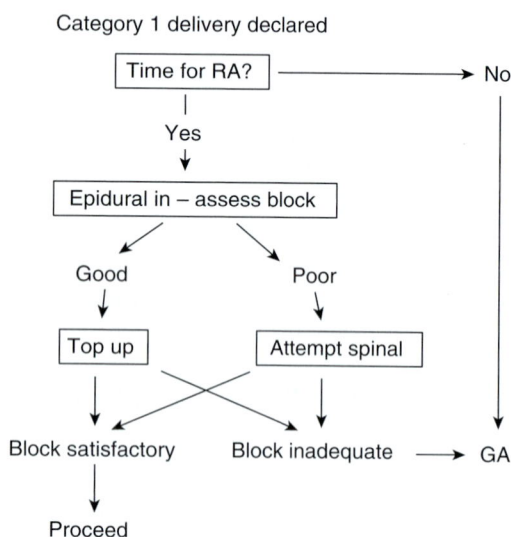

Category 1 delivery declared

Time for RA? → No

Yes

Epidural in – assess block

Good / Poor

Top up / Attempt spinal

Block satisfactory / Block inadequate → GA

Proceed

Figure 24.3 Flow diagram illustrating suggested choice of regional anesthesia for Category I delivery (RA, regional anesthesia; GA, general anesthesia)

of the full epidural top-up. The standard total volume for top-up is 20 ml. However, a reduced dose of 15 ml should be considered if the block is high or dense or the woman is of short stature.

The anesthetist should remain with the woman, observing her and monitoring pulse and blood pressure, maintaining communication, and ready to deal with any problems such as a high block or hypotension. Free-flowing IV fluids such as Hartmann's solution and immediate access to vasopressors, oxygen, and equipment to ventilate the lungs should be available.

In our institution, if a patient is having a trial of instrumental delivery in the OR, then the epidural is topped up as for an emergency cesarean delivery. The rationale is that if the trial fails, a Category I cesarean delivery may be necessary.

Regional Anesthesia in the Absence of Established Epidural Anesthesia

Fetal bradycardia may occur soon after initiation of epidural or CSE analgesia during labor, leading to a decision for cesarean delivery. The anesthetist in such cases may not be confident that there is enough time to top up the epidural.

It is possible to insert a spinal anesthetic in a comparable time to administration of general anesthesia, but the onset time of an acceptable block adds to the total time required.[13,14] Should spinal anesthesia be contemplated for Category I cesarean delivery, the technique of *rapid-sequence spinal* may be considered. This includes using a no-touch technique (gloves only and skin preparation with a wipe of 0.5% chlorhexidine), avoidance of spinal opioids requiring small volumes or dilution (e.g., diamorphine and morphine), and starting surgery before full development of the surgical block (i.e., accepting a level of T10 for loss of cold sensation).[13] There must be only a limited number of attempts at spinal insertion, and preoxygenation of the woman may be started to reduce delay in the event of failure and subsequent general anesthesia.

In the event of administering a spinal after epidural analgesia or failed epidural surgical top-up, there is an increased chance of high sensory block, which in severe cases may require respiratory support, compared with a spinal alone[15] (see also Chapter 30). This is likely to be worse after recent large-volume top-ups and concentrated local anesthetic in the top-up, in which case a reduced dose of 0.5% hyperbaric bupivacaine may be appropriate (e.g., 1.5–2 ml). However, if no attempt has been made to top up the epidural for surgery, then the standard dose of bupivacaine is likely to be preferable.

Learning Points

- Many Category I cesarean deliveries do not mandate general anesthesia, but sustained severe fetal bradycardia, especially accompanied by hemorrhage, umbilical cord prolapsed, or uterine scar dehiscence, is a red flag that indicates the likelihood of having to provide general anesthesia.
- Intrauterine resuscitation ensures optimal fetal oxygenation and may "buy time" for safer anesthesia and surgery.
- A well-functioning epidural during labor is a good indicator that it can be topped up rapidly for cesarean delivery.
- Multicompartment block is always possible. Spinal misplacement may only be detected by careful assessment. IV misplacement may be minimal until a forceful high-volume epidural injection is given. The anesthetist should never give a large dose without careful assessment before and during administration and must always be in a position to manage complications of misplacement.
- Spinal anesthesia may be required if the establishment of surgical block with the epidural fails, but it is preferable that concentrated local anesthetic top-ups have not been given before a spinal.
- If regional anesthesia is attempted for the Category I case, always have a backup plan for general anesthesia.

References

1. Panni MK, Segal S. Local anesthetic requirements are greater in dystocia than in normal labor. *Anesthesiology* 2003; **98**:957–63.
2. Alexander JM, Sharma SK, McIntire DD, et al. Intensity of labor pain and cesarean delivery. *Anesth Analg* 2001; **92**:1524–28.
3. Royal College of Obstetricians and Gynaecologists. Classification of urgency of caesarean delivery: a continuum of risk. GP11, 2010. Available at www .rcog.org.uk/classification-of-urgency-of-caesarean -section-good-practice-11 (accessed August 10, 2016).

4. Thurlow JA, Kinsella, SM. Intrauterine resuscitation: active management of fetal distress. *Int J Obstet Anesth* 2002; **11**:105–16.

5. National Institute for Health and Clinical Excellence (NICE). Intrapartum care: care of healthy women and their babies during childbirth, CG190, 2014. Available at www.nice.org.uk/guidance/cg190 (accessed August 10, 2016).

6. Russell IF. Epidural top-ups for Category I/II emergency caesarean section should be given only in the operating theatre. *Int J Obstet Anesth* 2004; **13**:259–65.

7. Moore P. Epidural top-ups for Category I/II emergency caesarean section should be given only in the operating theatre. *Int J Obstet Anesth* 2004; **13**:257–59.

8. Donnelly K, Stonley F, Patel K, et al. Epidural catheter migration during patient controlled epidural analgesia: two cases. *Anaesthesia* 2014; **69**(Suppl 4):26.

9. Gardner IC, Kinsella SM. Obstetric epidural test doses: a survey of UK practice. *Int J Obstet Anesth* 2005; **14**:96–103.

10. Scrutton M, Kinsella SM. Obstetrics, in K. Allman, A. McIndoe, I. Wilson, eds., *Emergencies in Anaesthesia*, 2nd edn. Oxford: Oxford University Press; 2009, pp. 145–78.

11. Hillyard SG, Bate TE, Corcoran TB, Paech MJ, O'Sullivan G. Extending epidural analgesia for emergency caesarean section: a meta-analysis. *Br J Anaesth* 2011; **107**:668–78.

12. Lam DTC, Ngan Kee WD, Khaw KS. Extension of epidural blockade in labour for emergency caesarean section using 2% lidocaine with epinephrine and fentanyl, with or without alkalinisation. *Anaesthesia* 2001; **56**:790–94.

13. Kinsella SM, Girgirah K, Scrutton MJL. Rapid sequence spinal for Category I urgency caesarean section: a case series. *Anaesthesia* 2010; **65**:664–69.

14. Kathirgamanathan A, Douglas MJ, Tyler J, et al. Speed of spinal vs general anaesthesia for Category I caesarean section: a simulation and clinical observation-based study. *Anaesthesia* 2013; **68**:753–59.

15. Stocks GM. Opposer: When using spinal anaesthesia for caesarean section after the epidural has failed, the normal dose of spinal anaesthetic should be used. *Int J Obstet Anesth* 2005; **14**:55–57.

Uterotonic Use

Chiraag Talati and Mrinalini Balki

Case Study

A healthy nulliparous woman was admitted to the delivery suite at 40 weeks' gestation for induction of labor of a postdates pregnancy. During her pregnancy, she developed gestational diabetes mellitus (GDM), managed with dietary control.

Labor was induced with the application of intravaginal dinoprostone gel. Six hours later, on examination, the cervix was 3 cm dilated, and the patient was contracting every 4–6 minutes. She requested labor analgesia, and an epidural was inserted by the anesthetist, which produced satisfactory analgesia.

Due to slow labor progression, augmentation was required, and the patient underwent artificial rupture of membranes (AROM). Following this, a continuous oxytocin infusion at 2 mU/min was started, which was doubled every 30 minutes until a maximum rate of 32 mU/min was administered. Labor progression remained slow, and 12 hours later, the patient's cervix was only 6 cm dilated. She also developed a temperature of 38.5°C and was treated with antibiotics for suspected chorioamnionitis.

A decision was made for cesarean delivery for failure to progress in labor, and the patient's epidural was topped up in the OR. Following delivery of the baby, the obstetrician commented that the uterus was "boggy," and there was active bleeding. Uterine atony was diagnosed. Oxytocin 5 units was administered intravenously as a bolus, and an infusion of 20 units/liter was started. The uterus remained atonic, and the estimated blood loss exceeded 1,200 ml. As a second-line agent, ergonovine 250 µg diluted in 10 ml normal saline, was given slowly intravenously. The obstetrician continued with uterine massage and administered carboprost 250 µg intramyometrially and misoprostol 1,000 µg rectally.

The patient's total blood loss was estimated at 2,000 ml, and she was resuscitated with fluid therapy and blood products. Her uterine tone improved, and her bleeding ceased.

Key Points

- Patients may experience uterine atony secondary to multiple factors, including prolonged augmented labor, GDM, and chorioamnionitis.
- Multiple pharmacologic uterotonics for management of uterine atony may be required, including resuscitative measures for the effective management of postpartum hemorrhage (PPH).

Discussion

Postpartum Hemorrhage and Uterine Atony

The World Health Organization (WHO) defines primary PPH as maternal blood loss of 500 ml or more within 24-hours following birth. PPH is a global problem, with an incidence affecting 2 percent of all deliveries and is responsible for nearly one-quarter of all maternal deaths. Furthermore, the morbidity associated with PPH can be severe and includes hemorrhagic shock, subsequent multiorgan failure, and long-term disability.[1]

The pathogenesis of PPH includes the four *T*'s: *t*one (uterine atony), *t*issue (retained placenta or clots), *t*hrombin (maternal coagulopathy), and *t*rauma (genital tract). Of these, uterine atony is the most common cause, accountable for approximately 75 percent of PPH cases. Numerous factors are associated with uterine atony, and often a parturient may have multiple predisposing conditions (Table 25.1).

Uterotonics

There is significant evidence[2] to suggest that *active management of the third stage of labor* (AMTSL) versus *expectant management* is important in reducing PPH, and this is advocated by several international organizations.[1,3,4] Expectant management is a conservative or *more* physiologic approach, which

Table 25.1 Factors Associated with an Increased Risk of Uterine Atony

Overdistension of uterus	Polyhydramnios
	Multiple gestation
	Macrosomia
Uterine muscle exhaustion	Rapid labor
	Prolonged labor
	High parity
	Intrapartum oxytocin administration
Intra-amniotic infection	Fever
	Prolonged rupture of membranes
Functional/anatomic distortion of the uterus	Fibroids
	Abnormal placentation
	Uterine anomalies
Uterine relaxing medications	Halogenated anesthetics
	Nitroglycerin

Source: Adapted from Society of Obstetricians and Gynaecology of Canada clinical practice guidelines.[3]

awaits the natural separation of the placenta. Conversely, active management requires clinician intervention and encompasses three components following delivery: the administration of prophylactic uterotonic agents, early cord clamping, and controlled traction of the umbilical cord.[2]

On delivery, contraction of the myometrium is essential to ensure that muscle fibers exert tension on the maternal vessels to cause vasoconstriction and limit excessive bleeding.[2] This process can be augmented by the use of uterotonic agents. The WHO guidance advocates that the active management of the third stage of labor, through the administration of prophylactic uterotonics, following *all births* is mandated, and this includes vaginal births and cesarean deliveries.[1]

There are three main classes of uterotonic agents in current clinical practice, all with different mechanisms of actions and adverse effects (Figure 25.1, Table 25.2):

1. Oxytocin and its analogues
2. Ergot alkaloids
3. Prostaglandins

Oxytocin and Its Analogues

Oxytocin is an endogenous hormone synthesized primarily in the hypothalamus and secreted by the posterior lobe of the pituitary gland. It has several roles in the process of reproduction and childbirth, but its effects on myometrial contractility in the peripartum period are of utmost significance. As a result, synthetic oxytocin can be administered exogenously for labor induction, augmentation, and prophylaxis or treatment of PPH. Due to its short duration of action, oxytocin is commonly delivered as a continuous IV infusion.

Carbetocin

This is a synthetic analogue of oxytocin with the advantage of a longer duration of action (4–10 times) than oxytocin and a similar side-effect profile. As a result of its prolonged effect, there is a reduced need for additional uterotonics.[5] The Society of Obstetricians and Gynaecology of Canada has recommended the use of carbetocin as an alternative to a continuous oxytocin infusion in *elective* cesarean deliveries and for vaginal deliveries in parturients with one risk factor for PPH.[3] Carbetocin is approved in 23 countries, including Canada and the United Kingdom, but not in the United States.

Mechanism of Action. Oxytocin and analogues are agonists at the oxytocin receptor (OTR) on the myometrial cell membrane. The OTR is a G protein–coupled receptor that activates phospholipase C (PLC), and this increases the production of inositol triphosphate (InsP3) and diacylglycerol (DAG). InsP3 stimulates release of calcium from the sarcoplasmic reticulum (SR), resulting in an increase in intracellular calcium concentration, and DAG leads to an increase in prostaglandin synthesis. The rise in intracellular calcium levels promotes the formation of the calcium-calmodulin complex and the subsequent interaction of myosin and actin filaments and thus smooth muscle contraction[6] (see Figure 25.1).

Administration. Oxytocin can be administered intravenously as a 5-unit slow bolus, repeated once more if required; intramuscularly (IM) 5–10 units; or as a continuous IV infusion of 20–40 units over a specified duration (2–8 hours depending on institutional policy or the clinical scenario). Carbetocin can be administered 100 µg intravenously as a slow bolus in elective cesarean deliveries or as 100 µg intramuscularly in vaginal deliveries with more than one risk factor for PPH.[3]

Table 25.2 Uterotonic Drugs, Administration Methods, Doses, Onset Time, Duration of Action, Side Effects, and Major Contraindications

Uterotonic drug	Administration	Onset	Duration of action	Side effects	Major contraindications
Oxytocin	IV slow bolus: 5 units over 1 minute (can repeat for a second dose)	IV: <1 minute	IV: 20 minutes	Reduction in SVR (hypotension, tachycardia, arrhythmia)	Hypotension
	IV continuous infusion: 20–40 units (rate as per local policy or clinical scenario)	IM: 3–5 minutes	IM: 30–90 minutes	Nausea and vomiting	Hemodynamic instability
	IM: 5–10 units				
Carbetocin	IV slow bolus: 100 µg over 1 minute	IV: 2 minutes	IV: 60 minutes	Reduction in SVR (hypotension, tachycardia, arrhythmia)	Hypotension
	IM: 100 µg	IM: 2 minutes	IM: 120 minutes	Nausea and vomiting	Hemodynamic instability
Ergonovine maleate	IV: 200–250 µg, slow, diluted over 1 minute	IV: <1 minute	IV: 45 minutes	Hypertension	Hypertension (pregnancy induced, preeclampsia, or preexisting)
				Nausea and vomiting	
	M: 200–250 µg (can repeat second dose after 2 hours)	2–3 minutes	3 hours	Increased risk of retained placenta	Myocardial ischemia
					Porphyria
Methylergonovine	IM: 200 µg	As per ergonovine maleate			
	IV: 200 µg, slow, diluted, over 1 minute				
Carboprost tromethamine (15-methyl PGF$_{2\alpha}$)	IM: 250 µg	IM: 3–5 minutes	IM: 60–120 minutes	Bronchospasm	Asthma
	Intramyometrial: 250 µg (unlicensed use) (Can repeat every 15 minutes; total of 8 doses; 2 mg maximum)	IMM: No data	IMM: No data	Nausea and vomiting	Caution in hepatic, renal, or cardiac disease
				Headaches	
				Shivering	
Misoprostol (PGE$_1$ analogue)	PO, SL, PV or PR: 600–1,000 µg	PO: 8 minutes	PO: 120 minutes	Pyrexia	
		SL: 11 minutes	SL: 180 minutes	Diarrhea	
		PV: 20 minutes	PV: 240 minutes	Nausea and vomiting	
		PR: 100 minutes	PR: 240 minutes	(All side effects less with PR)	
Syntometrine	IM: oxytocin 5 units + ergonovine 500 µg	As per oxytocin and ergonovine			

Abbreviations: IV, intravenously; IM, intramuscularly; IMM, intramyometrial; SVR, systemic vascular resistance; PO, per oral; SL, sublingual; PV, per vagina; PR, per rectum.

Sources: Data from refs. [13–21]

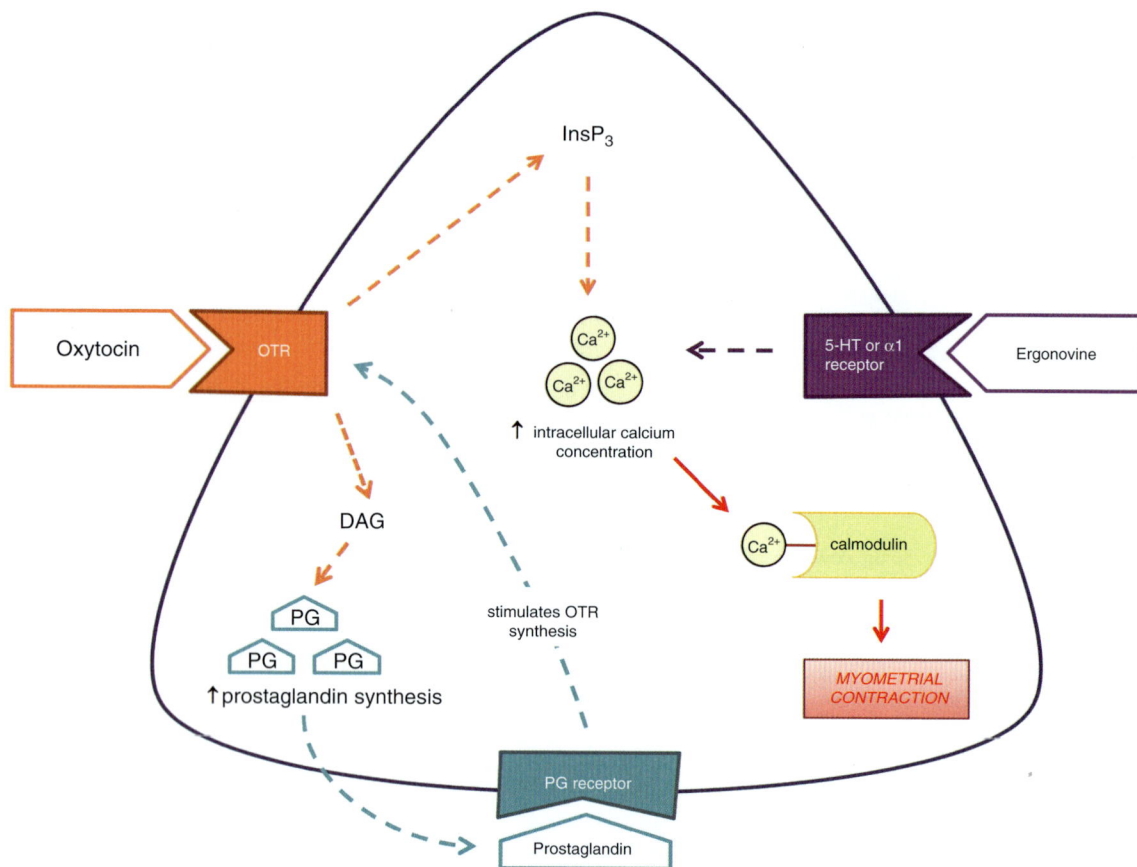

Figure 25.1 Schematic illustration of uterotonic mechanisms leading to myometrial cell contraction. Oxytocin binds to the OTR, which leads to an increase in the production of InsP3 and DAG. InsP3 stimulates the release of calcium from internal stores, and this promotes the formation of the calcium–calmodulin complex and ultimately smooth muscle contraction. DAG increases PG synthesis. Prostaglandin analogues bind to the PG receptor, which stimulates synthesis of the OTR. Ergonovine binds to either the 5-HT or α_1-receptor, which leads to a rise in intracellular calcium.

Abbreviations: OTR, oxytocin receptor; InsP3, inositol triphosphate; Ca^{2+}, calcium; PG, prostaglandin; 5-HT, 5-hydroxytryptamine; α_1, alpha-1.

Common Side Effects. Oxytocin and analogues can cause several unwanted cardiovascular effects, usually secondary to a reduction in systemic vascular resistance (SVR), including hypotension, tachycardia, myocardial ischemia, arrhythmias, and rarely, cardiac arrest. It can also cause free water retention, nausea, and vomiting.

Ergot Alkaloids

Ergonovine maleate and methylergonovine are ergot alkaloid derivatives[7] that have the ability to initiate strong tonic contractions of the uterus.

Mechanism of Action. This is poorly understood, although is likely to be a combination of its actions as an agonist at α-adrenoceptors and 5-HT receptors

on the myometrium, resulting in a rise in intracellular calcium.[7]

Administration. Ergonovine maleate 200–250 μg and methylergonovine 200 μg can be administered either intramuscularly or slowly and diluted intravenously. Ergot alkaloids need to be refrigerated at 2–8°C and protected from sunlight for better stability.

Common Side Effects. Most notably hypertension and severe nausea and vomiting are common.

Prostaglandins

Prostaglandins are endogenous lipid compounds derived from fatty acid precursors. Carboprost tromethamine, a methylated synthetic analogue of

$PGF_{2\alpha}$, and misoprostol, a synthetic analogue of PGE_1, are used commonly in clinical practice.

Mechanism of Action. Prostaglandins exert their effects via prostaglandin receptors found in the myometrium, which are G protein–coupled receptors. Prostaglandins stimulate the production of the OTR and a rise in intracellular calcium concentration.

Administration. Carboprost 250 µg can be administered intramuscularly or intramyometrially (unlicensed route) every 15 minutes if required, up to a total of 2 mg maximum. Misoprostol can be given 600–1000 µg via the oral, sublingual, rectal or vaginal routes.

Common Side Effects. Most notably shivering, headaches, and bronchospasm are seen with carboprost and pyrexia and diarrhea with misoprostol.

What, Where, and When?

The WHO guidance indicates that as a first-line agent, prophylactic oxytocin should be offered to all women following delivery to prevent PPH. If oxytocin is not available, provided that there are no major contraindications, either ergonovine or a combination of oxytocin/ergonovine should be administered.[1] In the home birth setting, where injectable uterotonics may not be accessible, misoprostol orally or rectally could be used, although this may not be as effective as oxytocin.[4]

In the setting of uterine atony and PPH, several steps need to be undertaken, including pharmacotherapy, surgical measures, and ongoing resuscitation. In terms of pharmacologic agents, more than one uterotonic drug may be required, and clinical judgment will need to be applied. However, a logical sequence, provided that there are no contraindications, would be as follows:[3,4]

- Oxytocin 5 units slow IV bolus over 1 minute; a second bolus may be required.
- Oxytocin 20–40 units IV infusion; range can vary depending on institutional policy or clinical scenario.
- Ergonovine 200–250 µg intramuscularly or a slow, diluted IV infusion; may be repeated after 2 hours (avoid in hypertension).
- Carboprost 250 µg intramuscularly or a direct intramyometrial injection; can be repeated at least eight times, with a minimum of 15-minute intervals (avoid in asthma).
- Misoprostol 600–1,000 µg rectally.

Current Controversies and Future Directions

Despite the existence of several uterotonic classes and agents, PPH continues to be a considerable determinant of maternal morbidity and mortality. Therefore, the subject of uterotonics remains an exciting area of research.

Oxytocin is typically the first-line agent in the prevention and treatment of PPH, but there is wide heterogeneity among physicians and institutions with regard to the choice of a second uterotonic. A recent retrospective nationwide study in the United States has confirmed this wide interhospital variation,[8] and a consensus is still awaited.

Recently, carbetocin, an oxytocin analogue, has been developed, with the advantage of providing sustained myometrial contractility when compared with oxytocin and therefore avoiding the need for a continuous infusion. A Cochrane review has concluded that when compared with oxytocin in cesarean deliveries, there is less requirement for further uterotonics with carbetocin, but there is no difference in the incidence of PPH.[9] Studies have shown that the adverse effects of carbetocin 100 µg IV are comparable with those of oxytocin 5 units IV.[10]

Furthermore, the exact dose and route of administration of uterotonic drugs also remain controversial. In elective cesarean deliveries and cesarean deliveries following labor arrest, the ED_{90} of an oxytocin IV bolus to produce effective uterine contractility was 0.35 unit (95% confidence interval [CI] 0.18–0.52 units)[11] and 2.99 units (95% CI 2.32–3.67 units),[12] respectively. As is evident, the dose can vary 10-fold depending on the type of patient population, and slow administration of a small 1- to 3-unit bolus should be sufficient during cesarean delivery for the prevention of uterine atony in most cases, with minimal adverse effects. However, despite this, most guidelines still recommend a slow IV bolus dose of 5 units. A recent study in elective cesarean deliveries demonstrated the ED_{90} of carbetocin as 14.8 µg (95% CI 13.7–15.8 µg),[5] which is less than one-fifth the current recommended dose (100 µg).[3] The use of carbetocin during cesarean delivery in laboring patients requires further investigation.

A final hot topic remains the phenomenon of OTR desensitization. Following prolonged exposure to oxytocin in an augmented labor, the oxytocin receptors undergo downregulation, and subsequent administration of oxytocin after delivery results in less effective uterine contractility. Certainly this is a significant risk factor for PPH, and the modification of labor augmentation regimens, with an aim toward attenuating OTR downregulation, requires further investigation.

Further research is required to investigate how different uterotonics compare with each other and whether they exhibit any synergistic effect.

Learning Points

- Uterine atony is the most common cause of PPH, and the etiology is multifactorial.
- There are several pharmacologic agents that can enhance uterine tone, and in severe PPH, a multimodal approach is indicated.
- Administration of individual uterotonic agents should be based on clinical judgment after careful consideration of benefits and adverse effects.
- There is no universal consensus on the selection of exact dosing, routes of administration, and second- or third-line uterotonic agents in the prevention or treatment of PPH. However, it is the authors' preference to consider a slow IV oxytocin bolus and continuous IV infusion as first line, ergonovine as second line, and carboprost and misoprostol thereafter, provided that there are no contraindications.
- Patients should be closely monitored for hemodynamic and respiratory changes during the administration of these medications. The important adverse effects include hypotension with oxytocin, hypertension with ergonovine, and bronchospasm with carboprost.

References

1. Gulmezoglu AM, Souza JP, Mathai M. *WHO Recommendations for the Prevention and Treatment of Postpartum Haemorrhage*. Brussels: World Health Organization; 2012.

2. Begley CM, Gyte GML, Devane D, et al. Active versus expectant management for women in the third stage of labour (review). *Cochrane Database Syst Rev* 2011; (11): CD007412.

3. Leduc D, Senikas V, Lalonde AB. Active management of the third stage of labour: prevention and treatment of postpartum hemorrhage. *J Obstet Gynaecol Can* 2009; **31**:980–93.

4. Mavrides E, Allard S, Chandraharan E, et al. on behalf of the Royal College of Obstetricians and Gynaecologists. Prevention and management of postpartum haemorrhage. *BJOG* 2016; **124**:e106–49. Available at www.rcog.org.uk/globalassets/docu ments/guidelines/gt52postpartumhaemorrhage0411 .pdf (accessed October 8, 2018).

5. Khan M,. Balki M., Ahmed I, et al. Carbetocin at elective cesarean delivery: a sequential allocation trial to determine the minimum effective dose. *Can J Anaesth* 2014; **61**:242–48.

6. Balki M, Tsen L. Oxytocin protocols for cesarean delivery. *Int Anesthesiol Clin* 2014; **52**:48–66

7. Rang HP, Dale MM, Ritter JM, et al. The reproductive system, in Rang HP, Dale MM, Ritter JM, et al., eds., *Rang and Dale's Pharmacology*, 7th edn. London: Churchill Livingstone; 2011, pp. 427–28.

8. Bateman BT, Tsen LC, Liu J, et al. Patterns of second-line uterotonic use in a large sample of hospitalizations for childbirth in the United States: 2007–2011. *Anesth Analg* 2014; **119**:1344–49.

9. Su LL,Chong YS, Samuel M. Carbetocin for preventing postpartum haemorrhage. *Cochrane Database Syst Rev* 2012; (4):CD005457.

10. Moertl MG, Friedrich S, Kraschl J, et al. Hemodynamic effects of carbetocin and oxytocin given as intravenous bolus on women undergoing caesarean delivery: a randomized trial. *BJOG* 2011; **118**:1349–56.

11. Carvalho JCA, Balki M, Kingdom J, et al. Oxytocin requirements at elective cesarean delivery: a dose-finding study. *Obstet Gynecol* 2004; **104**: 1005–10.

12. Balki M, Ronayne M, Davies S, et al. Minimum oxytocin dose requirement after cesarean delivery for labor arrest. *Obstet Gynecol* 2006; **107**:45–50.

13. Gizzo S, Patrelli TS, Di Gangi S, et al. Which uterotonic is better to prevent postpartum hemorrhage? Latest news in terms of clinical efficacy, side effects and contraindications: a systematic review. *Reprod Sci* 2013; **20**:1011–19.

14. Langsam Y. Oxytocin, 2012. Available at http://eilat .sci.brooklyn.cuny.edu/newnyc/DRUGS/OXYTOCIN .HTM (accessed December 15, 2014).

15. Canadian Pharmacist Association. e-Therapeutics, 2014. Available at www.e-therapeutics.ca/home .whatsnew.action (accessed December 15, 2014).

16. Herbert WNP, Zelop CM. ACOG practice bulletin: clinical management guidelines for obstetrician-gynaecologists. *Obstet Gynecol* 2006; **108**:1039–47.

17. Anderson LA, Stewart J, Thornton P, et al. Drugs.com, 2000. Available at www.drugs.com (accessed December 15, 2014).

18. Tang OS, Gemzell-Danielsson K, Ho, PC. Misoprostol: pharmacokinetic profiles, effects on the uterus and side effects. *Int J Gynecol Obstet* 2007; **99**: S160-67.

19. Schimmer BP, Parker KL. Contraception and pharmacotherapy of obstetrical and gynecological disorders, in Brunton L, Chabner B, Knollman B., eds., *Goodman & Gilman's the Pharmacological Basis of Therapeutics*, 12th edn. New York, NY: McGraw-Hill Medical; 2011.

20. Lexicomp Online, Hudson, OH, 2014. Available at http ://online.lexi.com/lco/action/home/switch (accessed December 15, 2014).

21. McEvoy GK, ed. *AHFS: Drug Information*. Bethesda, MD: American Society of Health-System Pharmacists; 2014. Available at www.ahfsdruginformation.com (accessed December 15, 2014).

Postpartum Sterilization/Tubal Ligation

Christopher R. Cambic

Case Study

A 36-year-old woman at 39 weeks' gestation presented in spontaneous labor. Her initial cervical examination showed 3 cm of dilation and 80 percent effacement, and she was contracting every 3 minutes. Her medical history was significant for two prior spontaneous vaginal deliveries, for which she received epidural analgesia. The rest of her history, physical examination, and airway examination were unremarkable.

Pain relief was requested, and an epidural technique was performed without difficulty. Patient-controlled epidural analgesia was started with an infusion of 0.1% bupivacaine and 2 µg/ml fentanyl, resulting in adequate labor analgesia. During the course of labor, the patient required one manual epidural bolus of 10 ml of 0.125% bupivacaine due to an inadequate sensory level. Twenty minutes after this bolus, the patient reported adequate analgesia and was found to have a T7 level to cold bilaterally.

The rest of the patient's labor course proceeded uneventfully, resulting in a vaginal delivery. One hour after delivery, the patient proceeded to the OR for a postpartum tubal ligation. The epidural catheter was incrementally dosed with a 20-ml mixture of 2% lidocaine, 1:200,000 epinephrine, and 2 ml sodium bicarbonate. Twenty minutes later, the patient had a T10 sensory level to pinprick bilaterally, and an additional 10 ml of the lidocaine, epinephrine, bicarbonate mixture was administered, resulting in a T7 sensory level to pinprick bilaterally. Because of the inadequate surgical anesthesia, a decision was made to proceed with general anesthesia. After administration of sodium citrate and preoxygenation, rapid-sequence induction was performed, and the patient was intubated. The rest of the procedure proceeded uneventfully.

Key Points

- Despite requiring one additional clinician-administered epidural bolus of medication, this patient's epidural catheter appeared to be functioning appropriately for labor analgesia.
- Because a functioning labor epidural catheter was a convenient option for providing a surgical level of anesthesia for this patient, the anesthesia provider bolused the catheter with an appropriate dose of local anesthetic.
- However, when surgical anesthesia was not achieved after epidural administration of 30 ml 2% lidocaine with epinephrine 1:200,000 and 2 ml sodium bicarbonate, general anesthesia was administered to enable completion of the procedure.

Discussion

Tubal sterilization is a highly effective form of female birth control, with a failure rate of less than 1 percent.[1] Performing tubal sterilizations during the postpartum period offers several surgical, anesthetic, and socioeconomic advantages, as well as some disadvantages[2–4] (Table 26.1). With the advantages outweighing the disadvantages, it is not surprising that more than 50 percent of tubal sterilizations are performed during the early postpartum period, resulting in obstetric anesthesia providers being frequently called on to provide care for this procedure.[2]

The American Society of Anesthesiologists (ASA) Task Force on Obstetric Anesthesia has published guidelines for the anesthetic management of obstetric patients undergoing postpartum tubal sterilizations[5] (Table 26.2). These guidelines are meant to assist the anesthesia provider in the optimal management of this patient population. In addition to these guidelines, all anesthesia providers should review each patient's peripartum course (including blood loss from delivery) prior to proceeding with the procedure because changes may have occurred in the interim. Finally, because pregnancy-induced physiologic changes persist into the postpartum period, anesthesia providers need to

Table 26.1 Advantages and Disadvantages of Postpartum Tubal Sterilization

Advantages	Disadvantages
• Fallopian tubes are located below the abdominal wall at the level of the umbilicus, allowing for easy access.	• Increased risk of regret, especially if the patient is 30 years old or younger or reports substantial conflict with her partner prior to the procedure.
• Abdominal wall laxity allows for manipulation of the incision to be located above each uterine cornu.	• May have inadequate time to allow for proper newborn assessment after vaginal or cesarean delivery.
• Lower failure rate (7.5 pregnancies/1,000 sterilizations) compared with procedures performed more than 6 to 8 weeks postpartum.	• May not be safe in some women with obstetric complications (e.g., uterine atony, postpartum hemorrhage) or comorbid medical conditions (e.g., peripartum cardiomyopathy, mitral stenosis).
• If parturient has a functioning epidural catheter in place for labor analgesia, it can be easily dosed to achieve a surgical level of anesthesia, eliminating the need for a second anesthetic.	
• Patient is already an inpatient, forgoing the additional inconvenience and cost of a second hospital visit.	
• Decreased socioeconomic burden if women who request a postpartum tubal ligation actually receive the procedure because women who request this procedure and do not receive it are more likely to become pregnant again within 1 year of delivery.	

Table 26.2 American Society of Anesthesiologist Guidelines for Optimal Management of Patients Undergoing Postpartum Tubal Sterilization[5]

- For postpartum tubal ligation, the patient should have no oral intake of solid foods within 6–8 hours of the surgery depending on the type of food ingested (e.g., fat content).
- Aspiration prophylaxis should be considered.
- Neuraxial techniques are preferred to general anesthesia for most postpartum tubal ligations. The anesthesia provider should be aware that gastric emptying will be delayed in patients who have received opioids during labor and that an epidural catheter may be more likely to fail with longer postdelivery time.
- If a postpartum tubal ligation is to be performed before the patient is discharged from the hospital, the procedure should not be attempted at a time when it might compromise other aspects of patient care on the labor and delivery unit.
- A basic preoperative evaluation should be performed for any obstetric patient before providing anesthesia care, including (a) maternal health and anesthetic history, (b) relevant obstetric history, and (c) baseline blood pressure measurement, as well as airway, heart, lung, and back examinations.

be aware of these changes and their impact on anesthetic management (Table 26.3).

Both neuraxial and general anesthesia may be used successfully for postpartum tubal sterilization. The decision of which anesthetic technique to use depends on several factors, including patient and provider preference, time interval between delivery and tubal sterilization, obstetric and anesthetic risk factors, and presence of a functioning epidural catheter.

Neuraxial anesthesia represents the most common anesthetic technique for postpartum tubal sterilizations in the United States.[6] Compared with general anesthesia, advantages of a neuraxial technique include the ability to maintain an intact airway reflexes to protect against gastric aspiration, avoidance of airway manipulation and maternal hypoventilation, and lack of volatile agent–induced uterine atony. For women who received labor epidural analgesia, additional benefits include use of the epidural catheter for surgical anesthesia and the ability to provide effective postoperative analgesia. Regardless of which neuraxial technique is used, a T4 sensory level is required to block visceral stimulation from fallopian tube manipulation.

The chief benefit of an epidural technique for these procedures is that a functioning labor epidural catheter can easily be augmented to a surgical level of anesthesia, obviating the need to perform another anesthetic technique. However, ASA guidelines suggest that epidural catheters placed for labor may be more likely to fail with longer delivery-to-reactivation intervals.[5] This observation is supported by several studies suggesting a lower likelihood of failed epidural catheter reactivation when the delivery-to-reactivation interval is less than 4–8 hours in

Table 26.3 Postpartum Physiologic Changes and Their Anesthetic Implications

Organ system	Physiologic changes	Anesthetic implications
Cardiovascular	• Immediately after delivery, cardiac output increases by as much as 75 percent of prelabor values due to relief of vena caval compression and an increase in central blood volume. • Cardiac output returns to prelabor values approximately 24 hours after delivery but does not return to prepregnancy values until 12–24 weeks postpartum. • Heart rate decreases significantly after delivery due to increased venous return and decreased sympathetic drive but does not reach prepregnancy values until 2 weeks postpartum.	• Patients who have cardiovascular disease (e.g., peripartum cardiomyopathy, mitral stenosis) may deteriorate in their hemodynamic status, making it unsafe to proceed with postpartum tubal sterilization. • Due to increases in central blood volume and cardiac output, postpartum patients are able to better tolerate larger blood losses compared with nonpregnant patients.
Respiratory	• Elevations in minute ventilation and oxygen consumption persist up to 6–8 weeks postpartum. • Functional residual capacity increases after delivery due to decreased impact of gravid uterus on the diaphragm but does not return to prepregnancy values until 1–2 weeks postpartum • Normal changes in Mallampati classification during labor can persist for up to 48 hours after delivery.	• Postpartum patients continue to have an increased risk of rapid oxygen desaturation during periods of apnea. • Increased risks of difficult mask ventilation and/or intubation persist during the postpartum period due to vascular engorgement and edema of the oropharynx, larynx, and trachea. • A smaller endotracheal tube size may be required due to edema of the vocal cords and glottic opening.
Gastrointestinal	• Pregnancy-induced decreases in lower esophageal barrier pressure do not resolve until 1–4 weeks postpartum. • Gastric emptying is likely delayed during the immediate postpartum period, especially if intrapartum opioids were administered. • The type of substance ingested (i.e., liquids versus solids) likely affects gastric volume and rate of gastric emptying.	• Parturients remain at increased risk for aspiration of gastric contents during the immediate postpartum period (18–24 hours). • Administration of aspiration prophylaxis (e.g., prokinetic agent, nonparticulate antacid, and/or H_2-receptor antagonist) is recommended, especially in patients with conditions known to increase the risk of gastric aspiration. • Adherence to an NPO requirement of 6–8 hours for solids and 2 hours for clear liquids is recommended.
Neurologic/metabolic	• Serum progesterone concentrations begin to decrease after removal of the placenta and reach nonpregnant levels by 24–72 hours postpartum. • Pseudocholinesterase activity decrease by 33 percent at 3 days postpartum and does not return to nonpregnant values until 2–6 weeks after delivery.	• Compared with pregnant patients, postpartum women require increased doses of local anesthetic for spinal and epidural anesthesia. • Increased minimum alveolar concentration requirements of volatile anesthetics are seen in postpartum parturients undergoing general anesthesia. • Increased duration of action of succinylcholine and mivacurium in the postpartum period may prolong recovery from neuromuscular blockade.

duration.[7–9] Overall, successful epidural reactivation is seen in 74–95 percent of catheters, with the highest success rate occurring when the block is extended less than 4 hours after delivery.[7–9]

One reason why epidural catheters reactivated at longer intervals have a higher failure rate is the larger incidence of catheter migration or dislodgement observed. In the peripartum period, significant catheter migration occurs in 36–54 percent of patients.[10,11] Single-orifice epidural catheters tend to have a higher rate of dislodgement when inserted 2 cm within the epidural space but a higher risk of unilateral block when inserted 6–8 cm.[12] For multiorifice epidural catheters, insertion of catheters 5 cm in the epidural space is associated with the highest incidence of satisfactory labor analgesia.[13] Therefore, to optimize the success rate of epidural catheter reactivation for postpartum tubal sterilization, insertion of the epidural catheter 4–6 cm within the epidural space is recommended. Additionally, securing the epidural catheter to the skin when the patient is in a nonflexed position is recommended, especially in obese parturients, because catheter position within the epidural space may change significantly when the patient moves from the flexed position.[14]

As demonstrated in the Case Study, some patients with functioning labor epidural catheters that are reactivated within a reasonable time interval may still not achieve a surgical level of anesthesia. Anesthetic options for this scenario include placement of a spinal anesthetic, replacement of the epidural catheter, a combined spinal-epidural technique, or general anesthesia. Each of these options has its own inherent benefits and risks.

Use of a spinal anesthetic technique after epidural catheter failure is controversial. Compared with an epidural technique, benefits of this technique include higher reliability, faster onset, denser sensory block, and lower local anesthetic doses. However, the exact dose of intrathecal local anesthetic required to achieve a surgical level of anesthesia in this scenario is difficult to predict and depends on several factors, including epidural space distension and its effect on intrathecal drug distribution, interpatient variability in response to intrathecally and epidurally administered medications, and patient body habitus.[15,16] Additionally, due to declining maternal progesterone levels, postpartum patients typically require higher doses of local anesthetics to achieve an adequate surgical level of anesthesia compared with pregnant patients.[17] Consequently, if the amount of intrathecal medication administered is not enough to achieve surgical anesthesia, the patient will likely need to undergo general anesthesia.

The more concerning issue with placement of a spinal anesthetic after failed epidural catheter reactivation is the occurrence of high or total spinal anesthesia. Several case reports have described the occurrence of total spinal anesthesia in this scenario, with a reported incidence of 0.8–11 percent.[15,18] Mechanisms for this increased risk include decreased size of the intrathecal space due to epidural space distension, passage of epidural medications through a dural hole from the subsequent spinal, and diffusion of epidural medications into the intrathecal space. Several techniques have been proposed to avoid high spinals in this scenario, but none has been demonstrated to decrease the incidence of total spinal anesthesia or conversion to general anesthesia.[19,20]

For situations in which reactivation of the epidural catheter has failed, replacement of the epidural catheter is another option. Benefits of this technique include extension of anesthesia for longer procedures and use of the epidural catheter for postoperative analgesia. However, these benefits are likely not to be clinically useful because postpartum tubal sterilizations are relatively short procedures compared with other operations, and postoperative pain requirements are moderate in intensity and often well controlled with systemic multimodal analgesia. The downsides of replacing the epidural catheter, however, are more clinically significant and potentially have a greater impact on patient safety. These drawbacks include increased risk of local anesthetic toxicity (especially if a large volume of local anesthetic has already been administered), failure of the replaced epidural catheter, and prolonged time to achieving adequate surgical anesthesia.

A combined spinal-epidural (CSE) technique using a lower intrathecal dose of local anesthetic is a third option. Use of this technique will likely decrease the risk of total spinal anesthesia but still allow for additional epidural dosing if the spinal component is inadequate for surgery or if the procedure lasts longer than expected. However, opponents of this technique voice concern about the presence of an "untested" epidural catheter. While this is a theoretical concern, evidence suggests a lower incidence of rescue analgesia with a CSE versus an epidural technique because the anesthesia provider is able to confirm placement of the epidural needle within the epidural space by obtaining CSF through the spinal needle.[21,22]

Although there is insufficient evidence to compare the benefits of neuraxial anesthesia versus general anesthesia for postpartum tubal sterilizations, there are certain situations (e.g., patient preference, coagulopathy) in which general anesthesia may be superior.[5] If general anesthesia is selected, several considerations must be taken into account. First, pregnancy-induced changes in pharmacokinetics are likely to still be present and affect anesthetic management. In particular, decreases in minimum alveolar concentration requirements, as well as changes in the response of postpartum patients to depolarizing and nondepolarizing neuromuscular blockers, will likely affect management of these patients under general anesthesia.[23,24] Second, changes in cardiopulmonary physiology not only may affect a patient's hemodynamics under general anesthesia but also may make mask ventilation and intubation difficult. Third, alterations in gastric physiology may increase a postpartum patient's risk of aspiration. As such, providers should treat the patient as a "full stomach" patient by adhering to NPO requirements, administrating gastric acid prophylaxis, and using a rapid-sequence induction technique with cricoid pressure, at least on the first postpartum day (gastric emptying appears to be normal on the second day). Finally, standard ASA monitors should be used for all patients, especially monitors for oxygenation and ventilation, to help decrease the morbidity and mortality associated with general anesthesia.

Propofol presents an excellent pharmaceutical option for the induction of general anesthesia in this patient population. With its reliable fast onset of action and rapid recovery, propofol has been shown to have similar pharmacokinetics during both the intrapartum and postpartum periods.[25] Thiopental also has a long history of efficacy and safety as an induction agent in the obstetric patient population, but its lack of access, especially in the United States, may limit its use.[26]

Maintenance of general anesthesia for postpartum tubal ligations can be done either by a total IV technique or with volatile halogenated agents. One significant downside of using volatile agents during the immediate postpartum period is their ability to cause uterine relaxation in a dose-dependent fashion, thereby increasing the risk of postpartum hemorrhage (PPH).[27] In order to minimize this risk, anesthesia providers could use 1.0 minimum alveolar concentration (MAC) or less of volatile agent and supplement with IV agents as needed to decrease the risk of intraoperative recall during these procedures. It is unclear how long after delivery the risk of volatile agent–induced PPH persists.

Succinylcholine is often used for muscle relaxation for postpartum tubal sterilization due to its rapid onset and offset of action. Compared with nonpregnant women, parturients show lower activity of pseudocholinesterase, which reaches its nadir around postpartum day 3.[28] Clinically, this results in a 25 percent prolonged recovery time from succinylcholine-induced muscle relaxation in postpartum women.[29] This prolonged recovery time may be especially important in "cannot intubate/cannot ventilate" scenarios, where rapid recovery from the effects of succinylcholine is essential. Conversely, nondepolarizing muscle relaxants exhibit a mixed response in postpartum patients. Compared with its use in nonpregnant control individuals, vecuronium

demonstrates greater than 50 percent prolongation of action during the postpartum period, whereas rocuronium shows no change in its duration of action, and cisatracurium has a shorter duration due to increased elimination and clearance from pregnancy-induced physiologic changes.[30–32]

Postoperative analgesia is ideally achieved with multimodal analgesia, typically using a combination of oral and/or parental opioids and nonsteroidal anti-inflammatory drugs. This method results in improved pain control and patient satisfaction, minimizes opioid-related side effects, and promotes earlier hospital discharge.[33] The use of neuraxial morphine for postoperative analgesia has also been shown to provide effective analgesia after postpartum tubal sterilizations.[34,35] However, the benefits of neuraxially administered morphine need to be weighed against the increased risk of nausea, vomiting, and pruritus, as well as the need for a 24-hour period of observation after administration to monitor for delayed respiratory depression.[34–36]

Learning Points

- Pregnancy-induced physiologic changes persist into the postpartum period and may have an impact on anesthetic management of patients undergoing postpartum tubal sterilizations.
- Although neuraxial and general anesthesia may be used for postpartum tubal sterilization, neuraxial techniques are preferred. A T4 sensory level is required to block visceral stimulation.
- Functioning epidural catheters are more likely to fail with longer delivery-to-reactivation intervals. Anesthetic management options for failed epidural catheters include replacement of the epidural catheter, spinal anesthesia, combined spinal-epidural technique, or general anesthesia.
- Pregnancy-induced changes in the MAC of volatile anesthetics and pharmacokinetic activity of neuromuscular blockers should be taken into account when using general anesthesia for postpartum tubal sterilization.
- Postoperative analgesia is ideally achieved with a multimodal technique, including opioids and nonsteroidal anti-inflammatory drugs.

References

1. Peterson HB, Xia Z, Hughes JM, et al. The risk of pregnancy after tubal sterilization: findings from the

U.S. Collaborative Review of Sterilization. *Am J Obstet Gynecol* 1996; **174**:1161–68.

2. Chan LM, Westhoff CL. Tubal sterilization trends in the United States. *Fertil Steril* 2010; **94**:1–6.

3. Hillis SD, Marchbanks PA, Tylor LR, et al. Poststerilization regret: findings from the United States Collaborative Review of Sterilization. *Obstet Gynecol* 1999; **93**:889–95.

4. Thurman AR, Janecek T. One-year follow-up of women with unfulfilled postpartum sterilization requests. *Obstet Gynecol* 2010; **116**:1071–77.

5. American Society of Anesthesiologists Task Force on Obstetric Anesthesia and The Society for Obstetric Anesthesia and Perinatology. Practice guidelines for obstetric anesthesia: an updated report by the American Society of Anesthesiologists Task Force on Obstetric Anesthesia and The Society for Obstetric Anesthesia and Perinatology. *Anesthesiology* 2016; **124**:270–300.

6. Pati S, Cullins V. Female sterilization: evidence. *Obstet Gynecol Clin North Am* 2000; **27**:859–99.

7. Vincent RD Jr, Reid RW. Epidural anesthesia for postpartum tubal ligation using epidural catheters placed during labor. *J Clin Anesth* 1993; **5**:289–91.

8. Viscomi CM, Rathmell JP. Labor epidural catheter reactivation or spinal anesthesia for delayed postpartum tubal ligation: a cost comparison. *J Clin Anesth* 1995; **7**:380–83.

9. Goodman EJ, Dumas SD. The rate of successful reactivation of labor epidural catheters for postpartum tubal ligation surgery. *Reg Anesth Pain Med* 1998; **23**:258–61.

10. Bishton IM, Martin PH, Vernon JM, et al. Factors influencing epidural catheter migration. *Anaesthesia* 1992; **47**:610–12.

11. Phillips DC, Macdonald R. Epidural catheter migration during labour. *Anaesthesia* 1987; **42**:661–63.

12. D'Angelo R, Berkebile BL, Gerancher JC. Prospective examination of epidural catheter insertion. *Anesthesiology* 1996; **84**:88–93.

13. Beilin Y, Bernstein HH, Zucker-Pinchoff B. The optimal distance that a multiorifice epidural catheter should be threaded into the epidural space. *Anesth Analg* 1995; **81**:301–4.

14. Hamilton CL, Riley ET, Cohen SE. Changes in the position of epidural catheters associated with patient movement. *Anesthesiology* 1997; **86**:778–84.

15. Furst SR, Reisner LS. Risk of high spinal anesthesia following failed epidural block for cesarean delivery. *J Clin Anesth* 1995; **7**:71–74.

16. Hogan QH, Prost R, Kulier A, et al. Magnetic resonance imaging of cerebrospinal fluid volume and the influence of body habitus and abdominal pressure. *Anesthesiology* 1996; **84**:1341–49.

17. Datta S, Hurley RJ, Naulty JS, et al. Plasma and cerebrospinal fluid progesterone concentrations in pregnant and nonpregnant women. *Anesth Analg* 1986; **65**:950–54.

18. Visser WA, Dijkstra A, Albayrak M, et al. Spinal anaesthesia for intrapartum caesarean delivery following epidural labor analgesia: a retrospective cohort study. *Can J Anaesth* 2009; **56**:577–83.

19. Portnoy D, Vadhera RB. Mechanisms and management of an incomplete epidural block for cesarean section. *Anesthesiol Clin North Am* 2003; **21**:39–57.

20. Dadarkar P, Philip J, Weidner C, et al. Spinal anesthesia for cesarean section following inadequate labor epidural analgesia: a retrospective audit. *Int J Obstet Anesth* 2004; **13**:239–43.

21. Simmons SW, Taghizadeh N, Dennis AT, et al. Combined spinal-epidural versus epidural analgesia in labour. *Cochrane Database Syst Rev* 2012; (10): CD003401.

22. Norris MC. Are combined spinal-epidural catheters reliable? *Int J Obstet Anesth* 2000; **9**:3–6.

23. Zhou HH, Norman P, DeLima LG, et al. The minimum alveolar concentration of isoflurane in patients undergoing bilateral tubal ligation in the postpartum period. *Anesthesiology* 1995; **82**:1364–68.

24. Chan MT, Gin T. Postpartum changes in the minimum alveolar concentration of isoflurane. *Anesthesiology* 1995; **82**:1360–63.

25. Gin T, Yau G, Jong W, et al. Disposition of propofol at caesarean section and in the postpartum period. *Br J Anaesth* 1991; **67**:49–53.

26. De Oliveira GS Jr, Theilken LS, McCarthy RJ. Shortage of perioperative drugs: implications for anesthesia practice and patient safety. *Anesth Analg* 2011; **113**:1429–35.

27. Chang CC, Wang IT, Chen YH, et al. Anesthetic management as a risk factor for postpartum hemorrhage after cesarean deliveries. *Am J Obstet Gynecol* 2011; **205**:462e1–7.

28. Shnider SM. Serum chlonesterase activity during pregnancy, labor and the puerperium. *Anesthesiology* 1965; **26**:335–39.

29. Leighton BL, Cheek TG, Gross JB, et al. Succinylcholine pharmacodynamics in peripartum patients. *Anesthesiology* 1986; **64**:202–5.

30. Khuenl-Brady KS, Koller J, Mair P, et al. Comparison of vecuronium- and atracurium-induced neuromuscular blockade in postpartum and nonpregnant patients. *Anesth Analg* 1991; **72**:110–13.

31. Gin T, Derrick JL, Chan MT, et al. Postpartum patients have slightly prolonged neuromuscular block after mivacurium. *Anesth Analg* 1998; **86**:82–85.

32. Gin T, Chan MT, Chan KL, et al. Prolonged neuromuscular block after rocuronium in postpartum patients. *Anesth Analg* 2002; **94**:686–89.

33. White PF, Kehlet H, Neal JM, et al. The role of the anesthesiologist in fast-track surgery: from multimodal analgesia to perioperative medical care. *Anesth Analg* 2007; **104**:1380–96.

34. Habib AS, Muir HA, White WD, et al. Intrathecal morphine for analgesia after postpartum bilateral tubal ligation. *Anesth Analg* 2005; **100**:239–43.

35. Marcus RJ, Wong CA, Lehor A, et al. Postoperative epidural morphine for postpartum tubal ligation analgesia. *Anesth Analg* 2005; **101**:876–81.

36. American Society of Anesthesiologists Task Force on Neuraxial Opioids and the American Society of Regional Anesthesia and Pain Medicine. Practice guidelines for the prevention, detection, and management of respiratory depression associated with neuraxial opioid administration: an updated report by the American Society of Anesthesiologists Task Force on Neuraxial Opioids and the American Society of Regional Anesthesia and Pain Medicine. *Anesthesiology* 2016; **124**:535–552.

Nondelivery Procedures

Alexandra Reeve, Selina Patel, and Adrienne Stewart

Cervical Cerclage

Case Study

A 28-year-old para 1 +3 woman presented for a cervical cerclage insertion at 16 weeks' gestation due to previous preterm labor. She weighed 55 kg and was otherwise fit and well, with no gastroesophageal reflux disease. On examination, she had a grade 2 Mallampati view, with good mouth opening, and a thyromental distance of greater than 6.5 cm. Her surgical history included several gynecologic procedures, for which she underwent general anesthesia uneventfully, although she experienced postoperative nausea and vomiting on each occasion.

For this procedure, the patient had a general anesthetic with an IV induction using fentanyl and propofol, after which a Supreme laryngeal mask airway (LMA) was inserted. She was maintained with an oxygen, air, sevoflurane mixture and allowed to breathe spontaneously. IV acetaminophen 1 g and ondansetron 4 mg were administered intraoperatively for analgesia and antiemesis. The procedure lasted 30 minutes. On emergence from anesthesia, the LMA was removed uneventfully, and the patient was taken to the post–anesthesia care unit (PACU).

In the PACU the patient experienced cramplike abdominal pains and received a further 150 µg fentanyl intravenously and 60 mg dihydrocodeine orally. She vomited once, an hour after eating a light meal. She was discharged home 8 hours postoperatively, feeling well. Discharge was delayed due to nausea and vomiting, for which the patient was treated with a further 4-mg dose of IV ondansetron and a 50-mg dose of IV cyclizine in the PACU.

Key Points

- This patient had a short procedure under general anesthesia. She experienced pain and postoperative nausea and vomiting that delayed her discharge home.
- If she had received a spinal anesthetic, it is likely she would have stayed a similar length of time to allow for the block to fully recede and for her to pass urine.
- In the past, passing urine and tolerating oral fluids were also required after general anesthesia before the patient could be discharged home, but this is no longer compulsory, as long as the patient and care givers have written information on where to access help should they need to.[1]

Discussion

Cervical cerclage is used to prevent preterm labor due to cervical insufficiency. It is characterized by shortening of the cervix or painless cervical dilatation, resulting in recurrent second-trimester pregnancy losses.[2] Decisions surrounding the management of cervical cerclage should be made with senior medical involvement and should also be performed by clinicians experienced with the technique.[3]

Indications for cervical cerclage include[3]

1. **History Indicated.** Cervical cerclage is offered to women with three or more previous preterm births and/or second-trimester miscarriages.
2. **Ultrasound Indicated.** Cervical cerclage is offered to women with a history of one or more spontaneous second-trimester miscarriages who have a cervical length of less than 25 mm before 24 weeks' gestation.
3. **Rescue Cerclage.** Cervical cerclage is offered to women with a dilated cervix on physical or speculum examination as a salvage measure in cases of premature cervical dilatation.

The operative procedure is generally no longer than 1 hour in duration but often requires a degree of Trendelenburg positioning, which can be uncomfortable for the patient if she is undergoing the procedure awake under spinal anesthesia.

Anesthetic Considerations

There is very little in the literature regarding the safety of one form of anesthesia over another. General anesthesia is considered safe before 18 weeks' gestation, with no increased risk of aspiration of gastric contents. Patients who undergo a general anesthetic for cervical cerclage can often be discharged home within a few hours postoperatively. Discharge criteria would be the same as for those undergoing any day-case procedure. Patients would require verbal and written instruction on discharge, should be warned of symptoms they may experience on discharge, and should have an escort suitable to care for the patient at home.

Because of concerns about the teratogenicity of certain drugs and their unlicensed use during pregnancy, clinicians are often reluctant to use multimodal antiemetic medications. This can sometimes present a challenge for the treatment of postoperative nausea and vomiting (PONV) and may delay discharge from hospital. Analgesia is limited to IV acetaminophen and short-acting opioids (e.g., fentanyl) for day-case surgery. Postoperatively, nonsteroidal anti-inflammatory drugs should be avoided because of their teratogenic effects, and a short course of a weak opioid, such as dihydrocodeine, in combination with acetaminophen is usually sufficient.

Uterine relaxation may be required intraoperatively if the fetal membranes are protruding. Trendelenburg positioning may be sufficient in some cases to reduce the herniated membranes. Volatile anesthetic agents may help further by causing a degree of uterine relaxation. Occasionally, tocolytic drugs may be required, especially if the cerclage is being carried out under a regional anesthetic.[2] In the case of an emergency rescue cerclage, it is even more important that the mother does not strain or cough (and potentially prematurely rupture the fetal membranes) during the procedure. Therefore, in these emergency cases, spinal anesthesia may be advantageous because it negates the risk of coughing on emergence from general anesthesia.

If a neuraxial anesthetic technique is chosen, a sensory block height of T10–L1 and S2–S4 is required to cover the cervical, vaginal, and perineal dermatomes.[2,4]

Safety of Drugs in Pregnancy

Despite the lack of published evidence, expectant mothers are often routinely informed of the potential risks associated with cerclage.[3] Risks such as iatrogenic rupture of membranes, infection, hemorrhage, and cervical stenosis[4] associated with the operative procedure are routinely discussed with the mothers preoperatively. The anesthetic technique, including any potential risks and benefits of one technique over another, is rarely discussed with the patient by the obstetrician. It is usually left to the anesthetist to consider and discuss. Many anesthetists, however, will inform patients that there is a potential small risk of miscarriage, regardless of technique used, and will reassure mothers that they will avoid any known teratogenic drugs.

The first trimester is the period when the fetus is most at risk of the teratogenic effects of drugs that cross the placenta because this is when organogenesis is taking place.[5] IV induction agents (e.g., thiopentone, propofol) and volatile anesthetic gases will cross the placenta because they are highly lipid soluble but will not cause any long-term effects in the undelivered fetus. Opioids such as fentanyl and morphine will cross the placenta and can cause neonatal respiratory depression but again should not have any long-term adverse effects in the unborn fetus. Local anesthetic drugs such as bupivacaine are lipid soluble and so will undergo placental transfer, but only after systemic absorption from the subarachnoid or epidural space.

Learning Points

- Aspiration is not considered to be a risk before 18 weeks' gestation in an appropriately fasted otherwise healthy parturient.
- Positioning and avoidance of straining may affect the choice of anesthesia.
- It is a short procedure, usually under 1 hour, and can be done as a day case.
- There is a lack of evidence regarding the safety of one form of anesthesia over another (often physician or unit preference).
- Use of known teratogenic drugs should be avoided.
- Usually the fetus is previable, negating the need for fetal monitoring intraoperatively.

Retained Placenta

Case Study

A 28-year-old low-risk multiparous woman presented for manual removal of placenta (MROP) in the OR. She had a spontaneous vaginal delivery 1 hour previously in the midwife-led birthing unit, but despite administration of syntometrine, the placenta had not been delivered. On arrival in the OR, there was ongoing bleeding from the placental site, and the estimated blood loss (EBL) in the delivery room was 800 ml. Initial monitoring in the OR demonstrated a heart rate of 105 beats/minute and a blood pressure of 96/64 mmHg. IV access with a 16-gauge cannula was in situ, via which the patient had received 1,000 ml Hartmann's solution prior to coming to the OR.

The patient had no significant past medical history and had undergone uneventful general anesthesia in the past. She was not starved, having eaten 4 hours previously, and had been drinking water throughout her labor. She was given gastrointestinal prophylaxis, with oral ranitidine and metoclopramide, prior to arriving in the OR. Airway examination revealed good mouth opening and a Mallampati grade 2 view. Her booking weight was 60 kg, and blood results prior to delivery were Hb 11.6 g/liter, platelets 268×10^9/liter, and white blood cell count 5.8×10^9/liter.

On arrival in the OR, the patient was placed in the left lateral position and given a spinal anesthetic (11 mg hyperbaric bupivacaine + 20 µg fentanyl). A phenylephrine infusion (50 µg/ml) was available, if required, to maintain hemodynamic stability. Once adequate anesthesia was established, the patient was placed in the lithotomy position, and surgery was started. During the operation, the patient bled a further 800 ml, and the major obstetric hemorrhage (MOH) protocol was initiated. A second large-bore cannula was inserted, and blood was taken for full blood count and clotting and fibrinogen analysis. The patient remained hemodynamically stable throughout as resuscitation continued with oxygen administration via a facemask and warmed crystalloid volume replacement. On delivery of the placenta, antibiotics and uterotonics were administered. Uterotonics consisted of a 5-unit syntocinon bolus, followed by an infusion of 40 units over 4 hours. The entire procedure lasted 40 minutes, with a total

Table 27.1 Risk Factors for Retained Placenta

History of previous retained placenta
Previous cesarean delivery/uterine surgery
Maternal age >35 years
Preterm labor
Induced labor
Multiparity
Preeclampsia

EBL of 1,600 ml. The patient was transferred to the obstetric high-dependency unit for close monitoring overnight, including hourly fluid balance, and made an unremarkable recovery. Blood results from the OR demonstrated normal clotting and platelet count, but hemoglobin had fallen to 8.2 g/liter, and the fibrinogen was 2.4 g/liter. Blood products were not required, and the mother was started on oral iron supplements.

Key Points

- This low-risk parturient had a retained placenta causing significant postpartum hemorrhage.
- Active resuscitation was started immediately, and the MOH protocol followed.
- Manual removal of the placenta was conducted successfully under spinal anesthesia.

Discussion

The *third stage of labor* is defined as the period between childbirth and complete expulsion of the placenta and membranes.[6] It can be managed physiologically (allowing the placenta to deliver spontaneously) or actively (using a prophylactic uterotonic, early cord clamping, and controlled traction). There is no international consensus on length of time allowed for the third stage of labor, but in the United Kingdom, the third stage is defined as prolonged if the placenta is retained after 30 minutes of active management or 60 minutes of physiologic management.[6]

Risk Factors and Complications

Retained placenta affects 0.5–3 percent of vaginal deliveries depending on the population studied,[7] and a number of risk factors have been identified (Table 27.1).

149

The most important complication of retained placenta is postpartum hemorrhage (PPH). The presence of a retained placenta causes contractile failure of the retroplacental myometrium. This prevents occlusion of blood flow through the placental arcuate and radial arteries, leading to potentially life-threatening hemorrhage. Although this is predominantly a primary PPH, secondary PPH due to retained placental fragments also can occur. After uterine atony, retained placenta is the second major indication for a blood transfusion in the third stage of labor, and several observational studies have shown that the risk of PPH increases with length of the third stage.[8] Other important complications of retained placenta include puerperal sepsis and uterine inversion.

Management

In the absence of increased bleeding, the initial management for retained placenta is often expectant and conservative. If this is insufficient, manual removal in the OR will be required. The optimal time for surgical intervention is a balance between risk of hemorrhage from leaving the placenta in situ, probability of spontaneous delivery, and risks associated with performing a manual removal itself (e.g., hemorrhage, trauma, and infection).[7] Following removal of the placenta, uterotonics should be administered, and the patient should be monitored for ongoing bleeding. Any significant hemorrhage requires prompt resuscitation and should be managed according to local protocols. Despite a lack of evidence on the use of prophylactic antibiotics for MROP, recommendations promoting a single dose have been published.[9]

Anesthetic Considerations

Choice of anesthesia for MROP will depend on the clinical situation, hemodynamic stability of the patient, and thorough clinical assessment, along with a discussion with the obstetric team. Sedation, regional anesthesia, and general anesthesia have all been used successfully. Irrespective of mode of anesthesia chosen, all patients should have precautionary airway assessments and gastrointestinal prophylaxis.

Although uncommon, judicious use of sedatives and short-acting opioids may be sufficient to allow examination and MROP by a skilled obstetrician. However, if uterine exploration is needed, definitive anesthesia should be offered and performed.[6]

Central neuraxial blockade is commonly used for MROP and should be considered in patients who are not bleeding severely and are hemodynamically

stable. Traditional recommendations for cold blockade to T10 have now been superseded, with evidence demonstrating that cold blockade to T6 significantly improves intraoperative maternal comfort and overall satisfaction.[10,11] Intraoperative hypotension associated with regional anesthesia for MROP has been attributed to blood loss rather than height of block.[10] Spinal anesthesia can be quickly established; alternatively, epidural analgesia started during labor can be extended or established de novo. Sacral anesthesia, however, will be less reliable with epidural than with spinal anesthesia.

In the presence of active hemorrhage or hemodynamic instability, it may be more prudent to conduct the case using a general anesthetic technique. Rapid-sequence induction and tracheal intubation are often required, and use of induction agents that maintain cardiovascular stability (ketamine or etomidate), along with short-acting opiates, should be considered in cases of cardiovascular collapse and severe hypervolemia. In a more stable patient, a standard rapid-sequence induction with thiopentone or propofol and a short-acting opiate can be considered.

Uterine Relaxation

In some instances, the obstetrician may require a degree of uterine relaxation to facilitate manual removal of the placenta. If the patient is under general anesthesia, maintenance with a halogenated volatile agent will cause dose-dependent uterine relaxation, aiding placental removal. The magnitude of uterine relaxation achieved is similar between sevoflurane, halothane, and desflurane, provided that equipotent doses are used. Isoflurane, however, has been shown to be less effective at uterine relaxation than the other volatile agents.[12] If uterine relaxation is required in the presence of regional anesthesia, nitroglycerin can be administered sublingually (two doses of 400 μg) or intravenously (50–100 μg). Nitroglycerin provides rapid onset and offset smooth muscle relaxation due to its short plasma half-life (2–3 minutes), making it an ideal choice.[13] Nitroglycerin's mechanism of action is via production of nitric oxide, which causes vascular smooth muscle relaxation. The resulting vasodilation can cause transient headache and hypotension in the mother that may require treatment with IV fluids and vasopressors.

Learning Points

- Retained placenta is a leading cause of PPH, and active resuscitation must be initiated early.

- Retained placenta often requires manual removal in the OR.
- Choice of anesthesia depends on the clinical situation and degree of hemorrhage.
- Regional anesthesia should ensure cold blockade to the level of the T6 dermatome.

References

1. Verma R. Day case and short stay surgery: 2. *Anaesthesia* 2011; **66**:417–34.

2. Chestnut DH, Wong CA, Tsen LC, et al., eds. *Chestnut's Obstetric Anesthesia: Principles and Practice*, 5th edn. New York, NY: Elsevier; 2014, pp. 348–51.

3. Royal College of Obstetritions and Gynaecologists. Cervical cerclage (Green-Top Guideline No. 60), RCOG, May 2011. Available at www.rcog.org.uk/guidelines.

4. Suresh MS, Segal BS, Preston R, Fernando R, Mason CL, eds. *Shnider and Levinson's Anesthesia for Obstetrics*, 5th edn. Philadelphia, PA: Lippincott Williams & Wilkins; 2013, pp. 220–22.

5. Griffiths SK. Placental structure, function and drug transfer. *BJA CEACCP* 2015; **15**(2):84–89.

6. National Institute for Health and Care Excellence (NICE). Intrapartum care: care of healthy women and their babies during childbirth (NICE Guideline CG190). London: NICE; December 2014.

7. Weeks AD. The retained placenta. *Best Pract Res Clin Obstet Gynaecol* 2008; **22**:1103–117.

8. Akinola OI. Manual removal of placenta: evaluation of some risk factors and management outcome in a tertiary maternity unit. A case controlled study. *OJOG* 2013; **3**:279–84.

9. World Health Organization (WHO). *WHO Guidelines for the Management of Postpartum Haemorrhage and Retained Placenta*. Brussels: WHO Library; 2009.

10. Broadbent CR. What height of block is needed for manual removal of placenta under spinal anaesthesia? *Int J Obstet Anaesth* 1999; **8**:161–64.

11. Adams L. Anaesthetic protocol for manual removal of placenta. *Anaesthesia* 2013; **68**:104–5.

12. Yoo KY. The effects of volatile anesthetics on spontaneous contractility of isolated human pregnant uterine muscle: a comparison among sevoflurane, desflurane, isoflurane, and halothane. *Anesth Analg* 2006; **103**(2):443–47.

13. Caponas G. Glyceryl trinitrate and acute uterine relaxation: a literature review. *Anaesth Intensive Care* 2001; **29**:163–77.

Preterm Labor

Errol R. Norwitz and Denis Snegovskikh

Case Study

A healthy nulliparous woman at 27 + 1 weeks' gestation presented with regular painful uterine contractions and cervical dilation to 2 cm. Her vital signs were normal, and the initial fetal heart rate tracing was Category I. A dose of betamethasone was administered, and IV magnesium sulfate therapy was initiated for fetal neuroprotection. An anesthesiology consult was requested. Early epidural placement was recommended and accepted by the patient. Two hours after an uneventful epidural placement, a Category III fetal heart rate tracing was observed. The tracing did not show any improvement with resuscitative measures, and the patient was transferred to the OR for an urgent cesarean delivery. Surgical T4 level of epidural anesthesia was achieved with 20 ml of a lidocaine, bicarbonate, and epinephrine mixture. Twelve minutes after skin incision, a viable baby boy was born via classical hysterotomy with Apgar scores of 5 and 7 and 1 and 5 minutes, respectively. The newborn was transferred to the NICU for further care. Uterine atony was noted, which failed to respond to an initial IV infusion of oxytocin and an intramuscular injection of methylergonovine 0.25 mg. Uterine tone improved after a single intramyometrial injection of carboprost 0.2 mg. The remainder of the surgery was uneventful, with an estimated blood loss of 1,300 ml. No blood transfusion was required. Morphine 3 mg was administered epidurally for postoperative pain control. The epidural catheter was removed, and the patient was transferred to the PACU in a stable condition.

Key Points

- A healthy patient in preterm labor in the absence of any identifiable risk factors commonly presents to the obstetric anesthesiologist for analgesia or anesthesia.
- Prompt anesthesiology consultation may allow for the early establishment of epidural analgesia, which can later be converted into epidural anesthesia for an urgent classical cesarean.
- Uterine atony initially refractory to IV oxytocin and methylergonovine can sometimes be corrected with prostaglandins such as carboprost.

Discussion

The mean duration of a singleton pregnancy is 40 weeks (280 days) dated from the first day of the last menstrual period. *Term* is defined as two standard deviations from the mean or, more precisely, 37 completed to 42 weeks (266–294 days) of gestation. *Preterm (premature) labor* is defined as labor occurring prior to 37 completed weeks of gestation. Preterm is further divided into extreme preterm (<28 weeks), very preterm (28–34 weeks), and late preterm (34–37 weeks).

According to the World Health Organization (WHO), complications of prematurity are the leading cause of death among children younger than 5 years of age worldwide. Preterm birth is also a major cause of perinatal morbidity, and delivery prior to 32 weeks of gestation frequently results in lifelong disability.[1] An estimated 15 million premature children are born each year worldwide. In 2010, 517,400 premature babies were born in the United States alone, which ranks sixth highest in the world in regard to the number of babies born too soon.[2] In 2013, 11 percent of all live-born babies in the United States were delivered preterm,[3] and half of those preterm babies were delivered via cesarean.[3] The high likelihood of operative delivery suggests that early anesthesia consultation should be a routine part of the peripartum management of preterm parturients.

Etiology of Preterm Labor

Preterm labor represents a syndrome rather than a single diagnosis because the etiologies are varied.

Approximately 20 percent of preterm deliveries are iatrogenic and are performed for maternal or fetal indications, including fetal growth restriction, preeclampsia, placenta previa, and nonreassuring fetal testing.[4] Of the remaining cases of preterm birth, around 30 percent occur in the setting of preterm premature rupture of the membranes, 20–25 percent result from intra-amniotic infection, and the remaining 25–30 percent are due to spontaneous (unexplained) preterm labor.

Anesthetic Management and the Preterm Neonate

Preterm babies may be more sensitive to the effects of medications than their term counterparts because they have decreased protein-binding capacity (secondary to hyperbilirubinemia), diminished hepatic clearance, and increased permeability of the blood-brain barrier. Although controversial, it is possible that the choice of anesthesia provided to the mother may affect neonatal outcome. In one prospective population-based cohort study conducted 18 years ago in France, neonatal mortality among 1,338 infants delivered via cesarean before 33 weeks of gestation was 10.1 percent with general, 12.2 percent with spinal, and 7.7 percent with epidural anesthesia. Even after adjustment for gestational age and potential confounding demographic and clinical factors, spinal anesthesia was still associated with a significantly higher risk of neonatal death than general anesthesia (odds ratio [OR] 1.7; 95% confidence interval [CI] 1.1–2.6).[5]

It was reported more than 20 years ago that compared with epidural anesthesia, general anesthesia at the time of cesarean will lower the Apgar score among preterm babies.[6] Similarly, for very preterm babies, cesarean delivery performed under general anesthesia is associated with an increased risk of neonatal intubation compared with spinal anesthesia (48.7 versus 25.2 percent, respectively; OR 2.8; 95% CI 1.8–5.1).[7] In addition to these short-term adverse events, much has been written about the potential long-term negative effects of general anesthesia on the developing brain. To specifically address this concern, a consortium called SmartTots (Strategies for Mitigating Anesthesia-Related Neurotoxicity in Tots) was established in 2009 by the Food and Drug Administration (FDA) and the International Anesthesia Research Society. Since that time, animal studies have confirmed that general anesthetic agents are indeed able to induce significant neurotoxicity, acting either via GABA receptors (e.g., propofol, etomidate, sevoflurane, desflurane) or NMDA receptors (e.g., ketamine).[8,9] In one study, for example, significant neuroapoptosis and impairment in synapse development were demonstrated in the brains of primates exposed to general anesthetic agents.[10] And data from small observational studies in children suggest that there may indeed be an association between exposure to general anesthesia and subsequent learning difficulties.[8,9] Taken together, these data suggest that epidural anesthesia is likely the safest mode of anesthesia for preterm cesarean deliveries. Well-designed studies in premature infants confirming an improvement in short- and long-term outcome measures with the use of epidural anesthesia are urgently needed.

Epidural administration of chloroprocaine has one additional benefit in that it is associated with a lower incidence of transient fetal heart rate abnormalities compared with bupivacaine or lidocaine.[11] It would therefore seem reasonable to use chloroprocaine when the fetus is preterm, especially if rapid induction of epidural anesthesia is required. Lidocaine and bupivacaine remain acceptable choices in nonemergent situations.

Preterm babies have decreased nonenzymatic antioxidant reserve.[12] As such, the potential benefit of increasing maternal oxygenation by increasing the percentage of oxygen in the inhaled gaseous mixture must be weighed against the potential harmful effects of increasing the release of oxygen free radicals within the fetoplacental unit.[13]

Anesthetic Management and the Preterm Parturient

Preterm birth is associated with an increased risk of retained placenta, uterine atony, and postpartum hemorrhage, often related to the underlying reason why the parturient is being delivered before term. Due to underdevelopment of the lower uterine segment, performance of a cesarean before 28 weeks' gestation often requires a high vertical (classical) uterine incision, which increases the risk of complications compared with a standard lower uterine segment hysterotomy.

Women in preterm labor prior to 34 weeks may be given a tocolytic agent in an effort to delay delivery for 24–48 hours. Administration of a tocolytic agent beyond 48 hours has not been shown to delay delivery or improve perinatal outcome and, as such, is not recommended. Such parturients are also typically given antenatal corticosteroids by SC injection in an effort to prevent respiratory distress syndrome, intraventricular hemorrhage, and necrotizing enterocolitis if indeed the fetus is born too soon. Prior to 32 weeks, a 12-hour course of magnesium sulfate given by IV infusion may be added for additional fetal neuroprotection. Magnesium sulfate should always be administered as an IV infusion. The typical loading dose is 4–6 g given over 20–30 minutes followed by a continuous infusion of 1–2 g/h. A steady state is usually reached 3–4 hours after the initial IV infusion. Serial clinical examinations with or without serum levels are used to monitor the effects of magnesium therapy. Recommended therapeutic plasma concentrations are 4.0–8.0 mEq/liter (4.8–8.4 mmol/liter), although patients may become symptomatic at lower serum levels. The first signs of toxicity (blurred vision and disappearance of deep tendon reflexes) may occur at serum levels as low as 3.5–5.0 mmol/liter, respiratory depression may occur at 5.0–6.5 mmol/liter, prolongation of the PR interval may occur at 7.5 mmol/liter, and cardiorespiratory arrest may occur at plasma concentrations in excess of 12 mmol/liter.[14] Magnesium sulfate is eliminated by the kidney, and caution must be exercised in the setting of renal insufficiency. In this setting, the same loading dose should be administered (because the volume of distribution has not changed), but the maintenance infusion should be reduced or discontinued entirely. Like calcium, magnesium is a cation and may interfere with calcium action. This anticalcium effect may interfere with neuromuscular transmission (which explains its effects on the muscles of the eye and the deep tendon reflexes) and can reduce uterine tone, leading to increased blood loss. Patients requiring general anesthesia also have reduced requirements for nondepolarizing muscle relaxant.

Learning Points

- Complications of preterm birth are the leading cause of mortality during the first 5 years of life. Eleven percent of births (1/9 deliveries) in the United States occur before 37 weeks' gestation.
- Almost half of preterm babies are delivered via cesarean.

- Spinal anesthesia may be associated with increased neonatal mortality compared with other types of anesthesia.
- General anesthesia at the time of cesarean results in lower Apgar scores, more frequent need for intubation, and might have negative long-term effects on neurodevelopment (although this remains controversial).
- High concentrations of inhaled oxygen given to mothers may increase the risk of complications related to free-radical toxicity within the fetoplacental unit, although this risk remains theoretical at this time.
- Preterm birth is associated with an increased risk of cesarean delivery (and especially classical cesarean), retained placenta, uterine atony, and postpartum hemorrhage.
- Magnesium sulfate given for fetal neuroprotection may result in magnesium toxicity and can prolong the effects of nondepolarizing muscle relaxants.

References

1. World Health Organization (WHO). Fact Sheet N363, updated November 2014. Available at www.who.int/mediacentre/factsheets/fs363/en/.

2. Blencowe H, Cousens S, Oestergaard MZ, et al. National, regional and worldwide estimates of preterm birth. *Lancet* 2012; **9**(9832):2162–72.

3. Martin JA, Hamilton BE, Osterman MJ, Curtin SC, Matthews TJ. Births: final data for 2013. *Natl Vital Stat Rep* 2015; **64**:1–65.

4. Tucker JM, Goldenberg RL, Davis RO, et al. Etiologies of preterm birth in an indigent population: is prevention a logical expectation? *Obstet Gynecol* 1991; **77**:343–47.

5. Laudenbach V, Mercier FJ, Roze JC, et al. Anesthesia mode for caesarean section and mortality in very preterm infants: an epidemiologic study in the EPIPAGE cohort. *Int J Obstet Anesth* 2009; **18**:142–49.

6. Rolbin SH, Cohen MM, Levinton CM, Kelly EN, Farine D. The premature infant: anesthesia for cesarean delivery. *Anesth Analg* 1994; **78**:912–17.

7. Burguet A, Pez O, Debaene B, et al. Very preterm birth: is maternal anesthesia a risk factor for neonatal intubation in the delivery room? *Arch Pediatr* 2009; **16**: 1547–53.

8. Rappaport BA, Suresh S, Hertz S, et al. Anesthetic neurotoxicity: clinical implication of animal models. *N Engl J Med* 2015; **372**:796–97.

9. Flick RP, Katusic SK, Colligan RC, et al. Cognitive and behavioral outcomes after early exposure to anesthesia and surgery. *Pediatrics* 2011; **128**:e1053–61.

10. Creeley C, Dikranian K, Dissen G, et al. Propofol-induced apoptosis of neurones and oligodendrocytes in fetal and neonatal rhesus macaque brain. *Br J Anaesth* 2013; **110**(Suppl 1):i29–38.

11. Abboud TK, Khoo SS, Miller F, Doan T, Henriksen EH. Maternal, fetal, and neonatal responses after epidural anesthesia with bupivacaine, 2-chloroprocaine, or lidocaine. *Anesth Analg* 1982; **61**: 638–44.

12. Buhimschi IA, Buhimschi CS, Pupkin M, Weiner CP. Beneficial impact of term labor: nonenzymatic antioxidant reserve in the human fetus. *Am J Obstet Gynecol* 2003; **189**:181–88.

13. Khaw KS, Wang CC, Ngan Kee WD, Pang CP, Rogers MS. Effects of high inspired oxygen fraction during elective caesarean section under spinal anaesthesia on maternal and fetal oxygenation and lipid peroxidation. *Br J Anaesth* 2002; **88** (1):18–23.

14. Lu JF, Nightingale CH. Magnesium sulfate in eclampsia and pre-eclampsia: pharmacokinetic principles. *Clin Pharmacokinet* 2000; **38**(4):305–14.

Accidental Awareness during General Anesthesia in Obstetrics

Fatima Khatoon and Mitko Kocarev

Case Study

A 24-year-old morbidly obese nulliparous parturient with an unremarkable medical and obstetric history presented at 39 weeks' gestation in active labor. On examination, her cervix was dilated 4 cm, and she was having regular uterine contractions. As per her plan of care, a combined spinal-epidural (CSE) technique was initiated for labor analgesia. Within 1 hour of initiation of the CSE, the patient was rushed to the OR because cardiotocography (CTG) showed persistent fetal bradycardia of 75 beats/min. During the transfer, the trainee anesthetist began topping up the epidural catheter using 20 ml 2% lidocaine with 100 µg epinephrine and 100 µg fentanyl. The repeat CTG in the OR showed persistent fetal bradycardia requiring immediate delivery of the fetus. Because the epidural block was found to be inadequate on testing, a decision was made to proceed with general anesthesia (GA). After preoxygenation using four vital capacity breaths, induction of GA was started using a standard rapid-sequence induction (RSI) technique with thiopental 375 mg and suxamethonium 100 mg. The first attempt at intubation with direct laryngoscopy using a Macintosh No. 3 blade revealed a Cormack Lehane view of Grade IIIb, leading to an unsuccessful intubation attempt. After face mask ventilation with 100% oxygen for 30 seconds while maintaining cricoid pressure, a second attempt at intubation was made with a Macintosh No. 4 blade using a conventional malleable stylet which was also not successful. Continuous face mask ventilation with 100% oxygen was maintained while a senior anesthetist from another OR attended the call for urgent help and successfully performed endotracheal intubation using a gum elastic bougie. The patient maintained her oxygen saturation levels above 95% at all times, but her heart rate and blood pressure showed higher than baseline readings. Surgery proceeded immediately after confirmation of the endotracheal tube position, and anesthesia was maintained with an end-tidal minimal alveolar concentration

(MAC) of 0.7 using sevoflurane with a mixture of 50% oxygen in nitrous oxide (N_2O). The surgery and anesthesia remained otherwise uncomplicated.

The next day, the anesthetist responsible for her original management was called by the ward nurse to assess the patient, who appeared to be in distress and claimed to remember events that took place during surgery. She looked terrified while recollecting her memory of "painful pressure on her throat" and a "feeling of suffocation." A Brice-modified questionnaire (Table 29.1) was used to make a diagnosis of intraoperative awareness. Using the Michigan classification of awareness instrument (Table 29.2), the intraoperative event was graded as Class 4D. The patient was counseled and had a detailed explanation about the series of events that could have been responsible for her postoperative distress. The anesthetist apologized for the unfortunate occurrence and offered reassurance with expert help. The patient eventually developed post-traumatic stress disorder (PTSD), which was managed by a psychotherapist using cognitive-behavioral therapy (CBT). She made a complete recovery within 3 years and went on to have another child by cesarean delivery under regional anesthesia.

Key Points

- Patients may experience accidental awareness during general anesthesia (AAGA) due to insufficient anesthesia.
- Multiple factors causing AAGA include inadequate doses of induction anesthetic agent and the absence of anesthesia maintenance during difficult airway management.
- Some patients may develop PTSD, which ideally should be managed with psychotherapy.

Discussion

Accidental awareness during general anesthesia (AAGA) is an infrequent but serious complication of general anesthesia occurring due to the inability to

Table 29.1 The Brice-Modified Questionnaire

1. What was the last thing you remember before going to sleep?

2. What is the first thing you remember after waking up?

3. Do you remember anything between going to sleep and waking up?

4. Did you dream during your procedure?

5. What was the worst thing about your operation?

Table 29.2 Michigan Awareness Classification Instrument

Class 0: No awareness

Class 1: Isolated auditory perceptions

Class 2: Tactile perceptions (e.g., surgical manipulation or endotracheal tube)

Class 3: Pain

Class 4: Paralysis (e.g., feeling one cannot move, speak, or breathe)

Class 5: Paralysis and pain. An additional designation of "D" for distress is included for patient reports of fear, anxiety, suffocation, sense of doom, sense of impending death.

D: Modifier that is added to signify emotional distress

achieve the intended level of unconsciousness throughout the whole procedure. It is believed to occur as a result of an imbalance between the depth of anesthesia and the stimulus to which a patient is exposed.

AAGA is classified based on the patient's ability to recall any intraoperative event. *Explicit awareness* refers to the conscious recollection of events, either spontaneously or on direct questioning. *Implicit awareness*, by contrast, refers to changes in performance or behavior that are produced by previous experiences but without any conscious recollection of those experiences.[1]

Owing to rarity and underreporting, the true incidence of AAGA remains unknown. Several multicenter studies using the Brice questionnaire consistently quote the incidence to be 0.1–0.2 percent[2–4] in the general population. It is three times more likely to occur in females than in males. A high incidence is observed in the obstetric population with a range varying between 0.4 and 1.3 percent.[5–7] According to the National Audit Project 5 (NAP5) activity survey (http://www.nationalau ditprojects.org.uk/NAP5report), which relied only on the self-reporting of awareness, cases from the obstetric population comprised of 0.8 percent of all general anesthesias (GAs) but accounted for 10 percent of all cases of AAGA.

Most cases of AAGA are inconsequential, but some patients experience unwanted psychological sequelae, particularly if it is accompanied by a painful memory of the surgery. These can range from short-term insomnia, anxiety disorders, and distressing flashbacks to irreversible fear of future surgery, depression, and posttraumatic stress disorder.[8–10] It may also have serious medicolegal implications for the anesthetist. A recent analysis by the American Society of Anesthesiologists' (ASA) Closed Claim Project revealed that 1.9 percent of all claims were for awareness under general anesthesia.[8]

Risk Factors

Intraoperative awareness is a multifactorial event. Available epidemiologic studies classify the risk factors into three main categories.

1. Patient Related

Young Age. The obstetric population represents a younger age group, and a higher incidence is described in young patients undergoing GA.[2,11] Resistance to anesthetic agents and the higher level of anxiety observed in this age group could be contributing factors.

Difficult Airway. The incidence of difficult airway in the pregnant population is eight times higher than in their nonpregnant counterparts.[12–14] Prolonged instrumentation due to a difficult airway remains one of the major predisposing factors of AAGA today.

Obesity. Obesity is frequently encountered during pregnancy, which, in turn, puts parturients at high risk of having a difficult airway and underdosing of anesthetic agents.

Fear and Anxiety. Most GAs are administered for emergency cesarean deliveries, which consequently elevates patients' anxiety levels.

Factors Associated with Resistance to Anesthetic Agents. Pyrexia, previous frequent exposure to anesthetics, hyperthyroidism, tobacco smoking, alcohol consumption, and chronic use of drugs (e.g., opioids, amphetamines, cocaine, and benzodiazepines) are all established causes of resistance to anesthetics.

Avoidance of Premedication.

Obstetric patients are not prescribed sedative or analgesic premedication because of the concern of causing unwanted side effects to the unborn baby.

Physiologic Changes of Pregnancy. The tachycardia in pregnancy may mask the clinical signs of inadequate anesthesia. At the same time, increased cardiac output not only decreases the duration of action of IV anesthetics but also prolongs the time to establish effective partial pressure of volatile agents, leading to a potential period of "light" or inadequate anesthesia and AAGA.

2. Anesthesia Related

Rapid-Sequence Induction (RSI). The tradition of using a RSI technique for induction of GA in the obstetric population remains unchanged. Frequently, due to the nature of the emergency, adequate time is not allowed for the anesthetic drugs to take full effect before airway manipulation or surgery is undertaken. Moreover, routine ventilation with volatile anesthetics is often avoided by some anesthetists before endotracheal intubation.

Choice of Induction Agents. The choice of propofol versus thiopental for induction of GA is still a subject of controversy in obstetrics. Some anesthetists favor the use of thiopental because it has a faster onset, has an easily detectable definitive endpoint indicating the onset of unconsciousness, and provides better hemodynamic stability than propofol. However, the optimal dose of thiopental is still controversial, and it has been suggested that the recommended maximum dose in adults may not be sufficient for the obstetric population.[15,16] More recently, propofol has been gaining popularity in obstetrics despite some earlier concerns about its slower onset and the effect on the compromised mother and fetus, the last being rare in clinical practice. Another reason for favoring the use of propofol is the well-known risk of thiopental–antibiotic syringe swap increasing the risk of AAGA (http://www.nationalauditprojects.org.uk/NAP5report).

Inappropriate Use of Volatile Agents and Nitrous Oxide. Previous practice advocated the use of a lower end-tidal MAC of volatile anesthetic agents in an attempt to minimize the occurrence of neonatal sedation and blood loss secondary to uterine atony. Moreover, a recurring theme called "mind the gap" has been emerging in the induction section of obstetric anesthesia. This gap is the period between rapid redistribution of the IV induction agent and slowly increasing partial pressure of the volatile anesthetic (Figure 29.1). Difficult airway management, delay in turning on the agent, and a slow increase in the ratio of inhaled anesthetic fraction due to low anesthesia gas-flow techniques are attributable factors causing a delay in achieving an effective partial pressure of a volatile agent such as sevoflurane. Furthermore, the practice of using a high concentration of oxygen until delivery of the fetus prevents the use of N_2O.

Avoidance of Opioids. Opioids are not routinely administered as a part of standard RSI because they readily cross the placenta and may cause neonatal respiratory depression. Their use also may delay the return of spontaneous ventilation in the mother in case of a failed intubation. However, these concerns lack scientific evidence, and opioids are increasingly being used as part of a balanced anesthetic technique for obstetric GA in the same manner as for nonobstetric procedures.

Difficulty in Monitoring the Depth of Anesthesia (DOA). Despite substantial advancements in anesthesia over several decades, unfortunately there is no single foolproof method of monitoring the DOA. Several studies[4] demonstrated that absolute reliance on either bispectral index (BIS) or end-tidal anesthetic concentration (ETAC) to be questionable. Over and above this, the physiologic signs of pregnancy, as mentioned earlier, add more uncertainty.

Malfunction or Failure of the Anesthetic Equipment. A breathing system failure, disconnection of an anesthesia circuit, faulty alarms within an anesthesia machine, and extravasation or blockage of the IV cannula are all associated with delayed, inadequate, or even no delivery of anesthetic agents, leading to AAGA.

3. Surgery Related

Emergency surgeries are responsible for up to 43 percent of cases of AAGA that occur in the general population.[5,17] Most GAs are administered for an emergency cesarean delivery. The overwhelming pressure of delivering a compromised fetus faced by the obstetrician makes the mother vulnerable to experience a period of insufficient anesthesia. Therefore, it appears that most of the cases of AAGA in obstetrics take place between the start of the skin incision and delivery of the fetus.

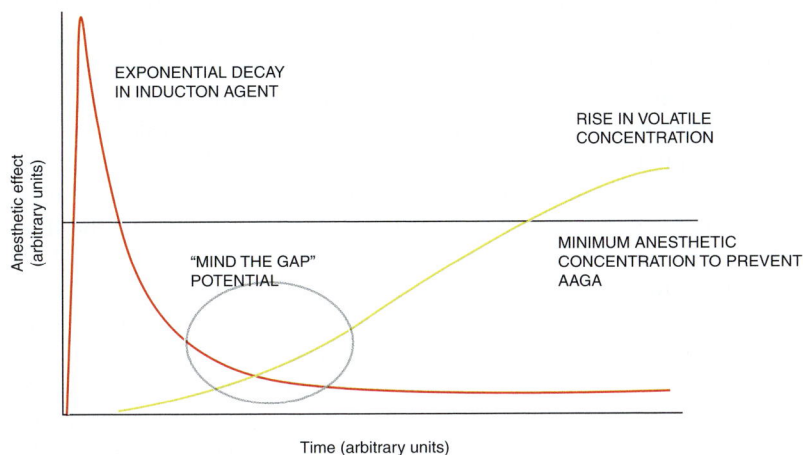

Figure 29.1 Mind the gap: diagrammatic representation of a gap that corresponds to the period between the rapid redistribution of the IV induction agent and the slowly increasing partial pressure of the volatile anesthetic.
Source: Reproduced with permission from the Royal College of Anaesthetists. Originally published in *Accidental Awareness during General Anaesthesia in the United Kingdom and Ireland: Report and Findings of the 5th National Audit Project*, September 2014.

Prevention of AAGA

The best approach for combating AAGA is prevention. Strict compliance with simple but rigorous measures can minimize the risk of AAGA.

Preoperative assessment with a focused history plays a fundamental role in identifying high-risk patients whose anesthetic needs should be modified. Specific attention must be paid in planning GA for an obese parturient with a potentially difficult airway. The 2006 American Society of Anesthesiologists (ASA) Task Force on Intraoperative Awareness recommends informing patients about the risk of AAGA (http://anesthesiology.pubs.asahq.org/article.aspx?articleid=1923386) and this is already included in the UK Royal College of Anaesthetists' patient information leaflet (http://www.rcoa.ac.uk/accidental-awareness). However, in an emergency situation when detailed discussion of AAGA is not feasible, the patient should be given a brief description of cricoid pressure and informed about the possibility of awareness of some sensations during the induction of anesthesia.[18]

Ensuring an efficient and fully functional operating suite around the clock to deal with any emergency surgery plays a pivotal role in preventing AAGA. Organized and regular maintenance of all the anesthetic equipment with a checklist is a must between patients. Special consideration must be given to mitigate the risk of drug errors by color coding, labeling, and physical separation of syringes, especially thiopental and antibiotics.

There is a lack of consensus among anesthetists regarding the choice of induction anesthetic agent. However, until concrete evidence emerges, it is prudent to ensure that every obstetric anesthetist has an understanding of the pharmacokinetics and pharmacodynamics of the drugs to be used in relation to pregnancy. Inadequate dosing of IV anesthetics is still a potential cause of AAGA. Current recommendations include a dose of no less than 5 mg/kg thiopental and 2–2.5 mg/kg propofol in a healthy parturient. In obese parturients, the doses of thiopental and propofol for induction should be calculated based on lean body weight (LBW).[19] Supplemental doses of induction agents should be administered when a difficult intubation necessitates a protracted period of multiple intubation attempts. It is important to remember that propofol has a slower onset of action and that the effect of thiopental wears off quickly because of its rapid redistribution.

As mentioned earlier, "mind the gap" addresses the period between rapid redistribution of the IV induction agent and slowly increasing partial pressure of the volatile anesthetic (see Figure 29.1). This interval is of particular concern in obstetrics because surgical intervention may take place during this period of inadequate anesthesia. Every effort should be made to build up the partial pressure of the volatile anesthetic agent as quickly as possible to avoid this gap. This can be done by turning on the vaporizer without any delay, using an initial high concentration of volatile anesthetic agents with high fresh gas flows,[18] and adding N_2O to facilitate faster onset via the second-gas effect. Also, ensuring a MAC of 0.7 or above throughout the surgery can help in reducing AAGA. Contrary to earlier beliefs, current available evidence does not suggest a relationship between a higher MAC of volatile anesthetic agents and neonatal sedation or increased blood loss due to a decrease in uterine tone.[6] As recommended by NAP5, appropriate use of uterotonics should allow the use of an adequate concentration of volatile anesthetic agent.

Unlike in other surgical specialties, N_2O still has a special role in cesarean delivery. Not only does it facilitates a faster onset of anesthesia, but it also has an analgesic property and the ability to reduce the requirement of volatile anesthetic agents. These positive effects, however, are offset by the common practice of giving a high oxygen concentration to the mother until delivery of the fetus. The practice of administering high oxygen concentration to parturients has failed to demonstrate any improvement in neonatal outcome; further research is needed to investigate the safe minimum inspired oxygen concentration in order to clarify the maximum concentration of N_2O that can be safely administered.

The routine use of any DOA monitor for cesarean delivery is uncommon. The most common method used by anesthetists is the continuous monitoring of physiologic variables such as tachycardia, hypertension, lacrimation, pupillary dilation, and sweating as signs of AAGA. However, the physiologic changes of pregnancy may mask some of these signs of light anesthesia. Nevertheless, ensuring an adequate ETAC or MAC of 0.7 or greater of volatile anesthetic agents has been associated with a dramatic decrease in AAGA.[4,20]

Some specialized electroencephalography (EEG)–based equipment has been developed to assist in monitoring DOA. The most commonly used is the BIS monitor, which has been shown to decrease AAGA by fivefold in high-risk populations undergoing GA.[21,22] Despite its popular use, studies indicating its precise accuracy and superiority over ETAC monitoring are equivocal.[22–24] More notably, the combined application of ETAC and BIS monitors using an alarm-triggering method for inadequate anesthesia has proven to be effective in reducing AAGA in high-risk nonobstetric populations.[11,21] In reality, though, it is almost never feasible to use these sophisticated monitors during a cesarean delivery, especially in an emergency, because of practical issues and the time factor involving their application. Moreover, it is likely that AAGA could already have occurred even before their application because clinical management of the mother and fetus takes priority.

The omission of opioids from a traditional RSI technique for a GA cesarean delivery because of fetal and maternal concerns is undoubtedly one of the most important attributable factors causing AAGA. However, these concerns are not evidence based. As recommended by the NAP5, research is needed to define the optimal dose and timing of opioids because it appears that incorporating them may reduce AAGA by shortening the "mind the gap" interval, improving intubating conditions, and providing analgesia for surgery.

Difficult airway leading to painful instrumentation and consequent delays in the delivery of volatile anesthetic agents were associated with two-thirds of the cases of AAGA in the NAP5 report. It is prudent for anesthetists to have a clear plan of action if a difficult airway is encountered. Recently published Obstetric Anaesthesia Association/Difficult Airway Society (OAA/DAS) guidelines provide algorithms for the safe provision of GA in obstetrics (http://www.oaa-anaes.ac.uk/ui/content/content.aspx?id=3447). Other strategies such as preparing a second syringe of an induction agent before induction to be used to maintain anesthesia, administering rocuronium instead of succinylcholine for intubation, and using a modified RSI in managing a potentially difficult airway are gaining increasing popularity among anesthetists.[25] There is a trend toward favoring the use of rocuronium, which at a dose of 1.2 mg/kg can provide similar onset and comparable intubating conditions to succinylcholine. If a decision to awaken the mother is made, reversing rocuronium using sugammadex can produce a faster return of neuromuscular function than the spontaneous offset of succinylcholine.[26] Another measure advocated by some anesthetists is to modify the classic RSI technique and ventilate the patient using a face mask before securing the airway.[27] Although research remains inconclusive about the effectiveness of cricoid pressure, there is a general agreement about reducing or removing cricoid pressure if faced with difficulty in intubation.

Intraoperative Management of Awareness

Anesthetists should have a high index of suspicion and low threshold for intervening when it comes to the diagnosis and management of AAGA. If clinical signs or DOA monitoring indicate that the patient may be experiencing AAGA, anesthesia should immediately be deepened without delay. Hypotensive patients should be managed with IV fluid, ventilatory modification, and vasopressors rather than by reducing the delivery of anesthetic agents. Although benzodiazepines lack retrograde amnesic effects, their use can be beneficial in reducing further recall through their anterograde amnesic effect.

Postoperative Management

Most claims of AAGA are genuine and credible.[28] Anesthetists must immediately respond to a patient claiming to suffer from AAGA. A detailed account of the event should be obtained in order to differentiate between genuine AAGA and dreaming or recall of events during emergence from anesthesia. A precise documentation of the event as described by the patient ("feeling of suffocation," "hearing conversation among the staff," or "shearing pain of the skin incision") should be made. The modified Brice questionnaire (see Table 29.1) to diagnose and the Michigan awareness classification instrument (see Table 29.2) to classify the degree of AAGA should be used. Denying the authenticity of a patient's claim may contribute to a worse psychological outcome.[29] A thoughtful approach and empathy must be offered. An apology should be made with a possible explanation of the events that occurred. The senior anesthetist, attending surgeon, and nursing staff should be notified. It is imperative that the patient receives the necessary psychological and psychiatric support with subsequent follow-up. The patient's record must include a detailed summary of the events in order to guide any future anesthetic management.

Learning Points

- AAGA is an infrequent complication of GA with potential detrimental psychological sequelae for the patient.
- Obstetrics remains as one of the surgical specialties with highest incidence of AAGA.
- Prevention is of paramount importance in combating AAGA.
- Ensure adequate DOA throughout the surgery by administrating recommended doses of induction anesthetic agents using an "overpressure" technique of volatile anesthetic agent delivery to minimize the IV induction-to-inhalation gap and ensuring a MAC of 0.7 or greater of a volatile anesthetic agent.
- In the event of prolonged instrumentation due to a difficult airway, supplemental doses of induction anesthetic agent should be administered.
- Application of DOA monitoring is highly recommended whenever feasible but should not take priority over safe management of the mother and fetus.
- Judicious use of opioids should be considered in patients with multiple risk factors for AAGA.
- Every obstetric patient must be informed about the risk of AAGA during preoperative assessment.
- A multidisciplinary approach is obligatory in managing a patient suffering from AAGA.

References

1. Schacter DL. Implicit memory: history and current status. *J Exp Psychol Learn Mem Cogn* 1987; **13**:501–18. Available at www.nationalauditprojects.org.uk/NAP5report.

2. Sebel BS, Bowdle A, Ghoneim MM, et al. The incidence of awareness during anesthesia: a multicenter United States study. *Anesth Analg* 2004; **99**(3):833–39.

3. Sandin RH, Enlund G, Samuelsson P. Awareness during anaesthesia: a prospective case study. *Lancet* 2000; **355**: 707–11.

4. Avidan MS, Jacobsohn E, Glick D, et al. Prevention of intraoperative awareness in a high-risk surgical population. *N Engl J Med* 2011; **365**:591–600.

5. Ghoneim MM, Block RL. Learning and memory during general anesthesia: an update. *Anesthesiology* 1997; **87** (2):387–410.

6. Lyons G, Macdonald R. Awareness during caesarean section. *Anaesthesia* 1991; **46**(1):62–64.

7. Paech MJ, Scott KL, Clavisi O, et al. A prospective study of awareness and recall associated with general anesthesia for cesarean section. *Int J Obstet Anesth* 2008; **17**(4):298–303.

8. Domino KB, Posner KL, Caplan RA, Cheney FW. Awareness during anesthesia: a closed claims analysis. *Anesthesiology* 1999; **90**:1053–61.

9. Samuelsson P, Brudin L, Sandin RH, Late psychological symptoms after awareness among consecutively included surgical patients. *Anesthesiology* 2007; **106**:26–32.

10. Lennmarken C, Sydsjo G. Psychological consequences of awareness and their treatment. *Best Pract Res Clin Anaesthesiol* 2007; **21**(3):357–67.

11. Mashour GA, Wang LYJ, Turner CR, et al. A retrospective study of intraoperative awareness with methodological implications. *Anesth Analg* 2009; **108** (2):521–26.

12. Kuczkowski KM, Reisner LS, Benumof JL. The difficult airway: risk, prophylaxis, and management, in Chestnut DH (ed.), *Obstetric Anesthesia: Principles and Practice*, 3rd edn. St Louis, MO: Mosby; 2004, pp. 535–62.

13. Hagberg CA: *Handbook of Difficult Airway Management*. Philadelphia, PA: Churchill Livingstone; 2000, pp. 301–18.

14. Barnardo PD, Jenkins JG. Failed tracheal intubation in obstetrics: a 6-year review in a UK region. *Anaesthesia* 2000; **55**:690–94.

15. Collis RE. Anaesthesia for caesarean section: general anaesthesia, in Collis RE, Plaat F, Urquhart J, eds., *Textbook of Obstetric Anaesthesia*. London: Greenwich Medical Media; 2002, pp. 112–32.

16. Yentis SM, Hirsch NP, Smith GB. *Anaesthesia and Intensive Care A–Z: An Encyclopaedia of Principles and Practice*, 3rd edn. London: Butterworth; 2004, pp. 81–83.

17. Bogetz MS, Katz JA. Recall of surgery for major trauma. *Anesthesiology* 1984; **61**(1):6–9.

18. Bogod D, Plaat F. Be wary of awareness: lessons from NAP5 for obstetric anaesthetists. *Int J Obstet Anesth* 2015; **24**:1–4.

19. Ingrande J, Lemmens HJ. Dose adjustment of anaesthetics in the morbidly obese. *Br J Anaesth* 2010; **105**(Suppl 1):i16–23.

20. Eger EI 2nd. Age, minimum alveolar anesthetic concentration, and minimum alveolar anesthetic concentration-awake. *Anesth Analg* 2001; **93**(4):947–53.

21. Punjasawadwong Y, Phongchiewboon A, Bunchungmongkol N, Bispectral index for improving anaesthetic delivery and postoperative recovery. *Cochrane Database Syst Rev* 2014; (**6**):Cd003843.

22. Myles PS, Leslie K, McNeil J, Forbes A, Chan MT. Bispectral index monitoring to prevent awareness during anaesthesia: the B-Aware randomized, controlled trial. *Lancet* 2004; **363**:1757–63.

23. Ekman, A, Lindholm, ML, Lennmarken, C, Sandin, R. Reduction in the incidence of awareness using BIS monitoring. *Acta Anaesthesiol Scand* 2004; **48**(1):20–26.

24. Avidan, MS, Zhang, L, Burnside, BA, et al. Anesthesia awareness and the bispectral index. *N Engl J Med* 2008; **358**:1097–108.

25. Chaggar RS, Campbell JP. The future of general anaesthesia in obstetrics. *BJA Educ* 2017; **17**(3):79–83.

26. Lee C, Jahr JS, Candiotti KA, et al. Reversal of profound neuromuscular block by sugammadex administered three minutes after rocuronium: a comparison with spontaneous recovery from succinylcholine. *Anesthesiology* 2009; **110**:1020–25.

27. Schlesinger S, Blanchfield D. Modified rapid-sequence induction of anesthesia: a survey of current clinical practice. *AANA J* 2001; **69**:291–98.

28. Moerman N, Bonke B, Oosting J. Awareness and recall during general anesthesia. *Facts Feelings Anesthesiol* 1993; **79**(3):454–64.

29. Heneghan C. Clinical and medicolegal aspects of conscious awareness during anesthesia: depth of anesthesia. *Int Anesthesiol Clin* 1993; **31**:1–11.

Failed Epidural Top-Up for Cesarean Delivery

Tauqeer Husain

Case Study

A fit and well low-risk nulliparous woman presented at 39 weeks' gestation to the delivery suite. She was contracting twice in 10 minutes, and at vaginal examination, her cervix was dilated 3 cm. Cardiotocography was unremarkable.

Pain relief was requested, and an epidural was inserted by the anesthetist. Patient-controlled epidural analgesia (PCEA) was started using a low-dose mixture (LDM) of 0.1% bupivacaine with 2 μg/ml fentanyl.

Subsequently, labor progression was slow, requiring augmentation with a syntocinon infusion. Although the labor pain was initially well controlled, as augmentation progressed, the patient became increasingly distressed due to pain and required multiple additional clinician-administered boluses of LDM.

After an extended period of augmentation, it was decided to deliver by cesarean due to a lack of labor progress. The patient was transferred to the OR, and an epidural top-up of 20 ml 2% lidocaine with 1:200,000 epinephrine and sodium bicarbonate was administered. Within 10 minutes, a block had been established bilaterally up to T6 to cold, when a prolonged fetal bradycardia necessitated urgent delivery. However, once the baby was delivered, uterine exteriorization resulted in the patient complaining of pronounced pain requiring conversion to general anesthesia (GA).

After rapid-sequence induction, the patient was successfully intubated, and surgery was continued. The patient went on to make an uncomplicated recovery.

Key Points

- This patient experienced intraoperative pain during cesarean delivery under epidural anesthesia.

- Her epidural required multiple clinician interventions for breakthrough labor pain, and cesarean delivery was expedited after epidural top-up due to fetal compromise.
- General anesthesia was administered after delivery to facilitate completion of surgery.

Discussion

Epidural analgesia (EA) is considered by many to be the "gold standard" for labor pain relief. UK audit data has consistently show that approximately 20% of all cesarean deliveries are performed under epidural anesthesia (Figure 30.1). Not only can it effectively relieve the pain of labor, but it also has the benefit of allowing conversion to anesthesia for urgent operative procedures such as cesarean delivery. Additionally, with the use of EA, the safety of obstetric anesthesia has improved markedly. This has been demonstrated by a reduction in airway and aspiration-related mortality and morbidity in serial obstetric safety audits.[1]

However, EA also present risks related to the procedure itself, the risk of failure, and the risks of subsequent general anesthesia (GA). The risk of failed epidural conversion for cesarean delivery (defined as the failure to induce and provide adequate anesthesia for the length of the procedure or the need for supplemental analgesia or GA) is variously quoted at between 7.1 and 24 percent.[2,3]

Risk Factors

A number of risk factors that might predict an increased risk of EA failure have been identified (Table 30.1). The effectiveness of EA in labor is linked to the effectiveness of the same epidural for anesthesia. Supplementation of labor analgesia with additional clinician-administered epidural boluses may be reflective of a suboptimal epidural catheter placement. As in the Case Study, this may then present

Table 30.1 Factors Associated with an Increased Risk of Epidural Conversion Failure

- Increased number of supplementary clinician boluses in labor
- Non-obstetric anesthetist providing care
- Urgency of cesarean delivery
- High maternal weight or height

during cesarean delivery as inadequate EA. If a patient is unable to obtain adequate relief from labor pain, without the need for supplemental epidural boluses, a low threshold for replacing the epidural catheter may reduce the risk of failed EA during cesarean delivery.

Increased maternal size, both height and weight, has been thought to be a risk factor for inadequate EA. The suggestion is that maternal obesity may be linked to increased epidural catheter movement due to increased variations in the distance between the skin and dural space with movement.[4] However, in practice, this might be offset by a greater intolerance of inadequate labor analgesia in this group of patients, leading to early replacement of poorly positioned epidural catheters.

Management of Failed EA

How inadequate EA is managed depends on the context of the situation. The choice of intervention should consider where in the process of cesarean delivery EA inadequacy has occurred. If it has not already taken place, the urgency of delivery should also be considered.

Before the Start of Surgery

Every effort should be made to ensure that the EA block has reached a satisfactory level prior to starting surgery. It is now commonly accepted that the best way to reduce the risk of intraoperative EA failure is to make sure that a block to light touch up to T5 is present.[5,6] If the block fails to achieve this, a decision should be made regarding the urgency of delivery. If time permits, optimization of EA anesthesia could be considered. This may include administering a top-up if an epidural catheter is in situ or insertion of further spinal anesthesia. Care should be taken when spinal anesthesia is administered after failed epidural top-up because of the risk of a high block or hypotension occurring. Although there is an argument for reducing the spinal dose given, the risk of further

inadequate anesthesia remains. It therefore may be reasonable to administer a "conventional" spinal dose, with care taken to manage hypotension expectantly with IV fluids, vasopressors, and positioning.

During Surgery (Before Delivery)

If surgery has started but delivery has not occurred, options for managing pain need to be balanced against the risk to the fetus. Both opioids and benzodiazepines have been used during elective cesarean delivery with no significant effect on fetal well-being.[7] However, the use of intraoperative remifentanil may be associated with significantly reduced Apgar scores.[8] Because of apparently contradictory evidence, it may be reasonable to avoid IV supplementation until delivery of the newborn has occurred. If 50% nitrous oxide is available, it may supply some analgesic benefit. However, the acute side effects, such as dose-dependent depression of respiratory function, dysphoria, and nausea, may limit its use. Additionally, although it may supply effective pain relief for minor procedures, the lack of effectiveness in severe pain means that it may be a temporary option at best.

As in the scenario of inadequate EA prior to the start of surgery, every effort should be made to optimize preexisting EA if a catheter is in situ.

During Surgery (After Delivery)

Once delivery of the newborn has taken place, concerns about the neonatal side effects of IV supplementation are removed, and so many more management options are available for inadequate EA. The use of 50% nitrous oxide, short-acting opioids, and low-dose ketamine has been described in managing intraoperative pain. If sensation is localized to small areas within the surgical field, local infiltration by the surgeon also may be considered. If anxiety appears to be an additional factor in maternal distress, a small titrated dose of anxiolytics such as a benzodiazepine also may be of use. However, the amnesic properties of this class of drug may not be acceptable to the patient, so alternatives such as propofol should be considered. In all situations where opioids, benzodiazepines, or propofol are considered, the benefits of administration need to be weighed against the risks of central, cardiovascular, and respiratory depression.

In all cases of inadequate EA, it is vitally important to maintain good communication with the patient. Clear explanation and reassurance not only will help to alleviate anxiety but also may act as a distraction

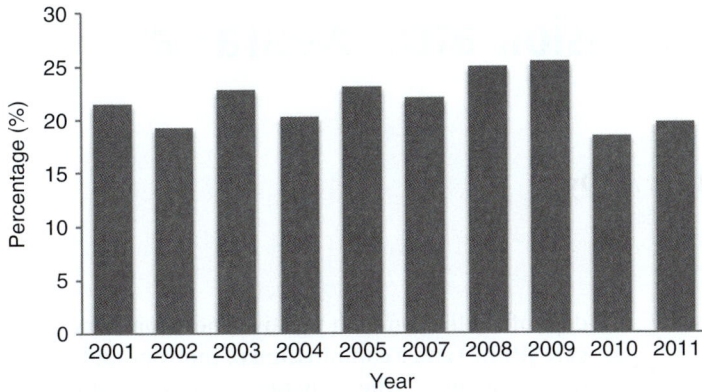

Figure 30.1 The percentage of cesarean deliveries performed under epidural anesthesia in the United Kingdom

Source: Taken from the National Obstetric Anaesthetic Database. Available at www.oaa-anaes.ac.uk/content.asp?ContentID=86 (accessed April 2014).

from the sensations. Additionally, the provision of GA, unless absolutely contraindicated, should always be an option that is considered in conjunction with the patient and birth partner. Where GA is required, attention should also be given to a plan of intra- and postoperative pain management.

Learning Points

- Risk factors for inadequate epidural anesthesia include the need for supplemental clinician-administered boluses during labor and large maternal size.
- An EA block up to and including T5 to light touch reduces the risk of intraoperative pain during cesarean delivery.
- Management of inadequate EA needs to take into account the urgency of delivery and the point during the surgery and delivery at which failure is evident.

References

1. Ngan Kee WD. Confidential enquiries into maternal death: 50 years of closing the loop. *Br J Anaesth* 2005; **94**: 413–16.

2. Kinsella SM. A prospective audit of regional anaesthesia failure in 5,080 caesarean sections. *Anaesthesia* 2008; **63**: 822–32.

3. Pan PH, Bogard TD, Owen MD. Incidence and characteristics of failures in obstetric neuraxial analgesia and anesthesia: a retrospective analysis of 19,259 deliveries. *Int J Obstet Anesth* 2004; **13**: 227–33.

4. Riley ET, Papasin J. Epidural catheter function during labor predicts anesthetic efficacy for subsequent cesarean delivery. *Int J Obstet Anesth* 2002; **11**:81–84.

5. Russell IF. Levels of anaesthesia and intraoperative pain at caesarean section under regional block. *Int J Obstet Anesth* 1995; **4**:71–77.

6. Russell IF. Assessing the block for caesarean section. *Int J Obstet Anesth* 2001; **10**:83–85.

7. Frölich MA, Burchfield DJ, Euliano TY, Caton D. A single dose of fentanyl and midazolam prior to cesarean section have no adverse neonatal effects. *Can J Anaesth* 2006; **53**:79–85.

8. Draisci G, Valente A, Suppa E, et al. Remifentanil for cesarean section under general anesthesia: effects on maternal stress hormone secretion and neonatal well-being: a randomized trial. *Int J Obstet Anesth* 2008; **17**:130–36.

Maternal Hypotension after Neuraxial Anesthesia

Ross Hofmeyr and Robert A. Dyer

Case Study

A 29-year-old gravida 2, para 1 woman at 34 weeks' gestation presented to the maternity center in labor. She had no previous medical history other than a cesarean delivery for early-onset preeclampsia during her previous pregnancy. In this pregnancy, she developed increasing dyspnea over the 3 days prior to admission. The cardiotocograph (CTG) indicated variable decelerations, and the obstetrician requested emergency operative delivery. Although the patient was tachycardic (heart rate 112 beats/min) and hypertensive (blood pressure 185/110 mmHg), with sparse crackles audible in the lower chest zones bilaterally, there was no known contraindication to neuraxial anesthesia. A standard spinal anesthetic (bupivacaine 9 mg and fentanyl 10 µg in 2 ml volume) was administered with 500 ml of colloid coload. After rapid onset of a T4 sensory block to cold sensation, the obstetrician proceeded with a lower segment cesarean delivery. Shortly after delivery, the patient's blood pressure fell from 150/95 to 85/40 mmHg, with worsening tachycardia (heart rate 130 beats/min).

As per routine practice, multiple titrated 50- to 100-µg boluses of phenylephrine were administered. Unexpectedly, the blood pressure and tachycardia did not improve, arterial oxygen desaturation was noted, and the patient became progressively more tachypneic, with the respiratory rate approaching 30 breaths/min. After preoxygenation, a rapid-sequence induction with etomidate and suxamethonium was performed, and the trachea was intubated. Rapid arterial oxygen desaturation occurred during intubation. Frank pulmonary edema was recognized when pink frothy sputum was seen in the endotracheal tube, and inotropic support and diuretic therapy using an epinephrine infusion and furosemide boluses were started. The patient was admitted to the obstetric high-dependency-care unit. Point-of-care transthoracic echocardiography (TTE) showed severe systolic heart failure (ejection fraction 15 percent). After 2 days of ventilation with positive end-expiratory pressure (PEEP) and a combination of inotrope and diuretic therapy, the patient was extubated. Echocardiography showed an improved ejection fraction of 30 percent with residual diastolic dysfunction, and full recovery was documented within 1 month.

Key Points

- Hypotension is a frequent complication of spinal anesthesia in healthy women. Typically, this develops in response to reduction in sympathetic outflow below the upper level of the block, with early-onset arteriolar dilatation and a decreased systemic vascular resistance, together with some degree of venodilatation.
- Prevention is most commonly achieved through coloading with IV fluids, and correction of hypotension by administration of phenylephrine.[1] However, not all hypotension during spinal anesthesia is due to the above-listed effects (Table 31.1).
- Increasing understanding of the cardiovascular effects of preeclampsia has lead to the appreciation of the varying pathologies that can occur in this disease.[2] In particular, ventricular hypertrophy in response to hypertension may result in decreased diastolic compliance and ultimately diastolic heart failure.
- Recent research has shown that patients with uncomplicated severe hypertension are less susceptible to spinal hypotension. In these patients, the usual response is mild afterload reduction.[3] Acute, rapid progression of hypertension, the rapid hemodynamic shifts during labor and delivery, and/or liberal fluid management may provide the tipping point from compensated to uncompensated cardiac failure.
- The obstetric anesthetist should be prepared to recognize and manage these complications.

Table 31.1 Recognition and Management of Hypotension during Spinal Anesthesia for Cesarean Delivery

Hemodynamic changes	Causes	Recommended management
Hypotension, increased heart rate	Decreased systemic vascular resistance and some venodilatation: • Sympathetic blockade due to spinal anesthesia • Drug effects (e.g. oxytocin)	Phenylephrine
Hypotension, bradycardia	Preload reduction: Bezold-Jarisch or inverse Bainbridge reflex	Anticholinergic; consider ephedrine
Severe persistent hypotension	Undiagnosed hypovolemia Undiagnosed cardiac disease: • Peripartum cardiomyopathy • Valvular heart disease • Rarely, preeclampsia	Fluids and inotropes if necessary
Cardiorespiratory collapse	High motor block Anaphylaxis Amniotic fluid embolism Sepsis	Full cardiopulmonary resuscitation

Discussion

Intrathecal anesthesia results in blockade of sympathetic innervation below the upper level of the spinal block. The resulting vasodilatation has a twofold effect. First, arteriolar dilatation dramatically reduces systemic vascular resistance to blood flow. Second, there is some increase in venous capacitance, effectively distributing the blood volume into a larger space and so directly reducing blood pressure. The increase in venous capacitance can be reduced by the administration of an IV fluid bolus at the time of onset of spinal anesthesia. This practice is referred to as *coloading*. Various studies have explored the value of crystalloid and colloid solutions, as well as the appropriate volume to be administered. While practices differ widely throughout the world, most practitioners are comfortable with administrating approximately 10–20 ml/kg of a crystalloid solution.

Techniques that attempt to improve venous return and limit aortocaval compression reduce, but do not prevent, spinal hypotension. Work done in the past 10 years suggests that early arteriolar dilatation is the major contributor to hypotension; this is usually accompanied by a partial compensatory increase in heart rate and cardiac output.[4] Therefore, pure alpha agonists are the logical choice to restore baseline heart rate, blood pressure, systemic vascular resistance, and cardiac output. Phenylephrine has been studied extensively in this role. It is easily titrated in small aliquots or by continuous infusion and may improve

fetal biochemistry and outcomes.[5] Ephedrine has also been commonly used. Its action is twofold: direct beta-adrenergic receptor agonism and delayed, indirect alpha-adrenergic effects by increasing the activity of norepinephrine at the postsynaptic alpha receptors. Because most patients with spinal hypotension respond with a reflex tachycardia, the beta-adrenergic stimulation is unnecessary.

Typically, for cesarean delivery, a spinal level of at least the T5 dermatome to pinprick and temperature is desirable.[6] Should spinal blockade extend above T4, progressive blockade of the cardiac accelerator fibers (T1–T4) may limit the tachycardic response to hypotension, although the baroreceptor reflex is usually well maintained. Occasionally, reflex bradycardia in response to spinal anesthesia may necessitate anticholinergic therapy.[7] The prophylactic use of anticholinergic agents to counter phenylephrine-induced bradycardia is not recommended.[8]

Preeclampsia is a life-threatening complication of pregnancy with a complex, incompletely understood etiology.[2] The pathognomonic hypertension has recently been shown through TTE to result in one of two patterns of cardiac dysfunction. This may be categorized by ventricular hypertrophy and diastolic dysfunction (heart failure with preserved ejection fraction) or occasional progression to severe systolic dysfunction and frank heart failure (heart failure with reduced ejection fraction).[9] In the former instance, whereas the hypertrophied ventricle is able to maintain adequate ejection and thereby systolic function

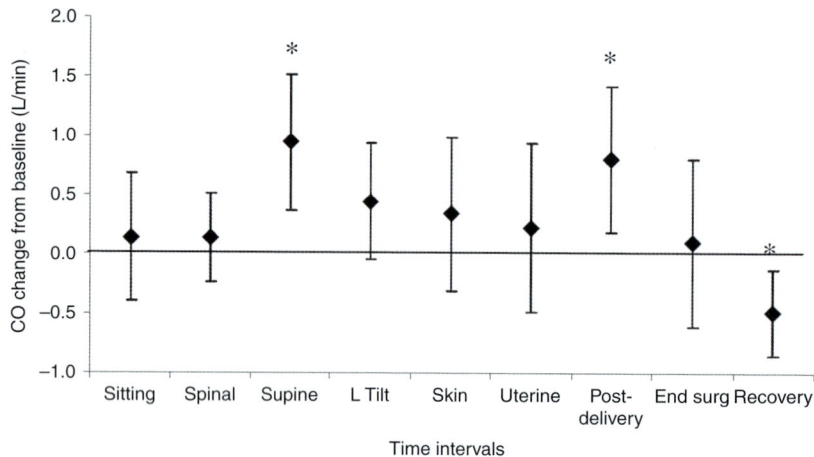

Figure 31.1 Changes in cardiac output during cesarean delivery under spinal anesthesia in severe preeclampsia
Source: Used with permission from Dyer RA, Piercy JL, Reed AR, et al. Hemodynamic changes associated with spinal anesthesia for cesarean delivery in severe preeclampsia. *Anesthesiology* 2008; 108(5):802–11.[2]

the reduction in compliance reduces diastolic filling. This diastolic dysfunction is often clinically subtle and unrecognized until decompensation due to disease progression or effects of anesthesia. In the latter instance, systolic heart failure occurs as a consequence of the inability of the hypertrophied ventricle to maintain adequate ejection. The recognition and correct management of these subtypes are essential in the avoidance of adverse outcomes. While rapid cardiac decompensation is an uncommon consequence of spinal anesthesia and cesarean delivery, understanding the pathophysiology is essential in the management of these rare events.

The importance of diastolic function in the etiology of cardiac failure cannot be underestimated. Typically, preeclampsia represents a hyperdynamic state with increased contractility, left ventricular hypertrophy, raised systemic vascular resistance, and diastolic dysfunction.[10] This produces abnormalities of left ventricular diastolic filling. The heart becomes progressively more dependent on atrial contraction to ensure adequate ventricular filling. The gradual increase in left ventricular end-diastolic pressure probably contributes to the development of pulmonary edema.

The incidence in preeclampsia of progression to heart failure with reduced ejection fraction is unknown; one previous paper described systolic heart failure in 4 of 16 patients with pulmonary edema.[11] Recognition of the cause of cardiac dysfunction (whether diastolic or systolic) is essential for the safe management of these patients.[2]

The vast majority of cases of uncomplicated severe preeclampsia with isolated diastolic dysfunction develop minimal spinal hypotension, and cardiac output is well maintained (Figure 31.1). Such spinal hypotension responds rapidly to conventional vasopressor therapy using phenylephrine, in preference to excessive fluid administration.[12] However, a poor or paradoxical response should prompt the obstetric anesthesiologist to search rapidly for an alternative cause. Volume overload will frequently be signaled by worsening respiratory function, desaturation, and the development of pulmonary edema. Failure of adequate contractile function and ejection should respond better to inotropic agents than to the use of phenylephrine, which as a pure alpha agonist increases afterload and may in this condition impair maternal cardiac output to a clinically significant extent. In the event that a patient continues to deteriorate despite the use of phenylephrine, undiagnosed cardiac dysfunction should be suspected, and inotropic agents such as epinephrine should be used. In the emergency setting, the obstetric anesthesiologist should follow the ABC approach, providing supportive care. Supplemental oxygen, rapid tracheal intubation, ventilation, and administration of adrenergic agents take precedence over the exact diagnosis and etiology.

TTE has been shown to be effective in the rapid recognition of cardiac dysfunction in obstetric patients. While this is not yet a standard of care, rapid point-of-care examinations such as the rapid obstetric screening echocardiography (ROSE) protocol have been developed in obstetrics that can be performed repeatedly and reliably within a few minutes.[13] Recently, the value of point-of-care TTE has been recognized and endorsed by several cardiology societies.[14] In the future, bedside echocardiography performed by anesthetists may become as commonplace as auscultation with a stethoscope.

Heart failure with reduced ejection fraction most commonly manifests as peripartum cardiomyopathy (PPCM). These patients often demonstrate symptoms of severe biventricular failure. Although the typical presentations of preeclampsia and PPCM are distinct, the conditions are more difficult to distinguish when preeclampsia is complicated by severe heart failure. The prevalence of preeclampsia has been found to be much higher in patients with PPCM than in the general population, and animal work may suggest pathophysiologic pathways common to both conditions.[15] The possibility exists that the development of preeclampsia in a patient with some degree of prior left ventricular systolic impairment due to PPCM may precipitate severe heart failure.

Should the anesthetist have delayed cesarean delivery in this patient with fetal distress in order to perform bedside TTE? Certainly, it may have rapidly provided critical information to guide definitive therapy more accurately. This case shows that the understanding and recognition of both common and rare causes of spinal hypotension are important (see Table 31.1) and that individualization of care is of paramount importance.

Learning Points

- Hypotension is a frequent complication of spinal anesthesia for cesarean delivery.
- Spinal hypotension is typically caused by reduction in sympathetic outflow, decreased systemic vascular resistance, and increased venous capacitance.
- Typical spinal hypotension responds rapidly to administration of alpha agonists such as phenylephrine.
- Hypotension unresponsive to phenylephrine or associated with associated symptoms of cardiac failure suggests an alternative etiology.
- The cardiovascular response to preeclampsia commonly represents diastolic dysfunction but may include systolic dysfunction and progression to severe heart failure.
- In the common scenario of diastolic dysfunction, maintenance of adequate preload without fluid overload is essential. Spinal anesthesia is usually well tolerated.
- In rarer cases of severe systolic dysfunction, there is a fine balance between maintenance of adequate preload and careful afterload reduction. This is usually best achieved through cautious, graded neuraxial blockade, but general anesthesia with inotropic support may be required.
- Preoperative point-of-care TTE is the ideal preoperative investigation when suitable skills exist.

References

1. Ngan Kee WD, Khaw KS, Ng FF. Prevention of hypotension during spinal anesthesia for cesarean delivery: an effective technique using combination phenylephrine infusion and crystalloid cohydration. *Anesthesiology* 2005; **103**(4):744–50.

2. Hofmeyr R, Matjila M, Dyer R. Preeclampsia in 2017: Obstetric and Anaesthesia Management. *Best Practice & Research Clinical Anaesthesiology* 2017; **31**(1):125–38.

3. Dyer RA, Piercy JL, Reed AR, et al. Hemodynamic changes associated with spinal anesthesia for cesarean delivery in severe preeclampsia. *Anesthesiology* 2008; **108**(5):802–11.

4. Langesaeter E, Dyer RA. Maternal haemodynamic changes during spinal anaesthesia for caesarean section. *Curr Opin Anaesthesiol* 2011; **24**(3):242–48.

5. Ngan Kee WD. Phenylephrine infusions for maintaining blood pressure during spinal anesthesia for cesarean delivery: finding the shoe that fits. *Anesth Analg* 2014; **118**(3):496–98.

6. Ousley R, Egan C, Dowling K, Cyna AM. Assessment of block height for satisfactory spinal anaesthesia for caesarean section. *Anaesthesia* 2012; **67**(12):1356–63.

7. Kinsella SM, Tuckey JP. Perioperative bradycardia and asystole: relationship to vasovagal syncope and the Bezold-Jarisch reflex. *Br J Anaesth* 2001; **86**(6):859–68.

8. Ngan Kee WD, Lee SWY, Khaw KS, Ng FF. Hemodynamic effects of glycopyrrolate pretreatment before phenylephrine infusion during spinal anesthesia for cesarean delivery. *Int J Obstet Anesth* 2013; **22**(3):179–87.

9. Dennis AT, Castro JM. Echocardiographic differences between preeclampsia and peripartum cardiomyopathy. *Int J Obstet Anesth* 2014; **23**(3):260–66.

10. Dennis AT, Castro J, Carr C, et al. Haemodynamics in women with untreated pre-eclampsia. *Anaesthesia* 2012; **67**(10):1105–18.

11. Desai DK, Moodley J, Naidoo DP, Bhorat I. Cardiac abnormalities in pulmonary oedema associated with hypertensive crises in pregnancy. *BJOG* 1996; **103**(6):523–28.

12. Dyer RA, Daniels A, Vorster A, Emmanuel A, Arcache MJ, Schulein S, Reed AR, Lombard CJ, James MF, van Dyk D. Maternal cardiac output response to colloid preload and vasopressor therapy during spinal anaesthesia for caesarean section in patients with severe pre-eclampsia: a randomised, controlled trial. Anaesthesia. 2018 Jan; 73(1):23–31. doi: 10.1111/anae.14040.

13. Dennis AT. Transthoracic echocardiography in obstetric anesthesia and obstetric critical illness. *Int J Obstet Anesth* 2011; **20**(2): 160–68.

14. Via G, Hussain A, Wells M, et al. International evidence-based recommendations for focused cardiac ultrasound. *J Am Soc Echocardiogr* 2014; **27**(7):683e1–33.

15. Bello N, Rendon IS, Arany Z. The relationship between preeclampsia and peripartum cardiomyopathy: a systematic review and meta-analysis. *J Am Coll Cardiol* 2013; **62**(18):1715–23.

Chapter 32

Management of an Anticipated and Unanticipated Difficult Airway in a Pregnant Patient

Mary C. Mushambi and Karunakaran Ramaswamy

Failed tracheal intubation is more frequent in obstetrics than in the nonobstetric population, and it has remained unchanged for many years at 1 in 390 for obstetric general anesthesia and 1 in 443 general anesthetics for cesarean deliveries.[1] Maternal physiologic and anatomic changes, comorbidities such as obesity, increasing maternal age, the remote location of most labor wards, the urgency of cesarean delivery, and finally the need for rapid-sequence induction for most obstetric general anesthetics[2] all add to the complexity of managing the obstetric airway. Most failed intubations occur during emergencies,[1,2] and the time pressure to deliver the baby often leads to poor preparation, planning, and performance of the rapid-sequence induction. The number of obstetric general anesthetics (GAs) is declining, leading to reduced experience for trainees.[3,4] It is therefore essential that teaching and training should focus on delivering a safe obstetric GA and aim to reduce adverse airway events and optimize the management of failed intubation should it occur. Careful planning and preparation prior to the administration of a GA are crucial in preventing serious untoward airway incidents. The aim of this chapter is to address first the management of the predicted difficult airway with emphasis on careful team planning and preparation and choice of a safe anesthetic strategy for the individual patient and secondly safe management of the unanticipated difficult airway.

Case Study

Anticipated Difficult Airway

This Case Study describes the management a 25-year-old pregnant woman (height 146 cm; weight 45 kg) with Klippel-Feil syndrome (KFS) who had a posterior placenta previa and a previous cesarean delivery. The patient had severe kyphoscoliosis (Figure 32.1) with significant back pain and was unable to lie flat owing to shortness of breath. A spinal anesthetic for her cesarean delivery 2 years previously had been extremely difficult, and she had found it difficult to breathe during surgery. She had a history of recurrent chest infections and shortness of breath walking 20 meters. On examination, her chest was clear, but she had obvious difficulty in breathing and very restricted rib movements. Airway assessment showed severely restricted neck movement from previous neck surgery (Figure 32.2) and a Mallampati grade 4. Pulmonary function tests showed restrictive lung disease with a FEV_1 of 1.2L, FVC of 1.3L, and FEV_1/FVC ratio of 92 percent. Her echocardiogram was normal.

The patient was discussed at a multidisciplinary team (MDT) meeting, and an agreement was reached for the obstetric and anesthetic management plans. An elective cesarean delivery under general anesthetic with awake fiberoptic intubation (AFI) was planned. The documented plan in the notes included a plan should the patient have an admission out of hours.

When the patient arrived in the OR, two 14-gauge cannulae were sited, and full monitoring was instituted, including a radial arterial line. Cell salvage and a Level 1 rapid infuser were set up. Glycopyrrolate 200 mcg was administered intravenously. The patient was asked to gargle with 3 ml 2% lidocaine gel (Instillagel) to help reduce the gag reflex. Further topical anesthesia to the mouth and oropharynx was achieved using 3 ml 4% lidocaine with a Mucosa Atomising Device (MAD). The supraglottic area, glottis, and infraglottic area were anesthetized using a spray-as-you-go (SAYGO) technique (total 3 ml 4% lidocaine). Supplementary oxygen was administered via nasal cannulae. Sedation was achieved using midazolam (1 mg) and a remifentanil infusion starting at 0.05 µg/kg/min. A cut Berman airway was used to prevent the patient biting on the fiberoptic scope

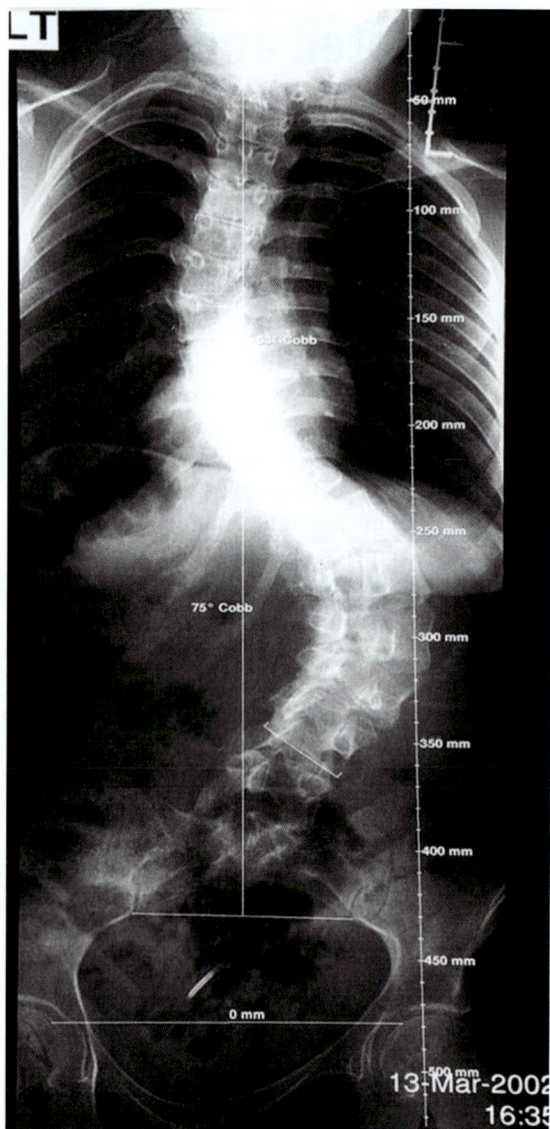

Figure 32.1 X-ray of patient showing severe kyphoscoliosis

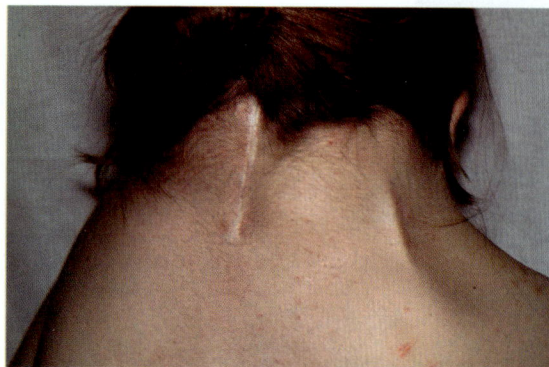

Figure 32.2 View of the back of patient's neck showing a scar from previous surgery and a webbed neck

inflated. Postintubation laryngoscopy revealed a Cormack and Lehane grade 4 view.

The baby's Apgar scores were 2 and 5 at 1 and 10 minutes with an umbilical venous and an arterial pH of 7.30 and 7.23. After an uneventful operation with a blood loss of 500 ml, the patient was transferred to the ICU and extubated after a few hours when she was awake, had good arterial blood gases, and was able to generate adequate tidal volumes.

Key Points

- Management of this patent involved an anticipated difficult airway and a potential risk of hemorrhage from a placenta previa.
- Regional anesthesia was not an option in this patient.
- General anesthesia following an awake fiberoptic intubation was therefore the technique of choice.

Discussion

Klippel-Feil syndrome (KFS) is an autosomal-dominant condition that leads to an abnormal fusion of cervical vertebrae. This may be associated with craniocervical junction anomalies (Figure 32.3), unstable cervical spine, kyphoscoliosis, and cardiac and genitourinary abnormalities.[5,6] My patient was of short stature and had severe symptomatic restrictive lung disease. Placenta previa, especially in a patient with a previous cesarean delivery, is associated with a possible risk of major hemorrhage at surgery.[7,8] This combination presents a dilemma of how to manage the anesthesia safely. Such patients

and to act as a conduit for the fiberscope. The gag reflex was difficult to suppress and was successfully obtunded with the injection of 1 ml 4% lidocaine through the cricothyroid membrane using a 20-gauge cannula. Once the fiberoptic scope was in the trachea, a size 6.0-mm reinforced cuffed endotracheal tube (ETT) was railroaded over the scope. After confirmation of correct placement of the ETT in the trachea with a capnograph, general anesthesia was induced using propofol and muscle paralysis with atracurium, and the endotracheal cuff was then

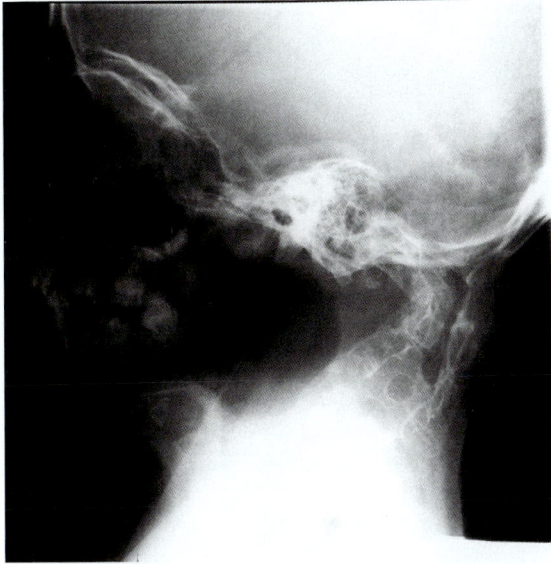

Figure 32.3 An X-ray of a patient with Klippel-Feil syndrome showing the abnormal cervical spine

should be discussed at MDT meetings in order to formulate a plan. The plan should be communicated to all labor ward staff and to the patient. A decision on the mode of delivery should be made based on what is the safest option for mother and baby. The only option for this patient was delivery by elective cesarean delivery. Regional anesthesia (RA) is considered by many anesthetists to be the anesthetic of choice in patients with a known difficult airway,[9] and it has been used in patients with KFS.[10,11] However, RA techniques can have significant drawbacks in such patients. It is difficult to estimate the local anesthetic volume in a single-shot spinal (SSS), particularly in a patient of such short stature, and there is a real risk of a high or total spinal anesthetic developing. Epidural anesthesia has a high intraoperative GA conversion rate (4.3 percent),[12] which is less desirable in a patient with a difficult airway. Combined spinal-epidural (CSE) anesthesia has been associated with inadequate intraoperative anesthesia in a patient with KFS.[11] Continuous spinal anesthesia (CSA) with a spinal catheter offers several advantages over SSS and CSE. It enables titration by injecting small volumes of local anesthetic through the catheter until the desired level of anesthesia is achieved. However, CSA is unfamiliar to many anesthetists and has a high failure rate and a high post–dural puncture headache rate.[13] For these reasons, and in

addition to the patient's previous experience, RA was considered unsafe in this patient.

Awake Fiberoptic Intubation (AFI) in a Pregnant Patient

AFI in a pregnant woman differs in many ways from that in a nonpregnant patient. The presence of a fetus means that any drugs administered to the mother can affect the baby. Neonatologists therefore should be made aware in advance. The nasal mucosa is congested and more vascular during pregnancy, and this makes oral intubation the preferred route of intubation. Occasionally, the oral route is not possible due to oral pathology. Cocaine is a very effective vasoconstrictor, but it is associated with reduced placental blood flow and therefore should be avoided during pregnancy.[14,15] Phenylephrine 0.5%/lidocaine 5% combination (Co-phenylcaine) and xylometazoline hydrochloride 0.1% spray are safer alternatives. However, vasoconstrictors should be used with care in preeclamptic patients because they may exacerbate the hypertension. Oral intubation is also more difficult than nasal intubation, and it requires more dense topical anesthesia in order to suppress the gag reflex.

It is important that aortocaval compression is avoided. Premedication should include an H_2 antagonist and 30 ml of 0.3 M sodium citrate immediately prior to starting sedation. An antisialogogue – glycopyrrolate 200 µg IV – will help to reduce secretions. Two experienced anesthetists are required, one to perform the endoscopy and the other to administer and monitor sedation. The help of an experienced anesthetic assistant is essential.

Some form of sedation such as midazolam, fentanyl, alfentanil, remifentanil, or propofol is recommended. Midazolam 0.5–1 mg is useful to ensure a degree of amnesia. Remifentanil is gaining popularity because it provides the best analgesia for the mother with conscious and cooperative sedation and suppression of the gag reflex, which gives good intubating conditions. Infusion rates of 0.05–0.5 µg/kg/min and a target controlled infusion (TCI) of 3–5 ng/ml have been used in nonobstetric patients with or without propofol (TCI 0.5–0.8 µg/ml).[16–18] TCI with propofol has been used for AFI in obstetrics with a target concentration of 0.6–1.0 µg/ml combined with midazolam 1 mg and topical anesthesia.[19]

Excessive sedation should be avoided because it reduces the protective laryngeal reflexes and increases

173

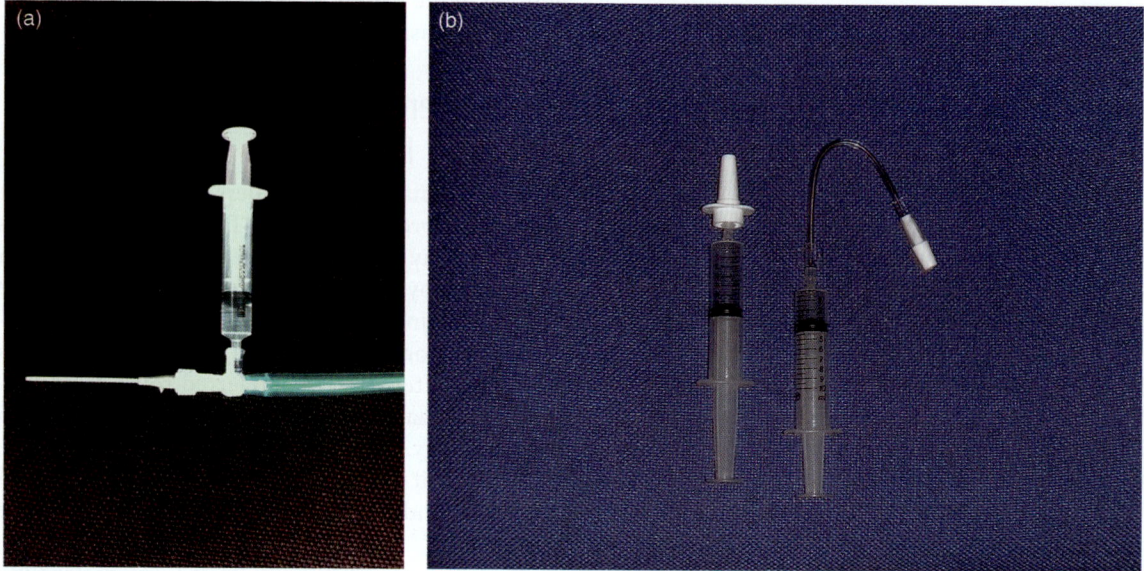

Figure 32.4 Two types of equipment used to administer local anesthetic to the upper airway: (a) Mucosa Atomising Device (MAD); (b) Mackenzie technique with 20-gauge cannula attached by a three-way tap to oxygen tubing, which is connected to 2 L/min oxygen supply.

the likelihood of aspiration. Antagonists such as flumazenil and naloxone should be readily available. Oxygen should be administered.

There have been concerns about the use of topical airway anesthesia in patients at risk of regurgitation and aspiration. However, studies have showed that the sedation provided is not excessive, and there is no evidence of an increased risk of regurgitation and aspiration.[20]

The nose, mouth and pharynx may be anesthetized by direct spray using a device such as the commercially produced Mucosal Atomising Device (MAD) (Figure 32.4a) or the Mackenzie technique, which uses an 18- or 20-gauge cannula attached by a three-way tap to oxygen tubing that is connected to 2 L/min oxygen (Figure 32.4b).[21] The patient may also be asked to gargle using 2% lidocaine gel (Instillagel). The remainder of the airway can be anesthetized using one of three techniques: the SAYGO technique, glossopharyngeal and superior laryngeal nerve blocks, and nebulized lidocaine. Nerve blocks are seldom carried out, and nebulized lidocaine, when used alone, does not provided sufficient topical anesthesia.

SAYGO is now the most commonly used method for anesthetizing the airway during AFI. This involves dripping local anesthetic into the airway via an epidural catheter fed through the working channel of the fiberoptic scope. Aliquots of 1 ml 4% lidocaine are

dripped into the supraglottic, glottis, and subglottic areas. A higher maximum dose of lidocaine of 9 mg/kg is allowable because most of it is swallowed and eliminated via first-pass metabolism.[22]

A small size tracheal tube, such as one 6 to 6.5 mm ID, should be used to reduce the chance of impingement on the arytenoids. The design of the tip of the tube may also make a difference, and the intubating LMA tracheal tube (LMA-Fastrach tracheal tube) with a Huber tip is the least likely to impinge. Following endotracheal intubation, the position of the tube must be confirmed with capnography before the patient is anesthetized and the cuff is inflated.

Learning Points

- Patients with Klippel-Feil syndrome have congenital anomalies that make airway management challenging.
- Patients with a difficult airway, restrictive lung disease, and a high risk of intraoperative bleeding present an anesthetic dilemma.
- These patients should be discussed at a MDT meetings to formulate and communicate the anesthetic and obstetric plans.
- Awake fiberoptic intubation in an obstetric patient requires the correct equipment and skills to safely secure an airway before general anesthesia is induced.

Case Study

Management of Unanticipated Difficult Airway in a Pregnant Patient

This Case Study describes the management of a 38-year-old Afro-Caribbean woman with a body mass index (BMI) of 48 kg/m^2 who presented for an elective cesarean delivery. The patient had three previous cesareans performed under spinal anesthesia. Airway examination revealed a Mallampati grade 2, good mouth opening, thyromental distance of 5 cm, and a short neck but otherwise unrestricted neck movement.

A CSE was performed with intrathecal injection of hyperbaric 0.5% bupivacaine 9 mg (1.8 ml) and 300 μg diamorphine. The patient was positioned supine with left uterine displacement using a wedge and Head Elevation Laryngoscopy Pillow (HELP, ALMA Medical). Blood pressure was maintained with IV crystalloid as a coload, and a phenylephrine infusion was titrated to the maintain patient's baseline systolic blood pressure of 120 mmHg. After testing the epidural catheter for the absence of CSF or blood, the epidural catheter was flushed with 2 ml saline.

A block to T3 and T4 to cold and touch, respectively, was achieved within 6 minutes of the spinal injection. At this point, the patient began to complain of feeling weakness in her arms and difficulty breathing. A high spinal block was suspected. The patient was reassured, and high-flow oxygen was administered using a bag-valve mask. However, the patient rapidly lost consciousness.

The OR team was alerted of the developing situation, and a decision to do a rapid-sequence induction (RSI) was made and additional help summoned. An attempt was made at intubation using a size 4 Macintosh blade and a 7.0 endotracheal tube after injection of a small dose of thiopental (50 mg) and suxamethonium (150 mg). A grade 4 Cormack and Lehane (C&L) view was obtained even with the release of cricoid pressure. The patient's lungs were ventilated successfully with a bag and facemask, and a second attempt was made with a McCoy No. 4 blade and bougie. A grade 3B C&L view was obtained. Attempts at intubation were abandoned, and a No. 4 I-gel (Intersurgical, Ltd) was inserted. Anesthesia was maintained with oxygen, nitrous oxide, and sevoflurane, and rocuronium was administered to facilitate ventilation.

Despite optimal left lateral tilt and IV fluid administration and phenylephrine infusion, the patient remained hypotensive (systolic blood pressure ≈ 70 mmHg, SpO$_2$ ≈ 95 percent), and therefore an epinephrine infusion (10 μg/ml at 15 ml/h) was administered. Surgery was difficult, and it took 45 minutes to deliver the baby. Once the baby was delivered, hemodynamic stability was restored and epinephrine was stopped.

The baby's Apgar scores were 7 and 9 at 1 and 5 minutes respectively. Total blood loss was 1.6L. At the end of surgery, the plan was to transfer the patient to the ICU. The decision was made to attempt to secure the airway with an endotracheal tube. A second experienced anesthetist attempted intubation. The first attempt with a McCoy No. 4 blade revealed a grade 3B laryngeal view. The attempt was abandoned, and after oxygenation, the next attempt with a McGrath videolaryngoscope was successful. The patient was successfully extubated within a few hours and had residual leg weakness from the spinal that resolved after a further few hours. At follow-up, the patient denied any episode of awareness. Both the parturient and her partner were debriefed on what had happened. A Difficult Airway Society alert form was completed, and one copy was given to patient, one sent to the family doctor, and another copy was put in the patient's medical notes.

Key Points

- This patient presented with a high BMI, a potentially difficult cesarean delivery, and a predicted difficult airway.
- An unanticipated total spinal meant that waking the patient following a failed intubation was not an option.
- Hence a decision to proceed with a second-generation supraglottic airway device (SAD) was made.
- Surgery was carried out by senior obstetricians, and uterine fundal pressure was minimized to reduce the risk of regurgitation.
- Cricoid pressure was removed once the second-generation SAD was in place.

Discussion

The Obstetric Anaesthetists' Association (OAA) and Difficult Airway Society (DAS) have developed the first national guidelines for difficult airway and intubation in obstetric patients[23] (Figure 32.5). The decision to either wake up the woman or proceed with surgery is critical, can be challenging, and is affected by multiple factors. The guidelines include

Master algorithm – obstetric general anaesthesia and failed tracheal intubation

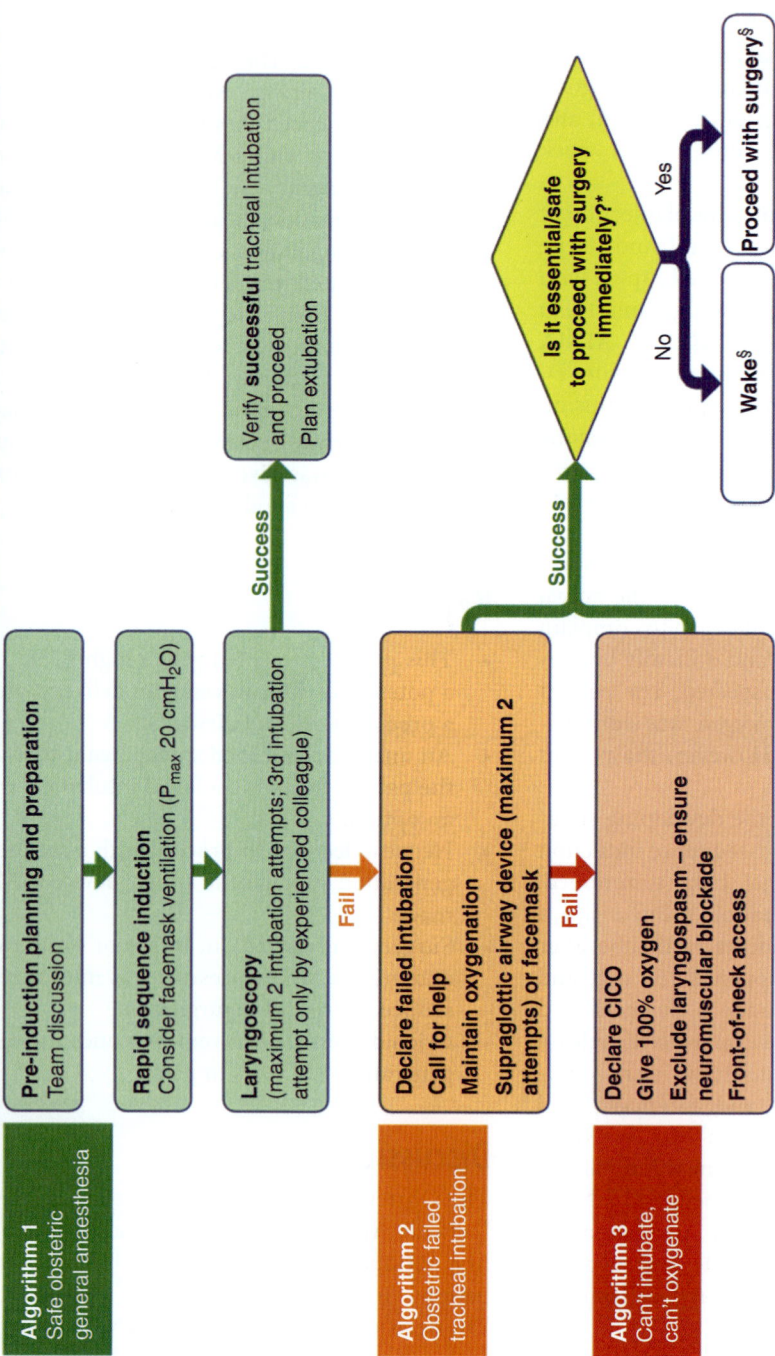

Algorithm 1
Safe obstetric
general anaesthesia

Pre-induction planning and preparation
Team discussion

Rapid sequence induction
Consider facemask ventilation (P_{max} 20 cmH$_2$O)

Laryngoscopy
(maximum 2 intubation attempts; 3rd intubation attempt only by experienced colleague)

↑ **Success** → Verify **successful** tracheal intubation and proceed
Plan extubation

Fail →

Algorithm 2
Obstetric failed
tracheal intubation

Declare failed intubation

Call for help

Maintain oxygenation

Supraglottic airway device (maximum 2 attempts) or facemask

Fail →

Algorithm 3
Can't intubate,
can't oxygenate

Declare CICO

Give 100% oxygen

Exclude laryngospasm – ensure neuromuscular blockade

Front-of-neck access

↑ **Success**

Is it essential/safe to proceed with surgery immediately?*

No → **Wake**§

Yes → **Proceed with surgery**§

Figure 32.5 Master algorithm – obstetric general anesthesia and failed tracheal intubation
Source: Reproduced with permission from the OAA.

Table 1 – proceed with surgery?

		WAKE ←	→ PROCEED		

Before induction

Factors to consider	WAKE			PROCEED
Maternal condition	• No compromise	• Mild acute compromise	• Haemorrhage responsive to resuscitation	• Hypovolaemia requiring corrective surgery • Critical cardiac or respiratory compromise, cardiac arrest
Fetal condition	• No compromise	• Compromise corrected with intrauterine resuscitation, pH < 7.2 but > 7.15	• Continuing fetal heart rate abnormality despite intrauterine resuscitation, pH < 7.15	• Sustained bradycardia • Fetal haemorrhage • Suspected uterine rupture
Anaesthetist	• Novice	• Junior trainee	• Senior trainee	• Consultant / specialist
Obesity	• Supermorbid	• Morbid	• Obese	• Normal
Surgical factors	• Complex surgery or major haemorrhage anticipated	• Multiple uterine scars • Some surgical difficulties expected	• Single uterine scar	• No risk factors
Aspiration risk	• Recent food	• No recent food • In labour • Opioids given • Antacids not given	• No recent food • In labour • Opioids not given • Antacids given	• Fasted • Not in labour • Antacids given
Alternative anaesthesia • regional • securing airway awake	• No anticipated difficulty	• Predicted difficulty	• Relatively contraindicated	• Absolutely contraindicated or has failed • Surgery started

After failed intubation

Factors to consider	WAKE			PROCEED
Airway device / ventilation	• Difficult facemask ventilation • Front-of-neck	• Adequate facemask ventilation	• First generation supraglottic airway device	• Second generation supraglottic airway device
Airway hazards	• Laryngeal oedema • Stridor	• Bleeding • Trauma	• Secretions	• None evident

Criteria to be used in the decision to wake or proceed following failed tracheal intubation. In any individual patient, some factors may suggest waking and others proceeding. The final decision will depend on the anaesthetist's clinical judgement.
© Obstetric Anaesthetists' Association / Difficult Airway Society (2015)

Figure 32.6 Wake or proceed with surgery?
Source: Reproduced with permission from the OAA.

Table 2 – management after failed tracheal intubation

Wake

- Maintain oxygenation
- Maintain cricoid pressure if not impeding ventilation
- Either maintain head-up position or turn left lateral recumbent
- If rocuronium used, reverse with sugammadex
- Assess neuromuscular blockade and manage awareness if paralysis is prolonged
- Anticipate laryngospasm/can't intubate, can't oxygenate

After waking

- Review urgency of surgery with obstetric team
- Intrauterine fetal resuscitation as appropriate
- For repeat anaesthesia, manage with two anaesthetists
- Anaesthetic options:
  - Regional anaesthesia preferably inserted in lateral position
  - Secure airway awake before repeat general anaesthesia

Proceed with surgery

- Maintain anaesthesia
- Maintain ventilation – consider merits of:
  - controlled or spontaneous ventilation
  - paralysis with rocuronium if sugammadex available
- Anticipate laryngospasm/can't intubate, can't oxygenate
- Minimise aspiration risk:
  - maintain cricoid pressure until delivery (if not impeding ventilation)
  - after delivery maintain vigilance and reapply cricoid pressure if signs of regurgitation
  - empty stomach with gastric drain tube if using second-generation supraglottic airway device
  - minimise fundal pressure
  - administer H_2 receptor blocker i.v. if not already given
  - Senior obstetrician to operate
  - Inform neonatal team about failed intubation
  - Consider total intravenous anaesthesia

© Obstetric Anaesthetists' Association
© Difficult Airway Society (2015)

Figure 32.7 Management after failed tracheal intubation
Source: Reproduced with permission from the OAA.

a table highlighting factors that need to be considered in the decision to either wake the woman up or continue with surgery should failed intubation occur (Figure 32.6). If intubation fails and the decision is made to proceed with surgery, a second-generation SAD with an esophageal port is recommended[23] (Figure 32.7). A muscle relaxant may be used to facilitate ventilation and prevent the possibility of laryngospasm and a can't intubate, can't oxygenate (CICO) situation developing.[23,24] It is important that a senior surgeon is available and anesthetic help is summoned immediately.

Should the patient need transfer to the ICU, the airway will need securing with an endotracheal tube using fiberoptic scope–guided intubation via the SAD or a percutaneous emergency front- of-the-neck airway access.[25] Intubation via a SAD must only be attempted using a technique familiar to the anesthetist.

Learning Points

- Failed intubation continues to be a common cause of maternal morbidity and mortality.[26]

- When failed intubation occurs, maternal oxygenation takes priority.
- If a pregnant woman cannot be woken up after failed intubation, the use of a second-generation SAD is recommended. If this fails, a front-of-the-neck airway access using surgical cricothyroidotomy should be performed.
- It is important that a senior obstetric surgeon performs the surgery and that all measures to reduce aspiration are taken.
- An adequate depth of anesthesia should be provided to prevent awareness.[27]
- All patients who have a failed intubation should be followed up by an anesthetist to assess any complications that may have occurred during the failed intubation, for debriefing, and for notification to future anesthetists using the DAS alert form (http://www.das.uk.com).

References

1. Kinsella SM, Winton ALS, Mushambi MC, et al. Failed tracheal intubation during obstetric general anesthesia: a literature review. *Int J Obstetc Anesth* 2015; **24**:356–74.

2. Quinn AC, Milne D, Columb M, Gorton H, Knight M. Failed tracheal intubation in obstetric anaesthesia: 2-year national case-control study in the UK. *Br J Anaesth* 2013; **110**:74–80.

3. Searle RD, Lyons G. Vanishing experience in training for obstetric general anesthesia: an observational study. *Int J Obstet Anesth* 2008; **17**:233–37.

4. Smith NA, Tandel A, Morris RW. Changing patterns in endotracheal intubation for anaesthesia trainees: a retrospective analysis of 80,000 cases over 10 years. *Anaesth Intensive Care* 2011; **39**:585–89.

5. Naikmasur VG, Sattur AP, Kirty RN, Thakur AR. Type III Klippel-Feil syndrome: case report and review of associated craniofacial anomalies. *Odontology* 2011; **99**:197–202.

6. Thomsen MN, Schneider U, Weber M, Johannisson R, Niethard FU. Scoliosis and congenital anomalies associated with Klippel-Feil syndrome types I–III. *Spine* 1997; **22**:396–401.

7. McShane PM, Heyl PS, Epstein MF. Maternal and perinatal morbidity resulting from placenta previa. *Obstet Gynecol* 1985; **65**:176–82.

8. Knight M, UKOSS. Peripartum hysterectomy in the UK: management and outcomes of the associated haemorrhage. *BJOG* 2007; **114**:1380–87.

9. Popat MT, Srivastava M, Russell R. Awake fibreoptic intubation skills in obstetric patients: a survey of anaesthetists in the Oxford region. Anaesthesia for predicted difficult airway. *Int J Obstet Anesth* 2000; **9**:78–82.

10. Dresner M, Maclean A. Anaesthesia for caesarean section in a patient with Klippel-Feil syndrome: the use of a microspinal catheter. *Anaesthesia* 1995; **50**:807–9.

11. Cavanagh T, Jee R, Kilpatrick N, Douglas J. Elective cesarean delivery in a parturient with Klippel-Feil syndrome. *Int J Obstet Anesth* 2013; **22**(4):343–48.

12. Pan PH, Bogard TD, Owen MD. Incidence and characteristics of failures in obstetric neuraxial analgesia and anesthesia: a retrospective analysis of 19,259 deliveries. *Int J Obstet Anesth* 2004; **13**(4):227–33.

13. Palmer CM. Continuous spinal anesthesia and analgesia in obstetrics. *Anesth Analg* 2010; **111**:1476–79.

14. Woods JR, Plessinger MA, Clark KE. Effect of cocaine on uterine blood flow and fetal oxygenation. *JAMA* 1987; **257**:957–61.

15. Addis A, Moretti ME, Ahmed Syed F, Einarson TR, Koren G. Fetal effect of cocaine: an updated meta-analysis. *Reprod Toxicol* 2001; **15**:341–69.

16. Puchner W, Egger P, Puhringer F, et al. Evaluation of remifentanil as a single drug for awake fibreoptic intubation. *Acta Anaesthesiol Scand* 2002; **46**:350–54.

17. Rai MR, Parry TM, Dombrovskis A, Warner OJ. Remifentanil target-controlled infusion vs propofol target-controlled infusion for conscious sedation for awake fibreoptic intubation: a double-blinded randomized, controlled trial. *Br J Anaesth* 2008; **100**:125–30.

18. Johnston KD, Rai MR. Conscious sedation for awake fibreoptic intubation: a review of the literature. *Can J Anaesth* 2013; **60**:584–99.

19. Popat M, Russell R. Awake fiberoptic intubation following previous failed intubation. *Int J Obstet Anesth* 2001; **10**:332–33.

20. Ovassapian A, Krejcie TC, Yelich SJ, Dykes MH. Awake fibreoptic intubation in the patient at high risk of aspiration. *Br J Anaesth* 1989; **62**:13–16.

21. Mackenzie I. A new method of drug application to the nasal passage. *Anaesthesia* 1998; **53**:309–10.

22. Williams KA, Barker GL, Harwood RJ, Woodall NM. Combined nebulized and spray-as-you-go topical local anaesthesia of the airway. *Br J Anaesth* 2005; **95**(4):549–53.

23. Mushambi MC, Kinsella SM, Popat M et al. Obstetric Anaesthetists' Association and Difficult Airway Society guidelines for the management of difficult and failed tracheal intubation in obstetrics. *Anaesthesia* 2015; **70**:1286–306.

24. Cook TM, Woodall N, Frerk C, Fourth National Audit Project. Major complications of airway management in the UK: results of the Fourth National Audit Project of the Royal College of Anaesthetists and the Difficult Airway Society, Part 1: Anaesthesia. *Br J Anaesth* 2011; **106**:617–31.

25. Kristensen MS, Teoh WHL, Baker PA. Percutaneous emergency airway access: prevention, preparation, teaching and training. *Br J Anaesth* 2015; **114**(3):357–61.

26. Cantwell R, Clutton-Brock T, Cooper G, et al. Saving mothers' lives: reviewing maternal deaths to make motherhood safer: 2006–2008. The Eighth Report of the Confidential Enquiries into Maternal Deaths in the United Kingdom. *BJOG* 2011; **118**(Suppl 1):1–203.

27. Pandit JJ, Andrade J, Bogod DG, et al. 5th National Audit Project (NAP5) on accidental awareness during general anaesthesia: summary of main findings and risk factors. *Br J Anaesth* 2014; **113**:549–59.

Major Obstetric Hemorrhage and Point-of-Care Testing

Rachel Collis, Lucy de Lloyd, and Simon Slinn

Case Study

A healthy primiparous woman with a body mass index (BMI) of 20 kg/m^2 presented at 41 + 5 weeks' gestation to the delivery suite following induction of labor for postdates. After a prolonged latent phase, her labor progressed slowly. She requested epidural analgesia, which was sited successfully without problems, after which labor was augmented with oxytocin. After a further 8 hours, the patient remained dilated at 9 cm despite adequate uterine contractions, and the decision was made to perform an emergency cesarean delivery.

Both the anesthesiologist and obstetrician had 5 years of specialty training, and consultants in both specialties were available to attend within 30 minutes from home because it was outside routine hours. The patient's baseline full blood count (FBC) showed a hemoglobin (Hb) of 101 g/liter, white cell count (WCC) of 18×10^9/liter, and platelet count of 220×10^9/liter. Two group and save samples had been sent to the blood bank earlier in the day, confirming blood group and no abnormal antibodies, which meant that should blood be required, it could be immediately issued without delay and further cross-matching.

The epidural block the patient had for labor analgesia was successfully topped up to provide anesthesia for her cesarean delivery using 20 ml 0.5% L-bupivacaine and 100 μg fentanyl. Following delivery, a slow IV bolus of 5 IU oxytocin was administered, and an oxytocin infusion was started at 10 IU/h. Almost immediately, the patient complained of feeling unwell, with a fall in blood pressure from 105/65 to 70/40 mmHg and an increase in heart rate from 105 to 125 beats/min noted. The anesthesiologist also noticed that there was already 1,200 ml of blood in the suction bottle and a number of heavily blood-soaked swabs, which had not yet been weighed, and blood

loss appeared to be continuing. Discussion with the obstetrician revealed that bleeding was mainly traumatic from an extension of the uterine incision with some uterine atony.

A major obstetric hemorrhage (MOH) was declared, alerting the blood bank to issue 4 units of packed red cells (PRCs) and to defrost fresh frozen plasma (FFP) but to delay transportation of the FFP until point-of-care (POC) testing results were available. Consultant anesthesiologist and obstetric staff were called from home. A second large-bore IV cannula was inserted and blood taken at the same time for a FBC, near-patient thromboelastometry FIBTEM, coagulation profile and venous blood gas analysis, including hemoglobin (Hb) and lactate estimation. Hb estimation on the blood gas analysis was 84 g/liter, lactate 3 mmol/liter, with a base deficit of –6 mmol/liter. The FIBTEM amplitude at 5 minutes (A5) was 25 mm, indicating adequate fibrinogen levels and implying normal coagulation despite the significant postpartum hemorrhage (PPH) of around 1,800 ml at this time. The local FIBTEM POC algorithm was followed (Figure 33.1), and the FFP was held in the blood bank rather than being delivered to the OR. The PRCs were available in the OR 15 minutes after request, and 2 units were transfused via a warming device. As part of the standard local practice 1 g tranexamic acid was given intravenously.

Surgical bleeding was brought under surgical control, and uterine atony was managed by repeating the 5-IU bolus of oxytocin, and after antiemetic prophylaxis with 8 mg ondansetron, 500 μg ergometrine (diluted in 20 ml saline) was given by slow IV injection. After the very brisk initial bleeding, 35 minutes after recognition of the major PPH, the bleeding slowed significantly, and after closing the uterus, hemostasis was secured. Most of the management was undertaken by resident medical staff, but attendance by the consultant obstetrician and anesthesiologist confirmed hemostasis and

---

* We thank Professor Peter Collins, consultant hematologist, for his role in developing our local FIBTEM-based MOH algorithm.

OBSCYMRU
Obstetric Bleeding Strategy for Wales

ROTEM Protocol
(For use in postpartum haemorrhage)

Blood loss >1000ml *Measured or suspected* or **Stage 2 activated***

Give Tranexamic Acid *(if not given already)*

TAKE BLOODS — POC: ROTEM, Lactate, Hb / Lab: FBC, Coag, +/- repeat Xmatch *(Alert lab staff)*

OPTIMISE PATIENT
Temp >36°C Hb >80g/L pH >7.2 Ionised Ca²⁺ >1mmol/L

REVIEW OTHER CAUSES OF BLEEDING
If coagulation normal, escalate obstetric & anaesthetic care

ONGOING BLEEDING or CLINICAL CONCERN?

NO *No blood products required*

CLINICAL MONITORING *Consider HDU care post-op*

ANY OF THE FOLLOWING?
Clinical concern
Suspected further bleeding *Inc. concealed bleeding*
>500ml further blood loss

YES   Only transfuse coagulation products if patient is bleeding

REVIEW FIBTEM A5 *(fibrin polymerisation)*

FIBTEM A5 ≥12mm or *Fibrinogen >2 g/L* → **No fibrinogen currently required**

FIBTEM A5 ≤11mm or *Fibrinogen <2 g/L* → **Give fibrinogen concentrate** A5 7-11mm = 4g / A5 <7mm = 6g

ANY OF THE FOLLOWING?
Any blood products given
> 500ml further blood loss
Clinical concern

If **FIBTEM A5 ≤11mm** after transfusing fibrinogen concentrate, or suspicion of abruption/AFE review EXTEM CT and FBC

REVIEW EXTEM CT *(thrombin generation)*

EXTEM CT <75sec or *normal PT/APTT* → **No FFP required**

EXTEM CT ≥75sec or *elevated PT/APTT* → **Give FFP** Booking Weight ≤ 50Kg = 3 Units / > 50Kg = 4 Units

REVIEW FBC *(platelet deficiency)*

Platelets >75 x10⁹/L → **No Platelets required**

Platelets ≤75 x10⁹/L → **Give Platelets** 1 adult unit

If you have any concerns discuss with haematologist

Haematologist
Blood Bank
Haematology Lab
Porters

NB: ROTEM does not reliably detect effects of: warfarin, aspirin, clopidogrel, reopro, direct oral anticoagulants, LMWH. It will not detect deficiency of von Willebrand factor.

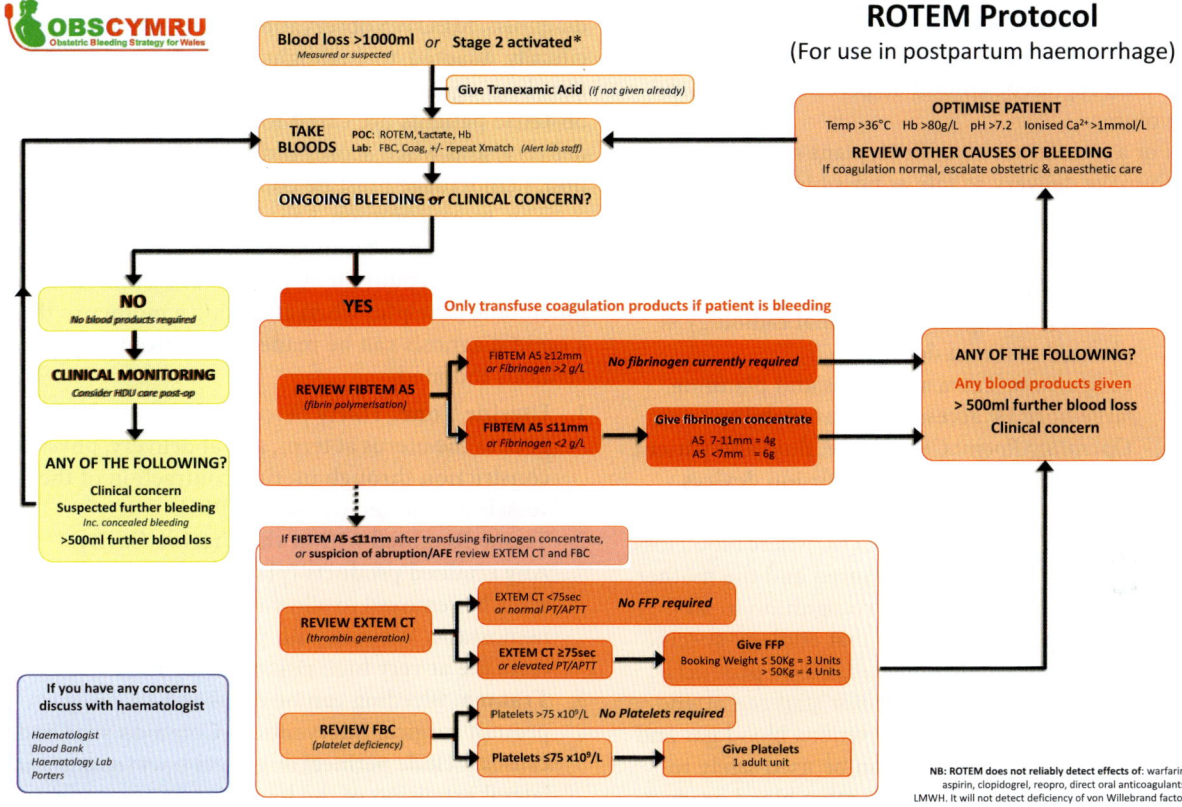

Figure 33.1 Algorithm for the use of FIBTEM during PPH; * Activation of PPH protocol when blood loss 1000- 1500ml

adequate resuscitation. The final measured blood loss was 2,600 ml. Initial fluid resuscitation was with 1 liter of balanced salt solution followed by 500 ml of a modified fluid gelatin in the first 25 minutes. Two units of PRCs were given when the blood loss was around 2 liters, followed by a further 1 liter of balanced salt solution over the next 30 minutes. After the initial dramatic fall in blood pressure, which was treated with fluid boluses and a 50-µg bolus of IV phenylephrine, the patient's systolic blood pressure remained above 100 mmHg. Her heart rate fell from the initial value of 125 beats/min to around 105 beats/min, probably reflecting mild hypoperfusion and anemia.

Repeat bloods taken toward the end of the procedure after transfusion of 2 units PRCs showed a Hb of 85 g/liter and a FIBTEM A5 value that had fallen to 14 mm, reflecting the significant bleed, but in the face of hemostasis still above the FFP FIBTEM transfusion trigger. The corrected calcium on blood gas analysis indicated a level of 0.9 mmol/liter, which was treated

by administering 10 ml 10% calcium gluconate by slow IV infusion

The patient was sent to a high-dependency area for recovery, with hourly urine output and observations recorded every 15 minutes on a modified early obstetric warning score (MEOWS) chart. She received one further unit of PRCs on the first postnatal day because she was symptomatic with a Hb of 76 g/liter, but otherwise recovered well.

Key Points

- Despite being healthy, this woman had multiple risk factors for significant postpartum hemorrhage (PPH). Her prolonged latent labor stage, pharmacologically augmented contractions with oxytocin, and obstructed labor put her at a high risk of uterine atony. She was additionally vulnerable to the effects of hemorrhage because of preexisting anemia and low BMI. Her estimated blood volume was around 5 liters, and total blood loss was therefore over 50 percent of her

181

circulating volume. This compares with a woman with a BMI of 24 kg/m^2 with an estimated blood volume of 6 liters, in whom the same blood loss would represent around 40 percent of her blood volume.

- For a woman at risk of PPH, plans should be made to make delivery as safe as possible. Such plans include

  - *Antenatal:* Identification and treatment of anemia. If very high risk (e.g., placenta accrete), arrange interventional radiology at planned cesarean delivery.
  - *Peripartum:* Team awareness and planning, large-bore IV access, blood availability.
  - *Operating Room:* Cell salvage, fluid and patient warming, and rapid fluid infusion devices.
  - Timely recognition of major PPH is comparatively easy in the OR, where blood loss should be routinely measured and the mother actively observed. Early recognition in all situations is essential so that etiology-specific treatments can be initiated, blood products ordered, and relevant senior staff can attend.
  - Near-side blood testing (venous blood gas and thromboelastometry) can be used safely to optimize use of blood and other blood products such as FFP, removing the need for formulaic replacement even in high-risk patients.

Discussion

Major obstetric hemorrhage (MOH) is classified as moderate (1,500–2,500 ml) or severe (>2,500 ml) blood loss. In the Scottish study of severe maternal morbidity, MOH was 80 percent of the reported maternal morbidity, with a rate of 5.8 per 1,000 births.[1] PPH remains a leading cause of maternal morbidity and mortality in the United Kingdom, and in 2014, the UK confidential enquiries into maternal deaths reported a mortality rate from obstetric hemorrhage of 0.49 per 100,000 maternities, where substandard care due to delayed recognition was frequently implicated.[2]

Late recognition of PPH may be due in part to the physiologic adaptations of pregnancy, which enable patients to compensate well for moderate levels of hypovolemia, and the fact that most pregnant woman are young and healthy. The classical signs of shock consequently may manifest only once substantial hemorrhage has already occurred, at around 30 percent of blood volume. Additionally,

hemorrhage may be concealed, further obscuring the diagnosis. MEOWS observation charts, which are specifically adapted to highlight physiologic deterioration in pregnant women, should be used whenever obstetric patients are cared for both before and after delivery, and when scores indicate clinical deterioration, hemorrhage must be considered.

The most common causes of PPH are uterine atony and trauma secondary to vaginal or cesarean birth, which account for 80 percent of cases. The 4 T's mnemonic is helpful when attending a mother so that a rapid diagnosis can be made and appropriate interventions initiated.

1. **Uterine Tone.** Thirty percent of blood volume goes to the uterus at term, and at delivery, physical constriction through uterine contraction of the vessels is required to prevent PPH.
2. **Tissue Retained within the Uterine Cavity.** Any retained products (placenta/membranes) must be removed to allow uterine contraction and hemostasis. Women with placenta accreta/percreta are at very high risk of major PPH.
3. **Trauma.** Bleeding can be rapid and requires prompt surgical intervention. Common sites and causes include perineal or genital tract trauma and lateral extension of the lower uterine segment at emergency cesarean, which is more common if the fetal head is engaged in the pelvis.
4. **Thrombin: Disorders of Coagulation.** Coagulopathy may precede hemorrhage and be causal or develop secondary to hemorrhage. Severe obstetric coagulopathy with consumption of clotting factors and platelets is associated with placental abruption, HELLP syndrome (hemolysis, elevated liver enzymes, and low platelets), severe sepsis, and amniotic fluid embolus. Dilution of coagulation factors by resuscitation with non-plasma-based fluids will also lead to coagulopathy, but this occurs late in obstetric hemorrhage because of increased baseline levels of fibrinogen and other clotting factors.

Management of Postpartum Hemorrhage

Early recognition is vital to allow a rapid structured response. When abnormal bleeding is noticed (>500 ml at vaginal birth and 1,000 ml after cesarean birth), medical staff should attend, if not already there, and therapeutic maneuvers should be initiated based on the cause of the PPH. This is facilitated by ensuring the routine weighing of all surgical swabs, pads, and bed linen because this correlates closely with a fall in hemoglobin. Visually estimating blood loss can lead to significant underestimation and subsequent delay in initiating interventions.[3] It is important to have a high index of suspicion because repeated small amounts of blood loss postpartum may be overlooked, and bleeding may be concealed.

Resuscitation should follow a structured ABC approach and identification and treatment of the cause using the 4 T's mnemonic. Adequate IV access should be established, with blood taken for FBC, laboratory-based coagulation, and blood bank specimens. POC measurements of Hb and lactate using a blood gas machine (which is available on many delivery suites) can be very helpful, allowing early recognition of anemia and metabolic acidosis, although a normal hemoglobin early in a PPH does not rule out a significant bleed. In addition, POC testing of coagulation using thromboelastography techniques can help the clinician make a decision about the administration of coagulation products based on actual rather than estimated need. Within 10 minutes it is possible to know if the bleeding is purely obstetric in origin and therefore will not improve until the underlying cause has been managed or if the bleeding is being caused or exacerbated by an underlying coagulation deficiency.

Fluid resuscitation should start immediately with warmed crystalloid, and efforts should be made to maintain normothermia because hypothermia can worsen coagulopathy. Blood products should be requested immediately so that they are ready for transfusion when required because there is often a significant delay. When bleeding is not rapidly controlled and the patient is in a delivery room, she must be moved urgently to the OR for examination under anesthesia.

The antifibrinolytic agent tranexamic acid has been shown to be of benefit in the bleeding trauma patient administered as a 1-g loading dose followed by subsequent infusion of 1 g, and its role in the bleeding parturient is under investigation.[4]

Use of POC Testing in Obstetric Hemorrhage

Hemoglobin Measurement

The decision to transfuse a woman during obstetric hemorrhage is ideally made in an informed manner because both over- and undertransfusion of red blood cells has implications for patient safety. Published guidelines on transfusion triggers advise that a Hb level of 80 g/liter is maintained.[5] POC Hb can be measured using a number of different devices, but Hb estimation, when taken in the context of the patient's acid-base balance, is particularly useful to assess the shock status of the patient and inform blood transfusion decisions. A venous blood sample taken at the same time as other bloods can be used. In the early stages of hemorrhage, a Hb determination can be falsely reassuring and should be rapidly repeated if there are signs of hemodynamic instability. A lactate level greater than 2 mmol/liter, even if the Hb appears normal, indicates a metabolic acidosis, and the Hb is likely to drop considerably once active resuscitation is started. In the Case Study, the initial blood gas sample showed a metabolic acidosis with a lactate of 3 mmol/liter, a base deficit of −6 mmol/liter, and a Hb of 84 g/liter. Based on the metabolic acidosis and the fact that bleeding was not controlled, this indicated that a Hb of 84 g/liter was not adequate, and PRCs were urgently required.

Coagulation Measurement

Coagulation testing in the laboratory takes 45–90 minutes and is therefore not available in a timely way when bleeding is rapid. It is clinically impossible to know the extent to which bleeding is exacerbated by a coagulopathy, which has led to the adoption of policies where FFP is routinely issued once a MOH protocol has been activated. National guidelines have previously recommended that FFP and PRCs should be given in a fixed ratio such as 1:1 if clotting results are not available, or if they are, then the activated partial thromboplastin time (aPTT) should be kept below 1.5 times normal and the fibrinogen level greater than 1 g/liter. These numbers are based on recommendations from nonpregnant populations, and increasingly, this approach is being questioned in PPH.[5]

In pregnancy at term, the normal range for fibrinogen increases to 4–6 g/liter, compared with 2–4 g/liter seen in the nonpregnant population.[6] Large placental abruptions and amniotic fluid emboli can cause rapid consumptive coagulopathy, and these patients may require early coagulation support. However, in the majority of cases of PPH, where the woman is otherwise well, coagulation remains adequate unless the PPH is not brought under control by obstetric interventions, where it may occur late in the course of the PPH due to dilution. Fibrinogen levels fall sooner than other coagulation factors,[7] and a fibrinogen of less than 3 g/liter, and especially less than 2 g/liter, at the onset of PPH appears to be a good predictor of progression to severe PPH.[8]

Most women will have normal clotting and a fibrinogen level of greater than 3 g/liter when PPH is recognized.[8] Giving FFP in a fixed ratio in this circumstance exposes women to risks such as volume overload and transfusion-related complications such as transfusion-related lung injury (TRALI) and alloimmunization. Furthermore, early transfusion of FFP can lead to the dilution of a previously adequate fibrinogen level because the mean fibrinogen level in FFP is 2 g/liter, much lower than the normal value for pregnancy.

However, waiting for conventional clotting results and waiting for these results to become significantly abnormal for pregnancy before giving FFP risks undertransfusion, worsening coagulopathy, and exacerbation of hemorrhage. Routine use of viscoelastic POC tests of coagulation in obstetric hemorrhage is controversial, although evidence supporting its role is mounting. At the current time, there are two commercially available semiautomated viscoelastic machines that use similar technology. ROTEM (TEM International, Munich, Germany), where a pin rotates in a stationary cup containing the sample (thromboelastometry), and TEG (Hemonetics Corp., Braintree, MA, United States), where the cup rotates around a stationary pin (thromboelastography). Both machines produce a real-time dynamic electronic readout as the rotation of the pin or cup slows as a blood clot forms. One manufacturer cannot be recommended above the other.[9] The POC test for fibrinogen, FIBTEM, is one way of estimating fibrinogen levels by extrinsically activating coagulation with tissue factor while inhibiting platelet activity and then measuring clot strength against time. Clot amplitude at 5 minutes (A5) shows moderate correlation with laboratory plasma fibrinogen levels,[7] with the A5 values of 15, 11, and 7 approximating to fibrinogen levels of 3, 2, and 1 g/liter, respectively. FIBTEM has the same predictive value as Clauss fibrinogen to predict severe ongoing PPH. An algorithm using FIBTEM A5 is shown in Figure 33.1 and has been used successfully used in over 500 PPHs of greater than 1,000 ml.

In the Case Study, a FIBTEM was taken on recognition of PPH. Given the rapidity of the bleeding, the sample was taken when the patient had bled approximately 1,800 mL but her A5 of 25 mm rapidly informed the team that her fibrinogen level was adequate for coagulation, and the transfusion of FFP could be safely withheld. Despite eventually losing approximately 50 percent of her blood volume, her coagulation was normal throughout, and PPH control was achieved entirely by surgical and pharmacologic intervention. It would be very difficult to predict this based on the clinical situation alone, and had her initial FIBTEM A5 been below 15 mm, the likelihood of her developing severe PPH that was difficult to control was considerable. If this had been the case, then FFP would have been given as quickly as possible and, with an A5 of less than 11 mm, consideration would have been given to the administration of fibrinogen concentrate or cryoprecipitate because they have been shown to improve outcome[10,11] (see Figure 33.1).

Learning Points

- Identify and plan ahead for high-risk cases, including ensuring the availability of blood.
- Appreciate the increased vulnerability of anemic and low-body-weight patients to hemorrhage.
- Use MEOWS charts and have a high index of suspicion in all obstetric patients. Bleeding can be overlooked or concealed – pregnant women manifest signs of shock due to hemorrhage late.
- Measure blood loss – an accurate ongoing assessment will inform clinical staff and guide subsequent care.
- Once abnormal bleeding has been identified, the major obstetric hemorrhage protocol should be activated early to alert key team members to attend the mother. This will enable appropriate obstetric intervention, resuscitation, and the timely ordering of appropriate blood and blood products.
- Early POC testing of Hb, acid-base status, and coagulation can inform care and help direct appropriate therapy.
- A Clauss fibrinogen level of less than 3 g/liter or FIBTEM A5 of less than 15 mm at the onset or recognition of PPH with ongoing bleeding predicts major PPH and can alert the team to high-risk cases. Aim to maintain a fibrinogen level of greater than 2 g/liter when bleeding is ongoing.

References

1. Lennox C, Marr L. Scottish Confidential Audit of Severe Maternal Morbidity, 9th Annual Report (data from 2011). Available at http://healthcareimprove mentscotland.org/his/idoc.ashx?docid=5fb640e2-d079 -48cc-ad49-a58f6929b685&version=-1.

2. Knight M, Kenyon S, Brocklehurst P, et al., eds., on behalf of MBRRACE-UK. *Saving Lives, Improving Mothers' Care: Lessons Learned to Inform Future Maternity Care from the UK and Ireland Confidential Enquiries into Maternal Deaths and Morbidity 2009–12.* Oxford: National Perinatal Epidemiology Unit, University of Oxford; 2014.

3. Lilley G, Burkett-St-Laurent D, Precious E, et al. Measurement of blood loss during postpartum haemorrhage. *Int J Obstet Anesth* 2015; **24**(1):8–14.

4. Novikova N, Hofmeyr GJ, Cluver C. Tranexamic acid for preventing postpartum haemorrhage. *Cochrane Database Syst Rev* 2015; (**6**):CD007872.

5. Royal College of Obstetrics and Gynaecology. *Postpartum Haemorrhage, Prevention and Management* (Green-top Guideline No. 52). London: Royal College; 2011.

6. Collis RE, Collins PW. Haemostatic management of obstetric haemorrhage. *Anaesthesia* 2015; **70**(Suppl 1):78–88.

7. de Lloyd L, Bovington R, Kaye A, et al. Standard haemostatic tests following major obstetric haemorrhage. *Int J Obstet Anesth* 2011; **20**(2):135–41.

8. Collins PW, Lilley G, Bruynseels D, et al. Fibrin-based clot formation as an early and rapid biomarker for progression of postpartum hemorrhage: a prospective study. *Blood* 2014; **124**(11):1727–36.

9. Solomon C, Collis RE, Collins PW. Haemostatic monitoring during postpartum haemorrhage and implications for management. *Br J Anaesth* 2012; **109**(6):851–63. Epub 2012 Oct 16. Review.

10. Mallaiah S, Barclay P, Harrod I, Chevannes C, Bhalla A. Introduction of an algorithm for ROTEM-guided fibrinogen concentrate administration in major obstetric haemorrhage. *Anaesthesia* 2015; **70**(2):166–75.

11. Ralph C. Use of ROTEM in major obstetric haemorrhage. *Anaesthesia* 2015; **70**(6):759–60.

Addendum

1. The Woman trial and a meta-analysis strongly support the early use of tranexamic acid 1g which should be repeated if blood-loss is ongoing after 30 minutes.

- Li C1, Gong Y, Dong L, Xie B, Dai Z. Is prophylactic tranexamic acid administration effective and safe for postpartum hemorrhage prevention?: A systematic review and meta-analysis. *Medicine* (Baltimore). 2017; **96**(1):e5653.

- WOMAN Trial Collaborators. Effect of early tranexamic acid administration on mortality, hysterectomy, and other morbidities in women with post-partum haemorrhage (WOMAN): an international, randomised, double-blind, placebo-controlled trial. *Lancet* 2017;**389**(10084):2105–2116.

2. The OBS 2 trial strongly supports the use of POC testing to safely withhold FFP and other blood coagulation products if the Clauss fibrinogen is >2g/L (POC testing equivalent). The OBS 2 trial also supports an intervention point with coagulation factors at a Clauss fibrinogen <2g/L with on-going bleeding (POC testing equivalent).

- Collins PW, Cannings-John R, Bruynseels D, et al. Viscoelastometry guided fresh frozen plasma infusion for postpartum haemorrhage: OBS2, an observational study. *Br J Anaesth* 2017; **119**(3):422–43.

- Cannings-John R, Bruynseels D, Mallaiah S, et al. Viscoelastometric-guided early fibrinogen concentrate replacement during postpartum haemorrhage: OBS2, a double-blind randomized controlled trial. Collins PW, *Br J Anaesth* 2017; **119**(3):411–421.

Cell Salvage for Cesarean Delivery with High Risk of Hemorrhage

Philip Barclay and Shubha Mallaiah

Case Study

A woman in her second pregnancy was booked for an elective cesarean delivery at 37 weeks' gestation. Her first pregnancy required a classical cesarean delivery due to a 10-cm lower uterine segment fibroid, and the patient had since undergone a myomectomy. Ultrasound examination showed a possible placenta accreta overlying the scar. Because her family was complete, she was consented for a potential cesarean hysterectomy in case an adherent placenta was found at delivery, which could lead to massive hemorrhage with persisting efforts to remove it. Her preoperative hemoglobin was 118 g/liter.

A combined spinal-epidural anesthetic technique (spinal dose 12.5 mg hyperbaric bupivacaine with 300 μg diamorphine) was used, with a crystalloid coload and a phenylephrine infusion to maintain blood pressure. Cell salvage was used from the start of surgery, with a separate suction catheter to remove amniotic fluid. After a healthy baby girl was delivered, 5 units of oxytocin was given slowly, followed by a 10 unit/h oxytocin infusion. At this point, the lower part of the placenta separated, and umbilical cord traction, in an attempt to detach the rest of it, produced dimpling of the uterus where the placenta remained adherent despite additional doses of uterotonics. A hysterectomy was subsequently performed as planned, with assistance from the attending gynecologist. Anesthesia was maintained with 5- to 10-ml boluses of epidural 0.5% levobupivacaine and 100 μg fentanyl. The patient remained hemodynamically stable throughout the procedure. The estimated blood loss was 1,500 ml, and most of this was collected both directly and by rinsing blood-soaked swabs. This was processed by the Cell Saver, and 477 ml of autologous blood was returned using a leukocyte depletion filter (LDF). The patient had a brief episode of symptomatic hypotension (BP 67/31 mmHg) on transfer to the high-dependency unit, but she recovered spontaneously and did not require further fluid boluses or vasopressor treatment. The patient received overnight high-dependency care. The postoperative hemoglobin concentration was 119 g/liter. The patient made an uneventful recovery and was discharged home on the third postoperative day.

Key Points

- Anticipation of problems during cesarean delivery in this patient due to her placenta accreta, fibroids, and previous uterine scarring resulted in a planned cesarean hysterectomy that avoided massive hemorrhage.
- Intraoperative cell salvage was used from the beginning of the procedure to collect most of the blood lost during surgery.
- The transfusion of autologous blood prevented postoperative anemia while avoiding the risks of allogeneic blood transfusion.

Discussion

It is routine practice to ensure that cross-matched blood is available for elective cesarean delivery patients at high risk of major obstetric hemorrhage. However, transfusion of allogeneic red cells is associated with many potential hazards for the parturient, with a 1 in 7,000 risk of acute transfusion reaction.[1]

In 2014, 3,017 adverse events were reported to the Serious Hazards of Transfusion (SHOT) group,[2] the majority of which were near misses due to error:

- 10 patients were given ABO-incompatible red cell transfusions due to clinical errors in either collection or administration, with one patient developing renal failure.
- 169 cases of major morbidity occurred, the majority due to acute allergic or febrile transfusion reactions and pulmonary complications.
- Transfusion-associated circulatory overload (TACO) accounted for 36 cases of major morbidity (two of which were obstetric) and six

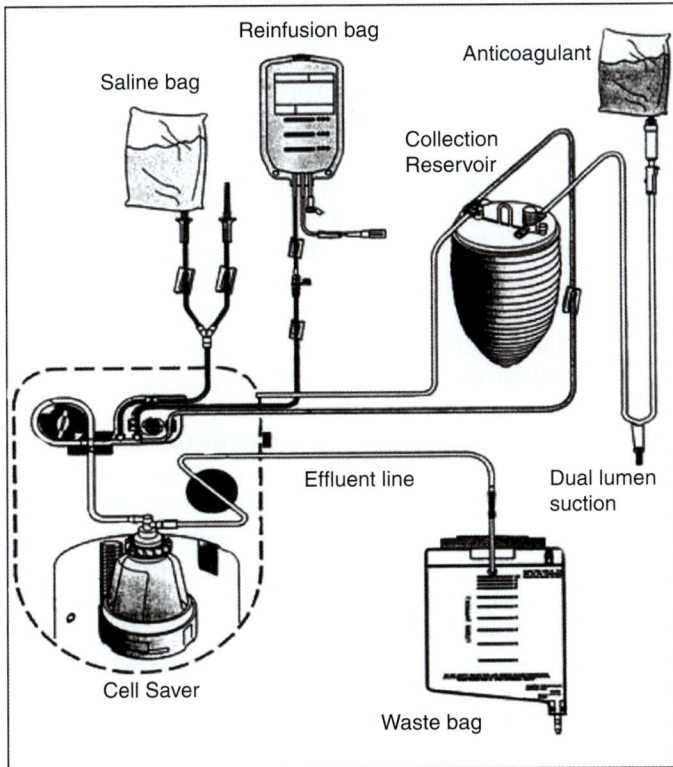

Figure 34.1 Cell salvage circuit
Source: Used with permission from Sorin, manufacturer of the Dideco Cell Salvage System.

deaths (none were obstetric). This is a particular hazard when several units of allogeneic blood are given to treat obstetric hemorrhage. Allogeneic blood from blood donors is also increasingly facing supply problems due to rising demand in the face of reducing number of donors.

Intraoperative cell salvage (IOCS) offers an effective alternative, providing a suitable supply of autologous blood from the patient in direct proportion to the magnitude of intraoperative hemorrhage, provided that no contraindications exist.

Autologous blood is fresh and warm, with red cells that maintain normal shape and deformability, resulting in an increased mean viability (88 percent compared with 70 percent for allogeneic blood).[3,4] Transfusion of autologous blood does not affect 2,3-diphosphoglycerate (DPG) levels in circulating blood, preserving oxygen transport capacity, unlike allogeneic blood, which reduced 2,3-DPG levels from 4.3 to 3.9 µmol/liter.[5] This has potential benefits in improving recovery and reducing postoperative

complications with little danger of immunomodulation, transmission of infections, hyperkalemia, or acidemia. It is also free from the dangers of incorrect blood transfusion because it is always started in a single-patient environment.

Mechanism of Cell Salvage

A dual-lumen anticoagulated suction tube is used to aspirate blood directly from the operative site or from blood-soaked swabs rinsed in saline (Figure 34.1). The collected blood is passed through a filter and collected in a reservoir. Once sufficient blood has been collected, the cell salvage machine can be set to manual or automatic to process the blood using a differential centrifugation bowl. This washes the cells and removes less dense elements, including platelets, activated clotting factors, and complement. The output contains red cells suspended in saline with a hematocrit of 0.5–0.8, which can be returned to the patient as an autologous transfusion within the next 6 hours.

IOCS Benefits in Nonobstetric Surgery

IOCS has become well established in nonobstetric surgery since the 1970s. A Cochrane review of 75 randomized, controlled trials in orthopedic and cardiac surgery found that IOCS reduced the requirement for allogeneic blood by 38 percent without adversely affecting mortality or morbidity.[6] Cell salvage is considered to be very safe and an essential standard of routine care in many specialties, such as vascular, orthopedic, and cardiac surgery.[2] Current guidelines from the Association of Anaesthetists of Great Britain and Ireland (AAGBI) for the use of blood components recommend that cell salvage be considered for high- or medium-risk surgery in nonobstetric adult patients when blood loss is likely to exceed 500 ml.[7]

Controversies Regarding IOCS in Obstetrics

For many years, IOCS was considered to be inappropriate for use in obstetrics for the following reasons.

1. Amniotic Fluid Contamination with IOCS

IOCS was thought to be contraindicated in cesarean delivery due to concerns about contamination of salvaged blood with amniotic fluid, potentially causing an amniotic fluid embolism (AFE). This syndrome was previously thought to be an embolic disease occurring when components of amniotic fluid entered the maternal circulation, causing hypoxia, collapse, coagulopathy, and a high mortality rate, with evidence of fetal squamous cells in postmortem maternal lung tissue. This may have been an erroneous explanation because there is evidence that amniotic fluid routinely enters the maternal circulation at the time of delivery.[8,9] The pathophysiology is now better understood, and it is thought that endothelin-1 plays a part in the early transient pulmonary hypertension, while amniotic fluid–derived tissue factor may be responsible for disseminated intravascular coagulopathy (DIC) as part of an anaphylactoid syndrome.[10]

Using a separate suction catheter for the amniotic fluid reduces the amount of contamination, and the wash process of cell salvage has been shown to completely remove active tissue factor from postwash samples.[11] However, some particulate components remain. The use of leukocyte depletion filters (LDFs) in obstetric patients significantly reduces the level of

particulate contaminants to a concentration similar to that seen in maternal venous blood at delivery.[12,13]

Leukocyte depletion of blood was described by Alexander Fleming in 1926 when he was investigating the effects of leukocytes on bacterial growth using cotton wool. Modern filters use a synthetic mesh made from a nonwoven web of microfibers. There is a coarsely woven prefilter, which screens out microaggregate debris. As the blood passes deeper through the filter layers, the effective pore size of the filter decreases. This physical barrier is supplemented by adhesion of leukocytes to the filter fibers.[14] LDFs are used to remove white cells from allogeneic blood transfusions to reduce the risk of adverse reactions and also have been shown to remove tumor cells when cell salvage is used for patients with malignancy.

There has only been one published case where AFE was claimed to have occurred following IOCS, in a Jehovah's Witness with HELLP syndrome who refused allogeneic blood products and received salvaged blood without an LDF. However, this diagnosis has been called into question in subsequent correspondence.[15]

2. Alloimmunization with IOCS

Alloimmunization is an additional consideration for Rhesus-negative mothers whose fetus may be Rhesus positive. This occurs when the mother's immune system is sensitized to foreign erythrocyte surface antigens by the transplacental passage of fetal red cells during delivery, trauma, or invasive obstetric procedures, stimulating the production of IgG antibodies. In subsequent pregnancies, these antibodies cross the placenta with potentially fatal consequences for the fetus, including hydrops fetalis. This can be prevented by antenatal Rhesus D immunoglobin prophylaxis

It has been shown that small amounts of transplacental hemorrhage (TPH) occur throughout pregnancy, peaking at delivery, with 1 percent of women having a TPH greater than 2.5 ml and 0.3 percent greater than 15 ml.[16] The quantity of fetal red cells that have entered the maternal circulation can be estimated by the Kleihauer test to determine the correct dose of anti-D. A dose of 500 IU within 72 hours of delivery is sufficient to neutralize up to 4 ml of fetal red cells.[17]

During cesarean delivery, fetal red cells may contaminate maternal blood aspirated during IOCS that are not removed by washing or using a LDF. The volume of fetal cells in reinfused blood may vary from 1 to 20 ml.[12,18] Current guidance from the British Committee for Standards in Haematology states that where the cord blood group is confirmed to be RhD positive (or unknown), a minimum of 1,500 IU of anti-D should be given after the reinfusion of salvaged red cells, and a maternal sample should be taken 30–45 minutes afterwards in case further anti-D is required. The transfusion laboratory must be informed so that the correct dose of anti-D is issued.[17]

Problems with LDF in Clinical Practice

The main problem with using a LDF in clinical practice is that it considerably slows the rate of reinfusion of salvaged blood, which is undesirable when treating hypovolemia associated with massive obstetric hemorrhage. The manufacturers advise that pressurized infusion bags must not be used to increase the rate of flow because the IOCS bags are weaker than standard blood bags and may rupture, which would defeat the purpose. There is also about 50–70 ml of air in the tubing that is pushed into the bag when it fills with processed blood, and pressurizing can result in air embolism. However, most reinfusion bags have two exit ports, and the speed of infusion can be doubled by spiking both ports.

There have also been several case reports of transient hypotension attributed to use of an LDF for the transfusion of salvaged blood in massive obstetric hemorrhage, which reversed when the transfusion was stopped.[19] In each case, pressure bags or syringes had been used to expedite the flow rate. This may have triggered a bradykinin burst within the negatively charged filter. Bradykinins are generated when plasma comes into contact with a negatively charged surface. This activates factor XII, which, in turn, activates the kinin-kallikrein system, resulting in the generation of bradykinin, a nonapeptide that causes vasodilation until it is rapidly broken down by kininases, including an angiotensin-converting enzyme inhibitor.[20]

Contraindications to IOCS

Sickle cell disease is a strong contraindication to IOCS because sickling of recovered red cells may occur in the hypoxic atmosphere of the Cell Saver reservoir. There have been two case reports of IOCS in patients with sickle cell trait with no deleterious effect, although a blood film of the salvaged blood from the first patient showed 15–20 percent sickled cells, whereas the second patient's film showed 20 percent altered but not sickled cells.[21]

Many relative contraindications to IOCS have been documented, mainly related to contamination of the collected blood with nontransfusable substances within the surgical field, such as bowel contents, infected material, bone cement, water, iodine, and so on.[22] Many cases of massive obstetric hemorrhage occur vaginally following procedures such as a trial of forceps delivery, manual removal of retained placenta, or repair of third- and fourth-degree tears. Currently, these losses are deemed unsalvageable because of the risk of bacterial contamination. This has been challenged by a recent case series in which women with ongoing bleeding after vaginal delivery were transferred to the OR, and a sterile under buttock drape with a pouch containing 200 ml of heparinized saline was used to collect blood before aspiration into a cell salvage system. Bacterial contamination was found in the postwash samples, but this was of a low level and likely to cause a similar level of bacteremia as occurs during dental procedures.[23]

Evidence of Benefits with IOCS in Obstetrics

A review of all clinical studies of outcomes with IOCS in obstetrics published from 1993 until 2013 with at least 30 subjects found only six articles suitable for systematic analysis. Of these, two were prospective controlled studies and four were case series.[24]

Both controlled studies were published in 1998. One was a multicenter cohort study that compared 139 patients who had received cell-salvaged blood with a historical cohort.[25] The study was underpowered to detect a difference between the two groups. The other study randomly allocated 34 patients in each group to IOCS or routine care during cesarean delivery.[26] This showed a large decrease in the number of patients requiring allogeneic transfusion, higher postoperative hemoglobin levels, and shorter hospital stays in the IOCS group.

Evidence of Benefit with IOCS in Placenta Accreta

Two recently published case series have examined the use of IOCS in patients with abnormal placentation. One prospective series described the use of IOCS in 18 women with placenta accreta who underwent cesarean hysterectomy under general anesthesia.[27] Fifteen of these patients (83 percent) received an autologous transfusion, and only two required allogeneic blood. The median blood loss was 2,900 ml, with a mean volume of 1,476 ml of salvaged blood returned to the patient.

Milne et al.[28] reported 103 cases of cesarean hysterectomy in their 8-year experience of 884 patients requiring IOCS. Of these, 75 (73 percent) had sufficient blood collected for reinfusion of salvaged blood, with a mean of 1.7 equivalent units of autologous packed red cells transfused per patient.

IOCS in Mothers Who Refuse Blood Transfusion

Deaths due to hemorrhage among mothers who refuse blood products have been shown to be a persistent problem in all the reports of confidential enquiries into maternal deaths since 2002. Most of these women will accept IOCS, and the availability of cell salvage can be helpful in preventing these deaths and is recommended.[29]

Cost Effectiveness

Brearton et al.[30] evaluated the costs of IOCS over a 5-year period between 2006 and 2011, where cell salvage collection was set up 587 times and blood was returned to 137 patients (23 percent). The total volume of blood returned to the 137 patients was 47,143 ml, equivalent to 189 units of packed red cells. The cost of cell salvage consumables required for collection and processing was found to be less than the equivalent cost of allogeneic red cells, showing that IOCS is cost effective.

Learning Points

- Cell salvage is an established standard of care in obstetrics and is recommended by the National Institute for Health and Care Excellence (NICE), the Association of Anaesthetists of Great Britain and Ireland (AAGBI), and the Confidential Enquiries into Maternal Deaths in the United Kingdom.[29]
- Use of cell salvage has been shown to reduce the need for allogeneic blood, particularly when placenta accreta is suspected and when cesarean hysterectomy is the last resort to control bleeding.[30]
- Cell salvage is an essential option when dealing with mothers who refuse blood products in whom a massive hemorrhage is anticipated.
- Although there is limited evidence to suggest that the routine use of cell salvage is both cost-effective and reduces the requirement for allogeneic blood,

this is from case series and cohort studies. The recently published SALVO trial showed that the routine use of IOCS was associated with a modest reduction in the need for allogeneic blood, but this was not statistically significant. In women with Rhesus-negative blood type who gave birth to Rhesus-positive babies, the use of IOCS resulted in an increased exposure to fetal blood.[31]

References

1. Norfolk D, ed. *Handbook of Transfusion Medicine*, 5th ed. Norwich: Stationery Office; 2013.

2. Bolton-Maggs PH, ed. *The 2014 Annual SHOT Report*. Manchester: Serious Hazards of Transfusion (SHOT); 2015.

3. Colwell CW Jr, Beutler E, West C, Hardwick ME, Morris BA. Erythrocyte viability in blood salvaged during total joint arthroplasty with cement. *J Bone Joint Surg Am* 2002; **84A**(1):23–25.

4. Ashworth A, Klein AA. Cell salvage as part of a blood conservation strategy in anaesthesia. *Br J Anaesth* 2010; **105**(4):401–16.

5. Schmidt H, Folsgaard S, Mortensen PE, Jensen E. Impact of autotransfusion after coronary artery bypass grafting on oxygen transport. *Acta Anaesthesiol Scand* 1997; **41**(8):995–1001.

6. Carless PA, Henry DA, Moxey AJ, et al. Cell salvage for minimising perioperative allogeneic blood transfusion. *Cochrane Database Syst Rev* 2010; (4):CD001888.

7. Klein AA, Arnold P, Bingham RM, et al. AAGBI guidelines: the use of blood components and their alternatives 2016. *Anaesthesia* 2016; **71**(7):829–42.

8. Liumbruno GM, Liumbruno C, Rafanelli D. Intraoperative cell salvage in obstetrics: is it a real therapeutic option? *Transfusion* 2011; **51**(10):2244–56.

9. Kuhlman K, Hidvegi D, Tamura RK, Depp R. Is amniotic fluid material in the central circulation of peripartum patients pathologic? *Am J Perinatol* 1985; **2**(4):295–99.

10. Campbell JP, Mackenzie MJ, Yentis SM, Sooranna SR, Johnson MR. An evaluation of the ability of leukocyte depletion filters to remove components of amniotic fluid. *Anaesthesia* 2012; **67**(10):1152–57.

11. Bernstein HH, Rosenblatt MA, Gettes M, Lockwood C. The ability of the Hemonetics 4 Cell Saver System to remove tissue factor from blood contaminated with amniotic fluid. *Anesth Analg* 1997; **85**(4):831–33.

12. Catling SJ, Williams S, Fielding AM. Cell salvage in obstetrics: an evaluation of the ability of cell salvage combined with leukocyte depletion filtration to remove amniotic fluid from operative blood loss

at caesarean section. *Int J Obstet Anesth* 1999; **8**(2):79–84.

13. Waters JH, Biscotti C, Potter PS, Phillipson E. Amniotic fluid removal during cell salvage in the cesarean section patient. *Anesthesiology* 2000; **92**(6): 1531–36.

14. Dzik S. Leukodepletion blood filters: filter design and mechanisms of leukocyte removal. *Transfus Med Rev* 1993; **7**(2):65–77.

15. Goucher H, Wong CA, Patel SK, Toledo P. Cell salvage in obstetrics. *Anesth Analg* 2015; **121**(2):465–68.

16. Ralph CJ, Sullivan I, Faulds J. Intraoperative cell salvaged blood as part of a blood conservation strategy in caesarean section: is fetal red cell contamination important? *Br J Anaesth* 2011; **107** (3):404–8.

17. Qureshi H, Massey E, Kirwan D, et al. BCSH guideline for the use of anti-D immunoglobulin for the prevention of haemolytic disease of the fetus and newborn. *Transfus Med* 2014; **24**(1):8–20.

18. Allam J, Cox M, Yentis SM. Cell salvage in obstetrics. *Int J Obstet Anesth* 2008; **17**(1):37–45.

19. Hussain S, Clyburn P. Cell salvage–induced hypotension and London buses. *Anaesthesia* 2010; **65**(7):661–63.

20. Iwama H. Bradykinin-associated reactions in white cell-reduction filter. *J Crit Care* 2001; **16**(2):74–81.

21. Okunuga A, Skelton VA. Use of cell salvage in patients with sickle cell trait. *Int J Obstet Anesth* 2009; **18**(1):90–91; author reply 91.

22. Esper SA, Waters JH. Intra-operative cell salvage: a fresh look at the indications and contraindications. *Blood Transfus* 2011; **9**(2):139–47.

23. Teare KM, Sullivan IJ, Ralph CJ. Is cell salvaged vaginal blood loss suitable for re-infusion? *Int J Obstet Anesth* 2015; **24**(2):103–10.

24. Dhariwal SK, Khan KS, Allard S, et al. Does current evidence support the use of intraoperative cell salvage in reducing the need for blood transfusion in caesarean section? *Curr Opin Obstet Gynecol* 2014; **26**(6):425–30.

25. Rebarber A, Lonser R, Jackson S, Copel JA, Sipes S. The safety of intraoperative autologous blood collection and autotransfusion during cesarean section. *Am J Obstet Gynecol.* 1998; **179**(3 Pt 1):715–20.

26. Rainaldi MP, Tazzari PL, Scagliarini G, Borghi B, Conte R. Blood salvage during caesarean section. *Br J Anaesth* 1998; **80**(2):195–98.

27. Elagamy A, Abdelaziz A, Ellaithy M. The use of cell salvage in women undergoing cesarean hysterectomy for abnormal placentation. *Int J Obstet Anesth* 2013; **22**(4):289–93.

28. Milne ME, Yazer MH, Waters JH. Red blood cell salvage during obstetric hemorrhage. *Obstet Gynecol* 2015; **125**(4):919–23.

29. Cantwell R, Clutton-Brock T, Cooper G, et al. Saving mothers' lives: reviewing maternal deaths to make motherhood safer: 2006–2008. Eighth Report of the Confidential Enquiries into Maternal Deaths in the United Kingdom. *BJOG* 2011; **118**(Suppl 1):1–203.

30. Brearton C, Bhalla A, Mallaiah S, Barclay P. The economic benefits of cell salvage in obstetric haemorrhage. *Int J Obstet Anesth* 2012; **21**(4):329–33.

31. Khan KS, Moore PAS, Wilson MJ, et al., on behalf of the SALVO Study Group. Cell salvage and donor blood transfusion during cesarean section: a pragmatic, multicentre randomised controlled trial (SALVO). *PLoS Med* 2017; **14**(12):e1002471.

Emergency Hysterectomy

Carolyn F. Weiniger, Neil Amison, and Doron Kabiri

Case Study

A 33-year-old gravida 4, para 3 woman was brought to the emergency room by her partner at 30 + 3/7 weeks' gestation with vaginal bleeding and sporadic painful uterine contractions. She previously had one normal vaginal delivery, followed by one cesarean delivery for breech presentation and a second cesarean delivery for failed attempted vaginal birth after cesarean delivery 16 months ago. Her 22-week ultrasound scan demonstrated central placenta previa with suspected signs of a placenta accreta. She was booked at 34 weeks' gestation for an elective cesarean delivery with hysterectomy, if needed, and was advised to come straight to hospital if she experienced vaginal bleeding.

Since the onset of vaginal bleeding 2 hours previously, she had used six heavy pads, and the bleeding had currently ceased. She was anxious and tired, and her contractions, although irregular (every 9–20 minutes) were very painful. In the emergency room, the resident obstetrician attached her to a continuous electrocardiogram monitor (heart rate 80 beats/min), noninvasive blood pressure monitoring (110/60 mmHg), pulse oximetry (SpO$_2$ 97% on room air), and fetal cardiotocography (normal). The obstetric trainee contacted the anesthesia team, who inserted a large-bore (14-gauge) IV cannula in her right antecubital fossa and sent blood for laboratory tests, including a complete blood count, coagulation profile, and blood cross-match. The anesthesia team assessed the patient, including airway, administered oxygen via a facemask, and administered 1 liter of crystalloid fluid. The patient was classed as American Society of Anesthesiologists (ASA) Class 1, body mass index (BMI) 24 kg/m^2, with an unremarkable airway.

The obstetric trainee contacted her obstetric consultant to inform him that a patient with bleeding placenta previa and suspected accreta was in the emergency room with normal vital signs and that emergency delivery was likely to be required.

A multidisciplinary team (MDT) gathered to discuss the optimal delivery strategy and timing for her cesarean delivery. This MDT comprised anesthesia, obstetrics, gynecology, neonatology, intensive care, interventional radiology, vascular surgery, urology, hematology, and nursing staff. Faced with this patient with a vaginal bleed and suspected placenta accreta with imminent labor, the decision was taken to perform an emergency cesarean delivery. The blood bank was alerted, and a postoperative ICU bed booked.

The obstetric trainee consented the patient for cesarean delivery and a hysterectomy, if needed. The anesthesia team discussed with the patient the advantages of general versus neuraxial anesthesia. The patient selected general anesthesia after discussion with her partner because she was very anxious and preferred to be "knocked out." She was transferred to the OR, connected to routine anesthesia monitors, and positioned supine with left uterine displacement. Under local anesthesia, her radial artery was cannulated for direct blood pressure measurements, and a large-bore (7 French gauge) peripheral catheter was inserted into her left antecubital fossa. Blood products (four units each of red blood cells, fresh frozen plasma, and platelets) were ordered to the OR; a Cell Saver unit and a rapid warming infuser were also primed. General anesthesia was performed using a rapid-sequence induction technique with tracheal intubation. A cystoscopy performed before surgery revealed placental intrusion into the bladder. Given the strong evidence of placenta percreta, the surgical plan included hysterotomy and delivery of the fetus, followed by hysterectomy.

Key Points

- A high index of suspicion is required for placenta accreta spectrum (PAS) in women with prior cesarean delivery and placenta previa.

- Management of PAS requires a multidisciplinary team and suitable support facilities such as the blood bank and the ICU.
- Cesarean hysterectomy may be planned and is associated with reduced blood loss, but uterine preservation strategies may be performed.
- Preparations are required for massive hemorrhage, including rapid infuser and Cell Saver.
- Patient blood management should include using a massive transfusion protocol and coagulation function assessments.
- Neuraxial anesthesia may be suitable for all but emergency cases, and conversion to general anesthesia may be required.

Table 35.1 Reasons for Hysterectomy

Emergency hysterectomy
Placenta previa causing uncontrolled bleeding
Placenta accreta causing uncontrolled bleeding
Uterine atony
Trauma/uterine rupture
Uterine inversion
Nonemergency hysterectomy
Menorrhagia due to fibroids
Pelvic pain due to endometriosis
Pelvic inflammatory disease (PID)
Adenomyosis or fibroids
Pelvic organ prolapse
Cancer of uterus
Cancer of ovaries
Cancer of cervix

Discussion

Emergency hysterectomy is an infrequent but distressing outcome of pregnancy. Hysterectomy may be anticipated in such a case of suspected placenta accreta as presented here or may be a lifesaving procedure in order to mitigate severe maternal morbidity or even mortality. This patient had clinical features of antenatal suspected placenta accreta, placenta previa, previous cesarean delivery, and ultrasound signs of accreta, but her premature presentation with antepartum hemorrhage disrupted the plan for elective cesarean delivery.

This chapter discusses the causes and risk factors for emergency hysterectomy, with a special focus on PAS as a major cause. It reviews the management of emergency hysterectomy, which includes assembling a multidisciplinary team, hemorrhage management including IV access, blood products massive transfusion protocol, and use of the Cell Saver. The anesthesia choice may be clear in favor of general anesthesia if the patient is unstable, but neuraxial anesthesia is supported for PAS cases even when hysterectomy may be performed.[1] Surgical and postoperative considerations are reviewed with a focus on material useful to the anesthesia practitioner managing an emergency hysterectomy.

Emergency Hysterectomy

The most common reasons for emergency cesarean hysterectomy are postpartum hemorrhage due to uterine atony and PAS (Table 35.1).

Risk Factors for Emergency Hysterectomy

1. **Uterine Atony.** Postpartum hemorrhage due to uterine atony accounts for 21–43 percent of emergency hysterectomy cases.[2,3] An overdistended uterus due to multifetal gestation, fetal macrosomia, or polyhydramnios, preeclampsia, prolonged first- and second-stage of labor, induction, and nulliparity are all risk factors for uterine atony.
2. **Uterine Rupture.** This is primarily a complication following previous cesarean delivery.[2]
3. **Placenta accreta spectrum.** Thirty-eight percent of emergency hysterectomies are performed for abnormal adherent placenta,[4] and cesarean hysterectomy is highly likely when placenta accreta is suspected. In one retrospective study, among 57 cases of antenatally suspected placenta accreta, 39 percent presented emergently with vaginal bleeding, and 98 percent underwent cesarean hysterectomy.[5] In this chapter, management strategies for placenta accreta are emphasized, and all abnormal adherent placentas are referred to as *placenta accreta* spectrum (PAS).

Placenta Accreta Spectrum

1. **Pathophysiology of Placenta Accreta Spectrum (PAS).** Placenta accreta is caused by a partial/complete lack of the deciduas basalis and a defective fibrinoid layer. The depth of invasion is

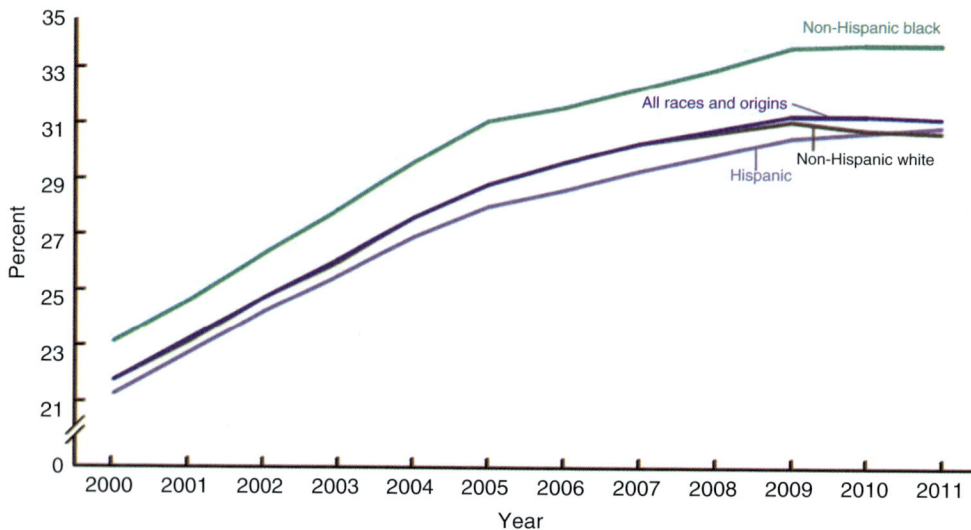

Figure 35.1 Cesarean delivery rate in the United States 2000–11
Source: From Martin JA, Hamilton BE, Ventura SJ, Osterman MJ, Mathews TJ. Births: final data for 2011. *National Vital Statistics Rep* 2013; 62:1–70[13] (all material in the report is in the public domain).

termed *placenta accreta* (placental villi attached to the myometrium), *increta* (invasion of placenta villi into the myometrium), or *percreta* (placental villi fully penetrating all layers of the myometrium to the serosal layer).[6]

2. **Risk Factors for PAS.** Women with PAS are usually asymptomatic,[7] and up to 20 percent of PAS cases have no discernible risk factors.[8,9] Among risk factors for PAS are cumulative prior cesarean deliveries,[10] placenta praevia, short time interval between cesarean deliveries, increasing maternal age, smoking, previous uterine surgery such as myomectomy or endometrial ablation, and prior dilatation and curettage.[10]

3. **Epidemiology of PAS.** In the United States over the last 30 years, a 10-fold increase in PAS cases has been reported, and in Western countries in general, the PAS rate ranges from 1 per 530 to 1 per 2,500 deliveries.[7,9,11] The PAS incidence correlates with the increase in cesarean delivery rate.[11,12] In 2008, the cesarean delivery rate in the United States reached a peak – 32.8 percent of all births – and it remains at this high rate[13] (Figure 35.1).

4. **Epidemiology of Placenta Accreta Spectrum.** Ultrasound as a tool for the diagnosis of PAS has a sensitivity of 77–86 percent and a specificity of 96–98 percent.[14] Additional benefits of MRI are unclear, with specificity and sensitivity similar to those of ultrasound.[6,10,15] Combining ultrasound findings with known clinical risk factors such as placenta previa and prior cesarean delivery improves the diagnostic sensitivity for PAS.[16,17] In the absence of a radiologic diagnosis (ultrasound or MRI), PAS is a clinical or pathologic diagnosis.[1]

Management Considerations for Emergency Hysterectomy

1. **Multidisciplinary Team Management.** The involvement of a multidisciplinary team (MDT) can reduce blood loss, transfusion requirements, and maternal mortality and morbidity.[10,18] Close working relationships between anesthesiologists, obstetricians, midwives, neonatologists, blood bank, radiologists, oncogynecologists and other surgical subspecialties are important to optimize teamwork, communication, and planning[7,10] (Figure 35.2). Drills to simulate team management of hemorrhage and emergency cesarean delivery may improve patient outcome and team performance.[19–21] A checklist may be useful to ensure that all MDT members are included and the necessary blood products ordered.[11] In our practice, we order 4 units of red blood cells and

		Transfusion in this pregnancy; if yes, give dates	yes/no
		Date of planned surgery	
Patient name		Planned surgery location and contact no.	
Medical record no.		Gestational age at planned delivery	
Estimated due date		Antenatal glucocorticoids; if yes, give dates	yes/no
Preoperative diagnosis of accreta; specify:	accreta/increta/percreta	Primary obstetrician; list name and contact no.	
Placenta location		Preoperative consultations and notifications[a]	If yes, list name and contact no.
Relevant ultrasound findings		Obstetric anesthesiologist/anesthesiologist	no/yes _____
Relevant MRI findings		Maternal fetal medicine specialist	no/yes _____
Obstetric history		Neonatologist/pediatrician	no/yes _____
No. of prior cesarean deliveries		Gynecologic oncologist/pelvic surgeon	no/yes _____
Other prior uterine surgery		Urologist	no/yes _____
Blood type		General surgeon	no/yes _____
Antibody screen		Vascular surgeon	no/yes _____
Date and value of most recent hematocrit/hemoglobin		Interventional radiologist	no/yes _____
Date and value of most recent creatinine		Blood bank specialist/hematologist	no/yes _____
Iron supplementation; if yes, specify type, dose	yes/no	Cell-saver specialist	no/yes _____
Epogen in this pregnancy; if yes, give dates	yes/no	Laboratory specialist	no/yes _____
		Intensive care specialist	no/yes _____

Figure 35.2 Example checklist for preparation of placenta accreta case
Source: Use with permission from Belfort MA. Placenta accreta. *Am J Obstet Gynecol* 2010; 203(5):430–39.[11]

4 units of fresh frozen plasma to the OR and check them prior to anesthesia in cases of suspected placenta accreta.

2. **Specialist Care Management.** Consider transfer to a tertiary care center if your center lacks expertise or logistics such as blood bank and ICU[1] (Table 35.2). Women managed with MDT in a tertiary center had reduced transfusion requirements and morbidity rates in one report.[5]

3. **Timing of Delivery.** Where possible, cesarean delivery is planned for PAS once the fetus has reached an appropriate gestational age – usually 34-36 weeks' gestation[22] – in order to avoid an emergency delivery with concomitant hemorrhage risk. The potential downside of early delivery is fetal immaturity, in particular lung development.[18] Some physicians in the United States wait for 37 weeks' gestation, considering that the risk of maternal hemorrhage is lower than fetal risk due to immaturity.[23]

Anesthetic Considerations

1. **Mode of Anesthesia.** Neuraxial anesthesia has fewer associated maternal complications such as failed intubation, aspiration of gastric contents,

hypoxia, awareness, and maternal death.[24–26] Regarding the anesthesia mode for PAS Lilker et al.[24] reported that over one-fifth of cases required conversion to general anesthesia due to patient discomfort and/or inadequate surgical conditions in a series of 23 placenta accreta cases.

2. **Emergency Obstetric Hemorrhage.** Bleeding placenta accreta or uterine atony may be an indication to consider general anesthesia due to the high risk of hypotension and coagulopathy.[9] Neuraxial anesthesia causes sympathectomy, potentially worsening hemodynamic instability from hemorrhage.[7] Factors that may influence the decision for neuraxial or general anesthesia include degree of placental invasion, predicted blood loss, length or difficulty of surgery, planned cesarean delivery versus attempted placental separation,[6] and difficult maternal airway. Regardless of anesthesia mode, blood products and vasoactive drugs such as phenylephrine, ephedrine, dopamine, and epinephrine should be available.[1] A plan for immediate conversion to general anesthesia should be in place, including a discussion with the patient to prepare her for the possibility that this may occur rapidly.

3. **Vascular Access.** We recommend insertion of two large-bore IV cannulas and invasive direct arterial

Table 35.2 Practice Surveys of Placenta Accreta Spectrum Management among Providers in the United States

	Jolley et al.[57]	Wright et al.[18]	Esakoff et al.[23]
Survey year	Survey collection period not reported; published 2011.	2011	2009
Survey population	Members of SMFM	Random sample of ACOG Fellows	Providers registered with SMFM
Number surveyed	1,759	994	1,861
Completed survey response	27%	51%	19%
Number of survey items	36	27	Not reported
Survey tool	Online tool (surveymonkey)	Written mailed survey	Written mailed survey
Annual number of accreta cases			
0	26%	18%	9%
1–3	45%	45%	69%[a]
4–9	30%	37%	17%[b]
≥10	3%	Not reported	5%§
Accreta patients not referred to tertiary unit	95%	33%	Not asked
Request for anesthesia consultation prior to surgery	87%	Not asked	Not asked

Anesthesia mode
  Spinal
  Epidural
  General
	Not asked	
		33%
		35%
		25%
			Not asked

Number that use cell salvage	50%	Not asked	Not asked
Number that use intravascular balloon catheters	35%	28%	36%

Abbreviations: SMFM = Society of Maternal-Fetal Medicine; ACOG = American College of Obstetrics and Gynecologists.

[a]Category was 1–5 cases per year.

[b]Category was 6–10 cases per year.

[c]Subset of the 4–9 cases per year respondents.

---

monitoring of blood pressure[9] for women at high risk for massive transfusion and hemodynamic instability. The internal jugular vein is in closer anatomic proximity to the carotid artery in a pregnant woman. In our practice, we insert a 14- and a 7F-gauge peripheral cannula and reserve central venous access for special cases. In women undergoing neuraxial anesthesia, we insert these lines under local anesthetic infiltration, but we may place the lines following induction in elective cases under general anesthesia.

Transfusion Considerations

1. **Blood Loss.** Increased plasma volume in pregnancy makes routine vital sign monitoring unreliable for blood loss assessments. An invasive arterial line allows beat-to-beat hemodynamic

assessments and serial point-of-care assessments for thrombolelastography and hemoglobin.[27–29] A recent survey of postpartum hemorrhage (PPH) management in the United States reported wide variation in blood loss estimation techniques. Visual estimates from suction bottles and the surgical field were used by 98 percent of the units, and only one-fifth added or used an objective measure of blood loss such as surgical swab weights or laboratory assessments.[30] Visual estimates are notably inaccurate, but training can improve the precision of these estimates.[31] The 2013 European guidelines for management of severe perioperative bleeding recommend performing coagulation assessments to guide blood management,[32] including a thromboelastogram. Normal fibrinogen levels in pregnancy are high, and therefore, a concentration below 2 g/liter is considered very low in pregnancy and may be associated with severe hemorrhage.[32]

2. **Massive Transfusion Protocol (MTP).** Recent transfusion policies stem from data on severely injured military personnel in armed conflicts. In 2005, the United States Army Institute of Surgical Research suggested a "damage control resuscitation" technique with a 1:1:1 red blood cell (RBC), fresh frozen plasma (FFP), platelets (PLTs) transfusion ratio.[7,10] Adherence to a MTP was associated with increased survival[33,34] and a drop in mortality from 65 to 19 percent. Similar figures have been published from civilian trauma centers.[35]

   Obstetric transfusion protocols are derived largely from trauma MTPs. A recent US survey reported that at least 20 percent of academic centers lack PPH protocols. Among units with a PPH protocol, 95 percent also had a MTP. Blood loss greater than 1,500 ml was the usual trigger to activate a MTP in obstetric hemorrhage management, and 35 percent of units use a predefined 1:1:1 RBC-FFP-PLT transfusion ratio.[30]

3. **Cell Salvage.** Cell salvage using a Cell Saver appears safe despite the potential risks of amniotic fluid embolization[36] and maternal alloimmunization[34,37] and may reduce allogeneic transfusion requirements.[37–39] In our practice, we use the Cell Saver for PAS cesarean delivery. In the United Kingdom, one-third of the labor and delivery units used the Cell Saver, and most of these promoted cell salvage in their PPH protocols.[40]

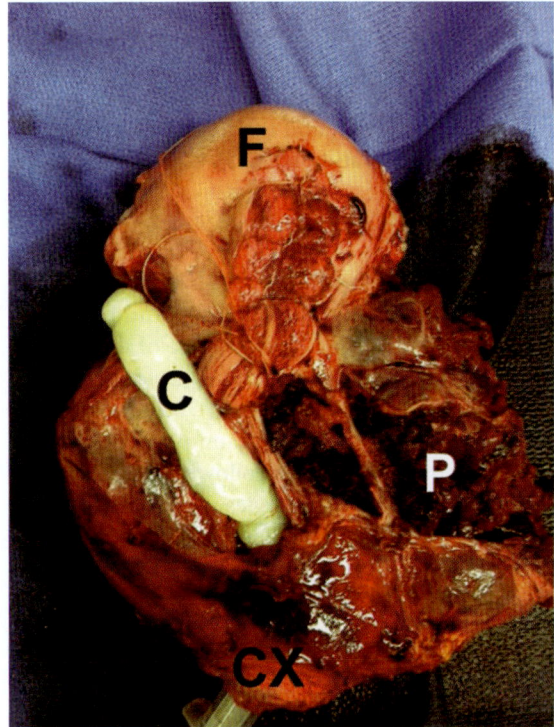

Figure 35.3 Hysterectomy specimen demonstrating placenta accreta. This placenta accreta was diagnosed prenatally. Following longitudinal incision and extraction of the fetus, cesarean hysterectomy was performed. The placenta had invaded the myometrium (left uterine wall) and could not be separated from the uterus. No planes of demarcation were identified. F = uterine fundus; C = umbilical cord; P = placenta; CX = cervix.
Source: Original photo attributed to Doron Kabiri (author).

Surgical Considerations

1. **Surgery Location.** In the United States, 60 percent of PAS cases are delivered in the main OR. A minority of physicians performs emergency hysterectomy for placenta accreta with only one consultant in the OR.[18] Most physicians in the United States reported underestimation of the hemorrhage potential for PAS.[18]

2. **Patient Positioning.** The low lithotomy position may be useful to assist with cystoscopy or vaginal bleeding assessment.

3. **Placenta Accreta Spectrum Diagnosed before Delivery.** Planned preterm cesarean hysterectomy is considered to be the safest and the most recommended treatment for suspected PAS

diagnosed before delivery to prevent massive hemorrhage and consequential morbidity[22] (Figure 35.3).

A multicenter review of emergency cesarean hysterectomy demonstrated 2.5 liters of average blood loss requiring 6.6 units of packed cells, whereas planned cesarean hysterectomy for placenta accreta may reduce the blood loss to 1.3 liters, requiring 1.6 units of packed cells.[41]

4. **Conservative Treatment for Placenta Accreta Spectrum.** Among women with a strong desire to maintain fertility, it may be possible to consider uterine preservation strategies.[5,22,42] This conservative approach of leaving the placenta and uterus in situ until spontaneous resorption occurs often requires complementary treatment such as uterine packing, oversewing of the placental bed, administration of prostaglandins, uterine or

hypogastric artery ligation, selective arterial embolization, administration of methotrexate,[43,44] or argon beam coagulation.[9,10,45–47] Complications including hemorrhage and infection may occur, and the reproductive benefit of uterine preservation is unclear.[42,48]

Hemorrhage Management

1. **Surgical Management.** Massive hemorrhage can lead to coagulopathy, tissue edema, and friability. Careful dissection and performance of the hysterectomy away from the site of placentation can reduce morbidity.[18] In severe coagulopathy, nonarterial diffuse bleeding cannot always be corrected by surgery, even following emergency hysterectomy. Other strategies used to control bleeding include Bakri balloon and B-Lynch suture.[27,49] Intractable hemorrhage following hysterectomy may require pelvic packing and intraabdominal drains such as a Jackson Pratt drain (a closed drain system).
2. **Nonsurgical Management of Hemorrhage.** Prior to hysterectomy, institutional PPH policies should guide management and may include pharmacologic modalities (e.g., oxytocin, methylergonovine, carboprost). Somewhat more contentious is tranexamic acid, recommended by the European Society of Anaesthesiologists to decrease hemorrhage and blood product requirements. Administration of tranexamic acid may be recommended prophylactically prior to cesarean delivery (a low-level recommendation based on poor evidence).[32] However, the 2016 French College of Gynaecologists and Obstetricians guidelines expressed a more conservative view on tranexamic acid: that it should not be used to prevent PPH, and furthermore, insufficient evidence exists to support its use and that clinicians should weigh up whether prophylactic administration is warranted.[50]

   Pelvic artery embolization and balloon occlusion catheters have been shown to reduce blood loss, but these techniques require skill and training to gain clinical experience, their use necessitates special preparation, and they are controversial.[51–53] Unless hemorrhage is anticipated, such as for suspected placenta accreta, it is unlikely that balloon catheters would be inserted prior to delivery. Logistical implications may deter the use of invasive radiology for hemorrhage control, and new hybrid operating suites may increase the use of these combined management strategies. Invasive radiology is only performed in approximately 33 percent of placenta accreta cases of respondents according to a US survey.[18] Internal iliac ligation may not reduce hemorrhage during cesarean hysterectomy for placenta accrete.[53]

Postoperative Considerations

1. **Intensive Care Unit (ICU).** It may be prudent to consider transfer of women with PAS if they present at an institution without an ICU; over 50 percent of emergency hysterectomy cases are admitted to the ICU.[54] Postoperative complications, most commonly infection, occur in almost 30 percent of women following emergency hysterectomy.[2,55,56] Antibiotics should be given as soon as possible and preferably before incision in accordance with patient sensitivities and local hospital policy. Hypotension, anemia, coagulopathy, and multiorgan failure may be detected through close monitoring.[9] Postoperative thromboprophylaxis in conjunction with surgical guidelines may be considered.
2. **Postoperative Surgical Considerations.** A low threshold for surgical reexploration should be anticipated due to the significant chance of hemorrhage or surgical complications such as urinary tract damage (29 percent).[55]

Conclusion

The case presented describes an emergency cesarean hysterectomy for bleeding placenta previa with suspected PAS. Neuraxial anesthesia is a recommended option, but emergency conversion to general anesthesia may be required. Patient blood management strategies include large-bore IV access, cell salvage, and the use of a massive transfusion protocol. To reduce maternal morbidity and mortality, elective cesarean hysterectomy in a tertiary care hospital with a MDT, suitable facilities for blood banking, and an ICU is considered to be the optimal management for PAS that is diagnosed or suspected prior to delivery. Postoperative complications include hemorrhage, and surgical reexploration may be required.

Learning Points

- Emergency hysterectomy risk factors include placenta accreta with or without previa.
- Multidisciplinary team work, emergency drill scenarios, and a checklist may improve maternal outcomes.
- Massive transfusion strategies include a protocol, adequate IV access, and cell salvage use to reduce allogeneic blood transfusion.
- The type of anesthesia used must take into account expectations of hemorrhage and the potential for difficult tracheal intubation.
- In cases of placenta accreta spectrum, attempted placental separation is associated with greater hemorrhage and other maternal morbidities than planned cesarean hysterectomy.
- Future fertility considerations may necessitate a plan for uterine preservation.

References

1. Kuczkowski KM. A review of current anesthetic concerns and concepts for cesarean hysterectomy. *Curr Opin Obstet Gynecol* 2011; **23**(6):401–7.

2. Machado LS. Emergency peripartum hysterectomy: incidence, indications, risk factors and outcome. *North Am J Med Sci* 2011; **3**(8):358–61.

3. Lee IH, Son JH, Shin YC, et al. Anesthetic review of emergency peripartum hysterectomy following vaginal and cesarean delivery: a retrospective study. *Korean J Anesthesiol* 2012; **63**(1):43–47.

4. Shellhaas CS, Gilbert S, Landon MB, et al. The frequency and complication rates of hysterectomy accompanying cesarean delivery. *Obstet Gynecol* 2009; **114**(2 Pt 1): 224–29.

5. Eller AG, Porter TF, Soisson P, Silver RM. Optimal management strategies for placenta accreta. *BJOG* 2009; **116**(5):648–54.

6. Wortman AC, Alexander JM. Placenta accreta, increta, and percreta. *Obstet Gynecol Clin North Am* 2013; **40**(1): 137–54.

7. Snegovskikh D, Clebone A, Norwitz E. Anesthetic management of patients with placenta accreta and resuscitation strategies for associated massive hemorrhage. *Curr Opin Anaesth* 2011; **24**(3):274–81.

8. Gielchinsky Y, Rojansky N, Fasouliotis SJ, Ezra Y. Placenta accrete: summary of 10 years. A survey of 310 cases. *Placenta* 2002; **23**(2–3):210–14.

9. Garmi G, Salim R. Epidemiology, etiology, diagnosis, and management of placenta accreta. *Obstet Gynecol Int* 2012; 2012:873929.

10. Eshkoli T, Weintraub AY, Sergienko R, Sheiner E. Placenta accreta: risk factors, perinatal outcomes, and consequences for subsequent births. *Am J Obstet Gynecol* 2013; **208**(3):219.e1–7.

11. Belfort MA. Placenta accreta. *Am J Obstet Gynecol* 2010; **203**(5):430–39.

12. Miller DA, Chollet JA, Goodwin TM. Clinical risk factors for placenta previa–placenta accreta. *Am J Obstet Gynecol* 1997; **177**(1):210–14.

13. Martin JA, Hamilton BE, Ventura SJ, Osterman MJ, Mathews TJ. Births: final data for 2011. *Natl Vital Stat Rep* 2013; **62**(1):1–70.

14. Warshak CR, Eskander R, Hull AD, et al. Accuracy of ultrasonography and magnetic resonance imaging in the diagnosis of placenta accreta. *Obstet Gynecol* 2006; **108**(3 Pt 1):573–81.

15. Lorenz RP. What is new in placenta accreta? Best articles from the past year. *Obstet Gynecol* 2013; **121**(2 Pt 1):375–76.

16. Comstock CH. The antenatal diagnosis of placental attachment disorders. *Curr Opin Obstet Gynecol* 2011; **23**(2):117–22.

17. Bowman ZS, Eller AG, Kennedy AM, et al. Accuracy of ultrasound for the prediction of placenta accreta. *Am J Obstet Gynecol* 2014; **211**(2):177.e1–7.

18. Wright JD, Silver RM, Bonanno C, et al. Practice patterns and knowledge of obstetricians and gynecologists regarding placenta accreta. *J Matern Fetal Neonat Med* 2013; **26**(16):1602–9.

19. Shoushtarian M, Barnett M, McMahon F, Ferris J. Impact of introducing practical obstetric multi-professional training (PROMPT) into maternity units in Victoria, Australia. *BJOG* 2014; **121**(13):1710–18.

20. Daniels K, Clark A, Lipman S, et al. Multidisciplinary simulation drills improve efficiency of emergency medication retrieval. *Obstet Gynecol* 2014; **123**(Suppl 1):143s–44s.

21. Lipman SS, Carvalho B, Cohen SE, Druzin ML, Daniels K. Response times for emergency cesarean delivery: use of simulation drills to assess and improve obstetric team performance. *J Perinatol* 2013; **33**(4): 259–63.

22. American College of Obstetricians and Gynecologists (AGOG). ACOG Committee Opinion No. 266: placenta accreta *Int J Gynecol Obstet* 2002; **77**(1):77–87.

23. Esakoff TF, Handler SJ, Granados JM, Caughey AB. PAMUS: placenta accreta management across the United States. *J Matern Fetal Neonat Med* 2012; **25**(6): 761–65.

24. Lilker SJ, Meyer RA, Downey KN, Macarthur AJ. Anesthetic considerations for placenta accreta. *Int J Obstet Anesth* 2011; **20**(4):288–92.

25. Sultan P, Hilton G, Butwick A, Carvalho B. Continuous spinal anaesthesia for caesarean hysterectomy and massive haemorrhage in a parturient with placenta increta. *Can J Anaesth* 2012; **59**(5): 473–77.

26. Hawkins JL, Chang J, Palmer SK, Gibbs CP, Callaghan WM. Anesthesia-related maternal mortality in the United States: 1979–2002. *Obstet Gynecol* 2011; **117**(1):69–74.

27. Ducloy-Bouthors AS, Susen S, Wong CA, et al. Medical advances in the treatment of postpartum hemorrhage. *Anesth Analg* 2014; **119**(5):1140–47.

28. Solomon C, Collis RE, Collins PW. Haemostatic monitoring during postpartum haemorrhage and implications for management. *Br J Anaesth* 2012; **109**(6):851–63.

29. Collis RE, Collins PW. Haemostatic management of obstetric haemorrhage. *Anaesthesia* 2015; **70**(Suppl 1): 78–86,e27–28.

30. Kacmar RM, Mhyre JM, Scavone BM, Fuller AJ, Toledo P. The use of postpartum hemorrhage protocols in United States academic obstetric anesthesia units. *Anesth Analg* 2014; **119**(4):906–10.

31. Zuckerwise LC, Pettker CM, Illuzzi J, Raab CR, Lipkind HS. Use of a novel visual aid to improve estimation of obstetric blood loss. *Obstet Gynecol* 2014; **123**(5):982–86.

32. Kozek-Langenecker SA, Afshari A, Albaladejo P, et al. Management of severe perioperative bleeding: guidelines from the European Society of Anaesthesiology. *Eur J Anaesthesiol* 2013; **30**(6):270–382.

33. Bawazeer M, Ahmed N, Izadi H, et al. Compliance with a massive transfusion protocol (MTP) impacts patient outcome. *Injury* 2015; **46**(1):21–28.

34. Holcomb JB, Tilley BC, Baraniuk S, et al. Transfusion of plasma, platelets, and red blood cells in a 1:1:1 vs a 1:1:2 ratio and mortality in patients with severe trauma: the PROPPR randomized clinical trial. *JAMA* 2015; **313**(5):471–82.

35. Duchesne JC, Hunt JP, Wahl G, et al. Review of current blood transfusions strategies in a mature level I trauma center: were we wrong for the last 60 years? *J Trauma* 2008; **65**(2):272–76; discussion 6–8.

36. American College of Obstetricians and Gynecologists (AGOG). AGOG Committee Opinion No. 529: placenta accreta. *Obstet Gynecol* 2012; **120**(1):207–11.

37. Malik S, Brooks H, Singhal T. Cell Saver use in obstetrics. *J Obstet Gynaecol* 2010; **30**(8):826–28.

38. National Institute for Health and Clinical Excellence (NICE). *NICE Interventional Procedure Guidelines 144: Intraoperative Blood Cell Salvage in Obstetrics*. London: NICE; November 2005.

39. Tevet A, Grisaru-Granovsky S, Samueloff A, Ioscovich A. Peripartum use of cell salvage: a university practice audit and literature review. *Arch Gynecol Obstet* 2012; **285**(2):281–84.

40. Teig M, Harkness M, Catling S, Clarke V. Survey of cell salvage use in obstetrics in the UK. *Int J Obstet Anesth* 2007; **16**(Suppl 1):30.

41. Zelop CM, Harlow BL, Frigoletto FD Jr, Safon LE, Saltzman DH. Emergency peripartum hysterectomy. *Am J Obstet Gynecol* 1993; **168**(5):1443–48.

42. Kabiri D, Hants Y, Shanwetter N, et al. Outcomes of subsequent pregnancies after conservative treatment for placenta accreta. *Int J Gynaecol Obstet* 2014; **127**:206–10.

43. Khan M, Sachdeva P, Arora R, Bhasin S. Conservative management of morbidly adherant placenta: a case report and review of literature. *Placenta* 2013; **34**(10): 963–66.

44. Sentilhes L, Ambroselli C, Kayem G, et al. Maternal outcome after conservative treatment of placenta accreta. *Obstet Gynecol* 2010; **115**(3):526–34.

45. Oyelese Y, Smulian JC. Placenta previa, placenta accreta, and vasa previa. *Obstet Gynecol* 2006; **107**(4): 927–41.

46. Dilauro MD, Dason S, Athreya S. Prophylactic balloon occlusion of internal iliac arteries in women with placenta accreta: literature review and analysis. *Clin Radiol* 2012; **67**(6):515–20.

47. Scarantino SE, Reilly JG, Moretti ML, Pillari VT. Argon beam coagulation in the management of placenta accreta. *Obstet Gynecol* 1999; **94**(5 Pt 2): 825–27.

48. Amsalem H, Kingdom JC, Farine D, et al. Planned caesarean hysterectomy versus "conserving" caesarean section in patients with placenta accreta. *J Obstet Gynaecol Can* 2011; **33**(10):1005–10.

49. Zhao Y, Zhang Y, Li Z. Appropriate second-line therapies for management of severe postpartum hemorrhage. *Int J Gynecol Obstet* 2014; **127**(2):180–82.

50. Sentilhes L, Vayssiere C, Deneux-Tharaux C, et al. Postpartum hemorrhage: guidelines for clinical practice from the French College of Gynaecologists and Obstetricians (CNGOF): in collaboration with the French Society of Anesthesiology and Intensive Care (SFAR). *Eur J Obstet Gynecol Reprod Biol* 2016; **198**:12–21.

51. Sadashivaiah J, Wilson R, Thein A, et al. Role of prophylactic uterine artery balloon catheters in the management of women with suspected placenta accreta. *Int J Obstet Anesth* 2011; **20**(4):282–87.

52. Bishop S, Butler K, Monaghan S, et al. Multiple complications following the use of prophylactic internal iliac artery balloon catheterization in a patient

with placenta percreta. *Int J Obstet Anesth* 2011; **20**(1):70–73.

53. Iwata A, Murayama Y, Itakura A, et al. Limitations of internal iliac artery ligation for the reduction of intraoperative hemorrhage during cesarean hysterectomy in cases of placenta previa accreta. *J Obstet Gynecol Res* 2010; **36**(2):254–59.

54. Silver RM, Fox KA, Barton JR, et al. Center of excellence for placenta accreta. *Am J Obstet Gynecol* 2015; **212**:561–68.

55. Yucel O, Ozdemir I, Yucel N, Somunkiran A. Emergency peripartum hysterectomy: a 9-year review. *Arch Gynecol Obstet* 2006; **274**(2):84–87.

56. Christopoulos P, Hassiakos D, Tsitoura A, et al. Obstetric hysterectomy: a review of cases over 16 years. *J Obstet Gynaecol* 2011; **31**(2):139–41.

57. Jolley JA, Nageotte MP, Wing DA, Shrivastava VK. Management of placenta accreta: a survey of maternal-fetal medicine practitioners. *J Matern Fetal Neonat Med* 2012; **25**(6):756–60.

Addendum

Markley et al published a retrospective analysis on 129 cases of PAS in a single centre within the United States. Among these, 122 (95%) had neuraxial block from the outset. There were a number of special features about this population with a very notably high frequency of neuraxial anesthesia:

1 – These were non-emergency cases.

2 – The conversion rate to general anesthesia was 20/122 (17%)

3 – 12/122 (10%) of the PAS cases had Mallampati airway score ≥3; three of these were converted to general anesthesia and difficult intubation was reported; one of these required a fibreoptic intubation. This study highlights that a decision for neuraxial block in a woman with suspected PAS and potential for hemorrhage should likely be limited to the few special centers with experience, equipment and staff to handle concurrently a massive hemorrhage and difficult intubation.

In our own clinical practice, women with a suspected difficult airway and suspected PAS will receive general anesthesia from the outset.

Reference

Markley JC, Farber MK, Perlman NC, Carusi DA. Neuraxial Anesthesia During Cesarean Delivery for Placenta Previa With Suspected Morbidly Adherent Placenta: A Retrospective Analysis. *Anesth Analg* 2018;**127**:930–938.

Interventional Radiology

Ian Renfrew and James Noblet

Case Study

A 33-year-old woman was listed first for an elective cesarean delivery due to a diagnosis of placenta previa. During surgery, almost no muscle was seen in the lower segment, with no evidence of transserosal placental invasion. The fetus was delivered in good condition, leaving an adherent placenta, which was detached piecemeal with bleeding from the placental bed, before the uterus was closed. In the postoperative care unit (PACU), the patient became hypotensive, progressing to a cardiac arrest with pulseless electrical activity (PEA). Fluid resuscitation and attempts at hemorrhage control using a Bakri balloon and uterotonics were sufficiently successful to restore cardiac output. However, the patient continued to bleed around the Bakri balloon, necessitating return to the OR and emergency subtotal hysterectomy. Continuing hemorrhage required further surgery later that afternoon, when the internal iliac arteries (IIAs) were dissected out and ligated with a clip, after which the abdomen and vagina were packed with surgical swaps. The patient was transferred to the ICU with significant hemodynamic compromise despite full inotropic support using infusions of norepinephrine to maintain cardiovascular stability. The interventional radiology (IR) service at a nearby specialist tertiary referral university hospital was contacted about undertaking a procedure to bring about hemostasis, ideally within the ICU at the host hospital. By this point, the patient had received a total of 52 units of packed red cells and other blood products, including platelets, fresh frozen plasma (FFP), and cryoprecipitate.

A radiologist from the specialist center went to the patient, and an ultrasound-guided right common femoral artery sheath and intraaortic balloon were inserted within the ICU. Hemodynamic parameters improved rapidly, allowing ambulance transfer to the regional interventional radiology center within the tertiary center.

A consultant anesthetist and obstetrician transferred the patient directly to the interventional radiology (IR) suite. Bilateral common femoral artery access was gained with ongoing hemorrhage demonstrated in the left internal iliac territories. Selective collateral vessel embolization of the proximal femoral and lumbar vessels supplying internal iliac territories was performed. This was necessary in view of the obstruction to the internal iliac arteries by the previously applied ligation clips.

Adequate hemostasis was finally achieved after a total of 75 units of packed cells, with a packed cell:fresh frozen plasma:cryoprecipitate:platelet ratio of 5:5:1:1, respectively, and full support by a specialist trauma anesthetist throughout.

The patient was transferred back to the ICU for stabilization, where she was found to have developed transient biochemical pancreatitis. The abdominal and vaginal packs were removed, and the patient was extubated on day 2. She was transferred back to her referring hospital on day 3. She was later discharged from hospital, being able to fully mobilize on day 8 postdelivery, with no significant morbidity.

Key Points

- This patient experienced major obstetric hemorrhage due to abnormal placentation in a unit without an IR service.
- Resuscitation management included damage-control IR in conjunction with massive blood component transfusion.
- Definitive embolization required transfer of the critically ill patient to the regional IR center.

Discussion

Location and Codependencies for Delivery of Patients at High Risk of Hemorrhage

In patients identified as at high risk of major peripartum bleeding, including abnormal placentation, deliveries should occur in institutions with experience in managing massive hemorrhage. The availability of the following services is desirable: intensive care, hematology, neonatology, interventional radiology, vascular surgery, and urology, as well as obstetrics and anesthesia. Increasingly, these specialties are colocated in major trauma and specialist centers.

The optimal location within each hospital that performs these complex cases will vary between institutions; with physical location, proximity to other services, space, and operator choice being important factors in the decision-making process. The pros and cons of using the obstetric ORs instead of the main ORs or the radiology suite must be discussed in advance, and rehearsals and drills should be undertaken regularly.

In our institution, patients believed to have abnormal placentation have their deliveries undertaken in one of the four dedicated IR suites. All elective patients have predelivery imaging with ultrasonography and MRI, with a multidisciplinary team meeting (MDT) outlining patient-specific strategies for both the intended elective delivery and any emergency presentation. When these cases are performed electively, the risks and benefits of general anesthesia (GA) can be balanced against those of regional anesthesia (RA) on an individual basis. In discussion with the patient, the mode of anesthesia can be planned, acknowledging the probable need to convert RA to GA in the event of major bleeding and the psychological distress this may cause the patient.

Our policy is to insert two large-bore sheaths, one in the common femoral artery and one in the femoral vein, once anesthesia has been achieved with a lumbar epidural block using a low-dose bupivacaine-fentanyl mixture. The arterial sheath allows rapid balloon occlusion of the aorta if massive hemorrhage occurs, whereas the venous sheath allows resuscitation via a rapid fluid transfuser system such as the Level 1 Fast Flow Fluid Warmer (Smiths Medical, Minneapolis, Minnesota, USA), while the epidural catheter is used to provide postoperative analgesia. In most cases, the patient is then given a general anesthetic according to local obstetric anesthetic practice, ensuring that surgery commences once the airway is secure following endotracheal intubation.

After delivery of the fetus, and in the event of significant bleeding, balloons may be used to occlude either the distal infrarenal aorta or common iliac or internal iliac arteries to achieve hemostasis and increase systemic vascular resistance. This helps to reduce the rate of blood loss, allowing treatment of profound hypovolemic shock, and provides an opportunity to consider the best strategy for further surgical or IR procedures. The more proximal the occlusion, the more likely hemostasis will be effective, because occlusion of the distal aorta will prevent in-line flow through the anterior division of the internal iliac arteries as well as collateral (retrograde) bleeding via the low lumbar and proximal thigh profunda femoris arterial branches. Clearly, this may cause ischemic injury and thrombosis, and one must consider this risk and balance it against the benefits occluding major blood vessels brings. There are multiple ramifications of effective further interventions beyond the scope of this chapter.

Transfer of Cardiovascularly Unstable Patients to Other Facilities Within or Beyond the Host Institution

The UK Royal College of Obstetricians and Gynaecologists (RCOG) outlines guidelines for management of major obstetric hemorrhage but does not deal with the transfer of cardiovascularly unstable patients. There is an acknowledgment that it is difficult to transfer a patient whose hemorrhage is uncontrolled, and it is a proposition even the most experienced anesthesiologist would find challenging. Anecdote supports the notion of non-image-guided balloon occlusion of the distal infrarenal aorta as a means of effecting temporary hemorrhage control. Clearly, this is a dramatic solution to a challenging problem but may provide the level of stability required to move a patient to an institution with the resources to achieve definitive hemorrhage control.

Arrangements for Management of Hemorrhage in Units Without Interventional Radiology

The Northwick Park Maternal Death Enquiry Healthcare Commission (August 2006) concluded:

> due to a shortage of suitably trained radiologists, it is not possible to provide full time cover for interventional radiology in all obstetric units. However, given the potential to save the lives of patients who have catastrophic postnatal bleeding, trusts with delivery units should, where feasible, engage with their neighbouring trusts to discuss the formation of networks. The aim should be to provide an emergency interventional radiology service that is responsive to patients' needs wherever and whenever they arise.[1]

The Department of Heath issued *Interventional Radiology: Guidance for Service Delivery 2010*, which noted that arterial embolization in the setting of

Table 36.1 Options for Management of Major Obstetric Hemorrhage

Pharmacologic
Uterotonics
Oxytocin analogues
Ergometrine
Synthetic prostaglandins
Drugs that may be useful in major hemorrhage with massive transfusion:
• Tranexamic acid
• Calcium
• Fibrinogen concentrate

Surgical
Uterine compression
Bakri balloon
B-Lynch suture
Vaginal or abdominal packing
Internal iliac artery ligation
Hysterectomy
Aortic cross-clamping

Radiologic
Balloon occlusion
• Aorta
• Common iliac arteries
• Internal iliac arteries
Embolization

postpartum hemorrhage (PPH) is safe, noninvasive, and reproducible with low complication rates and allows patients a subsequent normal pregnancy. It went on to state that hospitals with obstetric services should provide an emergency IR service to save the lives of patients with catastrophic PPH.[2]

Network arrangements are desirable, but for this to occur there are a number of important considerations, including the facilities and ability to transfer an unstable patient as well as critical care bed availability at the receiving hospital.

Treatment Options in PPH

The treatment of PPH can be pharmacologic, surgical, and radiologic (Table 36.1). The pharmacologic and surgical resources are more readily available than radiologic; therefore, radiologists tend to become involved with many of these patients when other treatment modalities have failed.

Accepting that the majority of patients with PPH are successfully managed with uterotonics and hysterectomy-sparing surgical intervention, a minority of patients will still remain without adequate hemorrhage control. Options in this scenario included

hysterectomy, arterial ligation, and radiologic embolization.

In this specific case, in view of ongoing bleeding and the presence of a large left retroperitoneal hematoma (and the absence of onsite interventional radiology), the internal iliacs were dissected out and ligated (this technique is reported to have a 39 percent failure rate).[3] Ligation of the proximal arterial inflow alone should not, and frequently will not, stop bleeding because the internal iliac arterial circulation collateralizes with the lumbar and proximal thigh arterial supply. Therefore, ligating the internal iliac arteries still allows bleeding in the internal iliac territory via back-bleeding but precludes the delivery of embolic material to the target territory via the "in-line" flow, consequently making the embolization procedure more difficult.

Embolization uses the blood flow to "carry" the embolic agent down the vessel to an arteriolar level, where it effects the "block," therefore allowing relative depressurization and clot formation. This effectively closes both the "front and back door" flow. The typical agent, spongostan, is generally reabsorbed at 2–3 weeks, allowing recanalization. Embolization is reported to be effective in 97 percent, with recognition in the Scottish Confidential Audit of Severe Maternal Morbidity for an increase in its utility.[3]

Balloon occlusion has been recently reused in major trauma (Resuscitative Endovascular Balloon Occlusion of the Aorta [REBOA]). The inflation of a compliant balloon in the appropriate area of the aorta increases afterload, central filling pressure, and therefore cerebral and myocardial perfusion. Additionally, occlusion of distal blood flow reduces perfusion to the area of hemorrhage. Placement of the aortic balloon in the infrarenal aortic zone III (Figure 36.1) allows for control of pelvic hemorrhage without disruption to the visceral arterial supply of the gastrointestinal tract, liver, and kidneys in aortic zone II.[4]

Anesthetic Considerations to Achieve Safe/ Timely Transfer

The rationale to transfer a woman with a PPH is to stop her bleeding with techniques unavailable in the institution in which she gave birth. It follows, then, that these women are likely to have lost a significant volume of blood and that this will be ongoing. As such, a degree of hypovolemia, anemia, hypothermia, and coagulopathy should be expected. Treating and/or avoiding these problems within an OR can be hard; doing it while moving

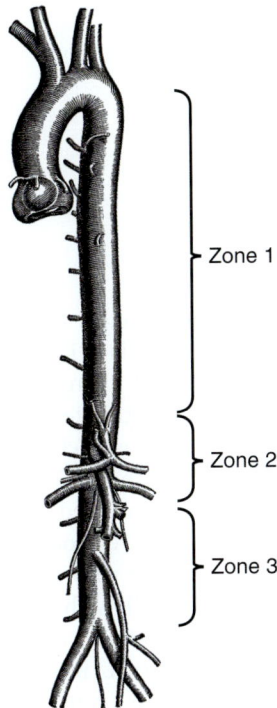

Figure 36.1 Aortic zones for resuscitative endovascular balloon occlusion of aorta (REBOA) placement.
Source: Image courtesy of Getty Images.

a patient to another hospital is even harder and should not be undertaken by teams that lack experience and training in this area. Measures to temporize the blood loss and to normalize physiology should be instituted prior to transfer and continued during the transfer, where feasible. This would include the transfusion of warmed blood products in the ratios described, forced air warming of the patient (top half only if there is occlusion of the aorta). and full monitoring. It is unlikely that the patient would not have already received a general anesthetic as part of the management of the PPH, but if not, then this should be considered prior to transfer if conversion to general anesthesia en route is a possibility.

The timing of the transfer is also tricky and often dictated by logistical issues as well as clinical decisions. The referral and acceptance process takes time and often needs experienced clinicians to ensure that communication is optimal. This may mean a key team member has to leave the "front line" or the referral is delayed until such a time that a pair of hands can be spared. Critical care beds to coincide with the radiologic resources may also be lacking, and ambulances can take time to arrive.

From a clinical perspective, it can be a fine balance with a narrow window in which to move the patient. Understandably, there is a reticence to fix hemorrhage by radiologic means in another hospital until all surgical avenues have been exhausted. Unfortunately, this often means that the patient has sustained considerable blood loss, along with its associated problems, by the time transfer becomes a necessity. A paradox exists then that the hemorrhage is not significant enough to warrant transfer until all local options have failed, at which time the patient has become too unwell to transfer at all. The solution to this problem is not obvious, but good situational awareness, clear lines of communication, and experienced personnel seem prudent.

Learning Points

- Be mindful of the highly effective radiologic options in the treatment of PPH – start the communication process early.
- Plans on how to manage PPH and patients identified with abnormal placentation/placental invasion should be formalized. Rehearse and train.

References

1. Investigation into 10 maternal deaths at, or following delivery at, Northwick Park Hospital, North West London Hospitals NHS Trust, between April 2002 and April 2005. Commission for Healthcare Audit and Inspection, 2006. Available at http://webarchive.nationalarchives.gov.uk/20060502043818/http://healthcarecommission.org.uk/_db/_documents/Northwick_tagged.pdf (accessed March 2018).

2. Interventional radiology: guidance for service delivery. A report from the National Imaging Board. Department of Health, 2010. Available at www.gov.uk/government/uploads/system/uploads/attachment_data/file/215929/dh_122191.pdf (accessed March 2018).

3. Mavrides E, Alalrd S, Chandraharan E, et al., on behalf of the Royal College of Obstetricians and Gynaecologists. Prevention and management of postpartum haemorrhage. *BJOG* 2016; **124**:e106–49.

4. Morrison J, Reva V, Lönn L, et al. Resuscitative endovacsular balloon occlusion of the aorta (REBOA), in DuBose J, Morrison J, Reva V, et al., eds., *The Art of Endovascular Hybrid Trauma and Bleeding Management*. Örebro: Örebro University Hospital; 2017, pp. 77–100.

Supplemental radiological images to complement this chapter are available from the editor by email (roshanagfernando@gmail.com)

Amniotic Fluid Embolism

Alison Gar-Pui Koo and Warwick D. Ngan Kee

Case Study

A healthy nulliparous 36-year-old woman presented at 41 weeks' gestation for postdates induction of labor. The progress of labor was slow, whereupon the patient became increasingly distressed and agitated and could not cooperate in order to receive epidural analgesia. Eventually, a Category I cesarean delivery for persistent fetal bradycardia was performed.

Standard general anesthesia with a rapid-sequence induction using propofol and suxamethonium was administered without complication. The patient was intubated and ventilated, and anesthesia was maintained with a mixture of oxygen, nitrous oxide, and sevoflurane. Lightly stained meconium liquor was noted at uterine incision, and a pediatrician was present to resuscitate the neonate. A 5-unit oxytocin bolus was given as standard at delivery. Following delivery, the patient's blood pressure decreased acutely to 72/40 mmHg with a heart rate of 52 beats/min and an oxygen saturation of 88 percent on 40% oxygen. There was equal air entry with no audible wheeze on auscultation, and ventilatory pressures were normal. Despite aggressive resuscitation with 1,000 ml crystalloid, 1000 ml colloid, 100% oxygen, and lung recruitment maneuvers, there was no significant clinical improvement. Initial estimated blood loss was 700 ml, and an oxytocin infusion (10 IU/h) was started. A bedside Hemocue was 7.8 g/dl. An arterial line was inserted, and a right internal jugular central venous catheter was placed under ultrasound guidance. The central venous pressure was elevated at 18 mmHg, and initial arterial blood gases were pH 7.28, PaO_2 9.6 kPa, $PaCO_2$ 6.2 kPa, base excess –10 mmol/L, and lactate concentration 5 mmol/L.

Surgery continued, during which escalating inotropic support with a norepinephrine infusion of up to 15 μg/min was required. The obstetricians noted a well-contracted uterus but ongoing abnormal oozing and suspected defective coagulation. A total of 4 units of packed red cells (PRCs), 4 units of fresh frozen plasma (FFP), and 4 units of platelets were transfused. The total estimated blood loss was 1.6 liters. The abdomen was packed and closed with an abdominal drain, and the patient was transferred to the ICU sedated and ventilated.

Immediate postoperative blood tests performed in the ICU were consistent with disseminated intravascular coagulation (DIC), with a hemoglobin concentration of 8.2 g/dl, platelet count of 63×10^9/L, white cell count of 10×10^9/L, international normalized ratio (INR) of 2.8, activated partial thromboplastin time (aPTT) of 59 s, and fibrinogen concentration of 0.6 g/liter. The chest x-ray showed bilateral interstitial infiltrates. Bedside transthoracic echocardiography showed left ventricular impairment with an ejection fraction of 30 percent. Right ventricular and pulmonary arterial pressures were normal.

The patient further received a transfusion of 2 units of PRCs, 4 units of FFP, 4 units of platelets, and 6 units of cryoprecipitate. Her coagulopathy was corrected and stable by postoperative day 1. Inotropic support was weaned off on day 3. However, the patient developed acute respiratory distress syndrome (ARDS) and required mechanical ventilation for 5 days. She was eventually extubated and discharged from the ICU on day 6.

Key Points

- This patient developed fulminant cardiovascular collapse during delivery.
- She exhibited premonitory symptoms, and the cardinal features of amniotic fluid embolism (AFE) syndrome: hypoxia, hypotension, and coagulopathy.
- Early aggressive resuscitation and postoperative ICU support were key to her survival.

Discussion

AFE is a rare but potentially devastating obstetric complication. Owing to rarity, variation in diagnostic criteria, and a range of symptoms and signs, it can be difficult to diagnose, and diagnosis is usually one of exclusion. The prospective UK Obstetric Surveillance System (UKOSS) estimated an incidence of AFE of 2.0 per 100,000 maternities.[1] It is among the top five leading causes of direct maternal death in the United Kingdom, with case-fatality estimates ranging from 11 to 61 percent.[2] High-quality supportive care is the mainstay for meaningful maternal outcome.

Risk Factors

There has been a plethora of associations with AFE, including advanced maternal age, multiparity, male fetus, induction of labor, assisted or cesarean delivery, placenta previa, placental rupture, and ethnic minority. However, no consistent data have yet proven any significant causation or, moreover, justified any prospective alteration of standard obstetric practice to reduce the risk of AFE.[1,3]

Pathophysiology

In 1941, Stiener and Lauschburg initially proposed the traditional concept of a simple obstructive mechanism of injury based on the finding of fetal debris in the pulmonary circulation of postmortem women who died from "obstetrical shock."[4] This has since been challenged; the close similarities between the manifestations of AFE and those of anaphylaxis and the systemic inflammatory response syndrome (SIRS) suggest a much more dynamic and complex picture. It has been suggested that the term *anaphylactoid syndrome of pregnancy* may better describe the pathophysiologic process and may be more suitable.

There first must be a breach of the maternal-fetal barrier and a favorable pressure gradient permitting transfer of amniotic fluid into the maternal circulation, perhaps via endocervical veins or a site of uterine trauma. Amniotic fluid contains many vasoactive and procoagulant substances, including arachidonic acid metabolites and cytokines. These components, however, have been demonstrated in pregnant women without clinical evidence of AFE. Therefore, it has been proposed that a secondary idiosyncratic humoral response must exist. This would subsequently trigger a pro-inflammatory cascade, a coagulation cascade, and potential deterioration to multiorgan failure in susceptible maternal-fetal pairs.[3,5]

Clinical Presentation

AFE classically presents during labor and delivery or in the immediate postpartum period. Hallmark findings are the triad of hypoxia, hypotension with cardiovascular collapse, and DIC. Outside of this triad, there also may be confusion and agitation, seizures, breathlessness, and evidence of fetal distress.

Both hypoxia and hypotension appear to follow a temporal pattern, representing the evolving mechanism of injury, from obstructive shock arising from embolic debris in the pulmonary vasculature to inflammatory shock. Early hypoxia is likely due to severe ventilation-perfusion mismatch. During this initial phase, severe pulmonary hypertension from pulmonary vasospasm can lead to acute right ventricular failure, impairment of left ventricular filling, severe left ventricular dysfunction, obstructive shock, and cardiogenic pulmonary edema.

In those who survive the initial insult, late hypoxia occurs primarily from noncardiogenic exudative pulmonary edema secondary to alveolar-capillary membrane damage. In this later phase, pulmonary hypertension is often not evident, and the ongoing left ventricular failure that is seen may be a result of myocardial ischemia or the presence of inflammatory myocardial depressants such as endothelin and other cytokines that are implicated in SIRS. During the later phase, although obstructive and cardiogenic shock may persist, a distributive pattern of shock predominates.

In both phases, severe hypoxic encephalopathy has been implicated in brain death and long-term neurologic sequelae. Cardiac arrhythmias including bradycardia, ventricular fibrillation, pulseless electrical activity, and asystole may also present and further complicate management[5] (Figure 37.1). Coagulopathy occurs in over 80 percent of cases and can itself lead to hemorrhagic shock and death. Although uncertain, it may be the result of a consumptive process or massive fibrinolysis.[6]

Diagnosis

Historically, AFE was diagnosed at autopsy by demonstrating the presence of fetal squames in the maternal pulmonary circulation. With improving survival rates and a better understanding of the

```
┌──────────────────────────────────────┐
│  Disruption of maternal fetal barrier │
│  and entry of immunologically active  │
│  amniotic fluid into maternal         │
│  bloodstream                          │
└──────────────────────────────────────┘
```

```
┌──────────────────────────────────────┐        ┌──────────────────────────────────────┐
│  Idiosyncratic SIRS-like activation   │        │  Activation of inflammatory cascade    │
│  of pro-inflammatory mediators in     │───────▶│  + Coagulopathy/DIC                    │
│  susceptible maternal-fetal pairs     │        │  + Bleeding                            │
└──────────────────────────────────────┘        │  + Hemorrhagic shock                   │
                                                 └──────────────────────────────────────┘
```

EARLY

```
┌──────────────────────────────────────┐        ┌──────────────────────────────────────┐
│  Stimulation of intense pulmonary     │        │  Ventilation/perfusion mismatch        │
│  vasoconstriction                     │        │  + Hypoxia and respiratory acidosis    │
│  + Severe pulmonary hypertension      │───────▶│  + Obstructive/cardiogenic shock       │
│  + RV failure & impaired LV filling   │        │  + Cardiogenic pulmonary edema         │
│  + Severe LV failure                  │        └──────────────────────────────────────┘
└──────────────────────────────────────┘
```

LATE

```
┌──────────────────────────────────────┐        ┌──────────────────────────────────────┐
│  Systemic inflammatory mediators and  │        │  Capillary leak syndrome               │
│  hypoxia                              │        │  + ARDS                                │
│  + Myocardial ischemia                │        │  + Non-cardiogenic pulmonary hypoxia   │
│  + Myocardial depression              │───────▶│  + Distributive shock                  │
│  + Continued LV failure               │        └──────────────────────────────────────┘
│  + Arrhythmias, PEA/asystolic arrest  │
│  + Multiorgan failure                 │
└──────────────────────────────────────┘
```

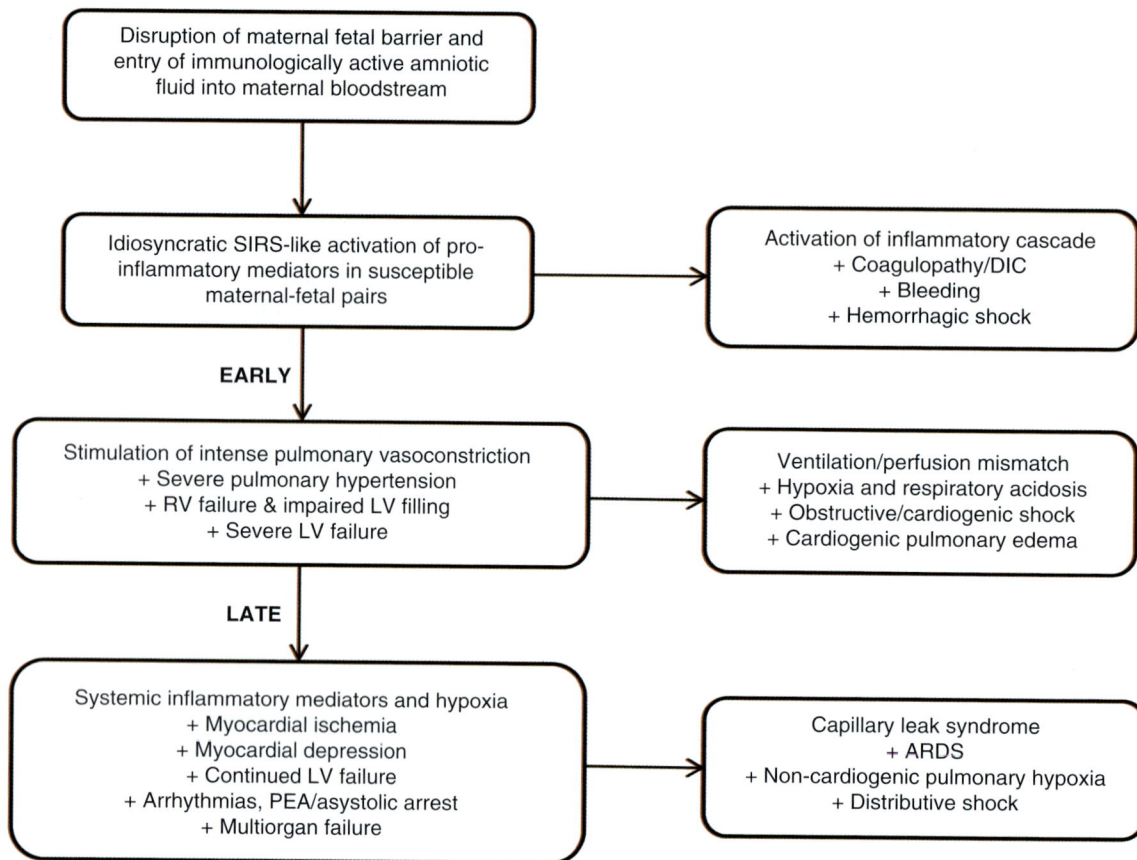

Figure 37.1 Proposed mechanisms for the pathophysiology of AFE. SIRS = systemic inflammatory response syndrome; DIC = disseminated intravascular coagulation; RV = right ventricle; LV = left ventricle; PEA = pulseless electrical activity; ARDS = adult respiratory distress syndrome. Adapted from: (i) Clark SL. Amniotic fluid embolism. *Obstet Gynecol* 2014; **123**:337–48 (ii) Moore J, Baldisseri MR. Amniotic fluid embolism. *Crit Care Med* 2005; **33**:S279–85

pathophysiology, this alone should no longer be considered a pathognomonic feature; detection should be primarily clinical. Key criteria for diagnosis are summarized by many AFE registries (Table 37.1).

In mothers who manifest AFE outside the classic triad, we must exercise caution and explore other potential obstetric and nonobstetric diagnoses. Obstetric differentials may include eclampsia, uterine or placental rupture, acute hemorrhage, and peripartum cardiomyopathy. Nonobstetric differentials are many and may include other emboli (fat, air, thrombus), anaphylaxis, transfusion reaction, sepsis, cardiomyopathy, myocardial infarction, and aspiration. In cases of regional anesthesia, high spinal and local anesthetic toxicity should also be considered.

Radiographic findings are not diagnostic, but patients with pulmonary edema will have bilateral interstitial and alveolar infiltrates. Routine blood tests will reflect the state of coagulopathy and end-organ dysfunction. Electrocardiography may show ischemia or arrhythmias. Echocardiography can highlight pulmonary hypertension, acute right ventricular failure, and diminished left ventricular contractility. Leftward deviation of the interventricular septum secondary to suprasystemic right-sided pressures or as the right ventricle dilates may also be evident.

There is currently no recognized laboratory test diagnostic for AFE. There has been interest in measuring immune markers such as complement and tryptase levels, but these have low sensitivity and specificity and should not be regarded as confirmatory tools. Newer tests include zinc coproporphyrin (Zn-CPI) and sialyl Tn (STN). The former is a component of meconium, and the latter is a fetal antigen present in both meconium and amniotic fluid. The clinical application of these assays has not yet been validated,

Table 37.1 Diagnostic Criteria for Amniotic Fluid Embolism

Excluding women with maternal hemorrhage as the first presenting feature, in whom there was no evidence of coagulopathy or cardiorespiratory compromise, and in the absence of other clear causes, AFE can be diagnosed by

I. Acute maternal collapse with one or more of the following features:

  - Premonitory symptoms such as restlessness, agitation, numbness, tingling
  - Shortness of breath
  - Seizures
  - Hypotension
  - Cardiac arrhythmias
  - Cardiac arrest
  - Coagulopathy
  - Maternal hemorrhage
  - Acute fetal compromise

OR

II. The finding of fetal squames or hair in the lungs of mothers during postmortem examination

Source: Adapted from the UKOSS Registry.[1]

but in the future they may be used to predict the severity or mortality from AFE.[7]

Management

Management of suspected AFE is supportive, and maternal cardiopulmonary stabilization is paramount. The vast majority of patients will need admission to the ICU. Clinical vigilance is vital because the speed of deterioration can be alarming; the time from collapse to death has been reported to be as rapid as 1–7 hours.[5]

The most important goal is to prevent hypoxia and subsequent end-organ failure. Because of clinical consistencies with ARDS, ventilation using lung protection strategies may be beneficial. Central venous catheter or pulmonary artery catheter placement and transthoracic or transesophageal echocardiography can all help guide fluid resuscitation and inotropic therapy, evaluate ventricular filling, and optimize hemodynamic management.

Coagulopathy will require correction with FFP, platelets, and cryoprecipitate, the administration of which can be guided by point-of-care devices such as thromboelastography. Antifibrinolytics such as tranexamic acid and aprotinin have both been used in AFE. In cases of hypofibrinogenemia, case reports have described fibrinogen concentrate as an effective addition to managing obstetric hemorrhage.[8] Routine use of recombinant factor VIIa has not been recommended, following reports of worse maternal outcome from massive intravascular thrombosis.[9]

Other management strategies have been reported anecdotally but are much more dependent on the availability of resources and expertise. Examples include intraaortic balloon counterpulsation, extracorporeal membrane oxygenation, cardiopulmonary bypass, plasma exchange transfusion, inhaled prostacyclin, and inhaled nitric oxide. Finally, in the event that catastrophic AFE occurs before delivery, early perimortem cesarean delivery offers the best chance for neonatal survival.

Outcome

There has been a significant improvement in prognosis and mortality since AFE was first described. This is largely due to advances in resuscitation and critical care. Greater awareness and earlier recognition have also meant detection of less severe cases that have survived and been included in AFE registries. For those who do survive, morbidity remains high with severe sequelae, particularly neurologic impairment. A recent study reported that cerebral injury occurred in 6 percent of women with AFE in the United Kingdom, and cerebral infarction occurred in 20 percent of women with AFE in Australia.[10] There are no data to support recurrence of this syndrome with subsequent pregnancies if the mother survives.[7]

Learning Points

- AFE is an unpredictable and unpreventable cause of sudden maternal collapse.
- Diagnosis is clinical, and it is important to exclude other common obstetric and nonobstetric causes of maternal hypoxia, hypotension, and coagulopathy.
- The exact pathogenesis is unclear but is likely to involve SIRS-like activation of an inflammatory cascade in susceptible individuals.
- Aggressive resuscitation and supportive care are the mainstay of treatment. Hypoxia, hypotension, and ventricular failure should be managed early with oxygen, respiratory support, fluids, vasopressors, and inotropic therapy. Coagulopathy and DIC should also be anticipated and corrected early.
- AFE should now be considered a survivable event.

References

1. Knight M, Tuffnell D, Brocklehurst P, et al. Incidence and risk factors for amniotic-fluid embolism. *Obstet Gynecol* 2010; **115**:910–17.

2. Knight M, Kenyon S, Brocklehurst P, et al., eds., on behalf of MBRRACE-UK. *Saving Lives, Improving Mothers' Care: Lessons Learned to Inform Future Maternity Care from the UK and Ireland Confidential Enquiries into Maternal Deaths and Morbidity 2009–12.* Oxford: National Perinatal Epidemiology Unit, University of Oxford; 2014.

3. Clark SL. Amniotic fluid embolism. *Obstet Gynecol* 2014; **123**:337–48.

4. Steiner PE, Lushbaugh CC. Maternal pulmonary embolism by amniotic fluid: as a cause of obstetric shock and unexpected deaths in obstetrics. *JAMA* 1941; **117**: 1245–54.

5. Moore J, Baldisseri MR. Amniotic fluid embolism. *Crit Care Med* 2005; **33**:S279–85.

6. Harnett MJ, Hepner DL, Datta S, Kodali BS. Effect of amniotic fluid on coagulation and platelet function in pregnancy: an evaluation using thromboelastography. *Anaesthesia* 2005; **60**:1068–72.

7. McDonnell NJ, Percival V, Paech MJ. Amniotic fluid embolism: a leading cause of maternal death yet still a medical conundrum. *Int J Obstet Anesth* 2013; **22**:329–36.

8. Bell SF, Rayment R, Collins PW, Collis RE. The use of fibrinogen concentrate to correct hypofibrinogenaemia rapidly during obstetric haemorrhage. *Int J Obstet Anesth* 2010; **19**:218–23.

9. Knight M, Fitzpatrick K, Kurinczuk JJ, Tuffnell D. Use of recombinant factor VIIa in patients with amniotic fluid embolism. *Anesthesiology* 2012; **117**:423–24.

10. Knight M, Berg C, Brocklehurst P, et al. Amniotic fluid embolism incidence, risk factors and outcomes: a review and recommendations. *BMC Pregnancy Childbirth* 2012; **12**:7.

Addendum

Since this content was written, further studies have suggested alternate and additional mechanisms for the actions of lipid emulsion in the treatment of local anaesthetic toxicity. An editorial by Picard and Meek highlights these issues.

Reference

Picard J, Meek T. Lipid emulsion for intoxication by local anaesthetic: sunken sink? *Anaesthesia* 2016; **71**:879–882

Local Anesthetic Toxicity

Rasha Abouelmagd and Tim Meek

Case Study

A 29-year-old 70-kg para 1, gravida 1 woman requested an epidural for labor pain relief at 5 cm of cervical dilatation. An epidural was inserted, and patient-controlled epidural analgesia (PCEA) was established using a low-dose epidural mixture of 0.1% bupivacaine with 2 µg/ml fentanyl.

The patient eventually delivered her healthy baby spontaneously but suffered a third-degree perineal tear that required repair in the OR. The patient was taken to the OR, and an epidural top-up of 15 ml 0.5% bupivacaine (75 mg) was administered after a negative aspiration test through the epidural catheter.

Moments after the injection, the patient became agitated and had a tonic-clonic seizure. Shortly after this, the ECG monitor showed runs of irregular rhythm with a noninvasive blood pressure monitoring system reading of 150/100 mmHg with a heart rate of 120 beats/min. Because of the clinical presentation and temporal association with the injection, local anesthetic systemic toxicity (LAST) was suspected.

An emergency (code blue) call for help was put out immediately. High-flow 100% oxygen via a bag-valve-mask system was administered, and 3 mg midazolam was given intravenously in increments, which stopped the seizure. A decision was made to intubate the patient's trachea to permit controlled ventilation, with a plan for expedited surgery. Thiopental 250 mg was given cautiously to prevent awareness, and succinylcholine 100 mg was given to facilitate intubation of the trachea using a rapid-sequence technique. *Lipid rescue* – treatment with an IV lipid emulsion – was initiated, using Intralipid 20% with a bolus dose of 1.5 ml/kg (105 ml) and an infusion starting at 15 ml/kg per hour (105 ml/h). Within 5 minutes, the patient's ECG showed sinus rhythm at a normal heart rate. Later aspiration of the epidural catheter showed free flow of blood, suggesting venous placement.

Surgery was performed under general anesthesia, and the patient was woken and her trachea extubated at the end of the procedure. No further seizures occurred, and the patient remained cardiovascularly stable postoperatively. She was discharged home 24 hours later.

Key Points

- This patient became unconscious and had a tonic-clonic seizure following an epidural top-up.
- A presumptive diagnosis of LAST was made.
- Venous blood was later aspirated through her epidural catheter, supporting IV placement or migration as a cause.
- Supportive resuscitation measures were instituted immediately.
- The early intervention with lipid emulsion could have possibly prevented the progression from cardiac toxicity to cardiac arrest.

Discussion

Local anesthetic systemic toxicity (LAST) is a potentially lethal complication of regional anesthesia and analgesia. A third of cases relate to epidural anesthesia, according to a large retrospective review of cases of LAST reported in the literature between 1979 and 2009.[1] After a single IV injection of a toxic local anesthetic (LA) dose, LAST occurs very rapidly, in less than 1 minute in 50 percent of cases and less than 5 minutes in 75 percent of cases. During a continuous infusion of local anesthetic solution, LAST can be delayed; it can occur days after initiation of the infusion.[1]

Normal Action and Toxic Action of Local Anesthetics

Anesthetists usually intend local anesthetic drugs (LAs) to act solely on peripheral neuronal tissue. LAs exist in both ionized acid and nonionized base forms. The nonionized form has the ability to cross the myelin sheath barrier and reach the axon. The low pH inside the cell facilitates the dissociation of the nonionized local anesthetic to the ionized form. It is the ionized fraction that has the ability to contact the sodium channels from the inside of the cells and consequently block them.[2] However, being sodium channel inhibitors, LAs can act in multiple locations in the CNS and the cardiovascular system, where sodium channels are widespread, causing undesirable effects. In excess, these undesirable effects may be regarded as toxicity. The development of symptoms and signs of LA toxicity relates directly to the concentration of the drug in the plasma. LAST is caused by a high circulating plasma concentration of LA, generally occurring as a result of either IV entrainment of LA or delayed absorption from the anesthetic depot at an injection site. The plasma concentration will depend on the rate of absorption from the injected site as well as inadvertent IV injection.[3]

Features of LAST

Most cases of LAST follow a broadly typical pattern of presentation, with a combination of CNS and cardiovascular system (CVS) signs and symptoms. The first signs or symptoms of LAST are often related to the CNS, with seizures being the most common sign.[1] The "classic" prodromal signs of agitation, metallic taste, circumoral numbness, and auditory changes occur in less than 20 percent of patients.[1]

The most frequent signs of CVS toxicity, occurring in about 50 percent of patients, are ECG abnormalities, including tachyarrhythmia, bradyarrhythmia, ventricular ectopics, conduction defects, or QRS complex widening. More ominous signs, such as malignant arrhythmia including ventricular tachycardia and fibrillation or asystole, occur in about 10 percent of patients.

Clinicians should note that in only 11 percent of cases of LAST do cardiovascular symptoms occur in the absence of CNS toxicity.[1] Because of the wide spectrum of presenting signs and symptoms and the fact that a "classic" presentation is uncommon in reality, vigilance and an index of suspicion of LAST should always be maintained.

CNS Toxicity

CNS toxicity is thought to occur in two stages, with initial blockade of sodium channels in inhibitory neurons, allowing the excitatory neurons to act

Table 38.1 Progression of Symptoms and Signs of LAST

Progression of CNS toxicity	Progression of CVS toxicity
Circumoral paresthesia	Hypertension
Tinnitus	Tachycardia (CNS excitation phase)
Confusion	Myocardial depression
Convulsions	Reduced cardiac output
Loss of consciousness	Hypotension
Coma	Peripheral vasodilatation
Respiratory depression	Severe hypotension
	Sinus bradycardia
	Conduction defects
	Dysrhythmias
	Cardiac arrest

Note: Patients may not exhibit all steps.

unopposed, resulting in seizures. Increasing concentration of local anesthetic then depresses all CNS neurons, manifesting ultimately as unconsciousness and coma. Electroencephalogram (EEG) recordings usually show slowing of activity and ultimately "silence" (inactivity). CNS depression in the brainstem can cause eventual collapse of the cardiovascular system. In most cases, convulsions can be managed successfully.[2]

Cardiovascular System Toxicity

Although the major pharmacologic effects of local anesthetics are mediated via blockade of sodium channels, they also can block potassium and calcium channels, contributing to cardiovascular toxicity. The enantiomers of LAs show differential ion channel blockade, the R-isomer having double the potency at sodium channels, 70 times the potency at potassium channels, and three times the potency at calcium channels.[4]

The channel blockade described has direct and indirect effects on the myocardium. Direct effects include negative inotropy and impaired conduction through cardiac conduction tissue. Abnormal conduction predisposes to reentry phenomena and dysrhythmias. Indirect effects may result from disruption to the autonomic outflow and direct effect on the cardiac center in the brain.[4]

Finally, LAs can also have effects on oxidative phosphorylation in the mitochondria and on intracellular cyclic AMP levels, both of which can disrupt cellular function[4] (Table 38.1).

LAST in Obstetrics

In obstetrics, the absolute and relative risk of LAST may be increased. Pregnant women form a large proportion of the patient population, and a disproportionately large number of them are subject to a regional anesthetic technique with potentially toxic LA doses. Hence the absolute risk is increased. Furthermore, it is accepted that obstetric care is increasingly complicated by rising maternal age, obesity, and other comorbidities.

Relative risk may be increased because there may be real differences in susceptibility to LA toxicity in the pregnant state. Several mechanisms may account for this. Epidural vein distension is said to make entrainment of local anesthetic and catheter migration more likely. Increased cardiac output may increase uptake of local anesthetic from the epidural space and increase delivery to target sites. Pregnancy-related decreases in protein binding may increase the availability of free drug in the vascular compartment.[5,6] The hormonal effects of estradiol[6] and progesterone[7] appear detrimentally to alter cardiomyocyte electrophysiology. Neurons may demonstrate increased susceptibility to local anesthetics during pregnancy, reducing the threshold for seizures.[8]

Cardiac arrest secondary to LAST remains a serious potential problem in obstetrics despite the use of low concentration LAs for labor analgesia and increased awareness of toxicity.[9,10] Clinicians would do well to remind themselves of the large dose of LA contained in an epidural top-up used to provide anesthesia (as opposed to analgesia) for surgery, whenever they administer one.

Prevention and Detection of LAST

Close monitoring is mandated during and after local anesthetic injection. Standard operating procedures for this should be agreed locally and adhered to. The patient must be continuously monitored after a single injection; it can take up to 45 minutes for blood concentrations of the local anesthetic to peak.[11] No single test or procedure is totally reliable in the prevention or detection of LAST. However, it is highly likely that a combination decreases the incidence of LAST.[11] In cases of continuous or intermittent LA infusion over a prolonged period (such as labor analgesia), continued vigilance is crucial, with appropriate training in recognition for allied healthcare professionals (Table 38.2).

Table 38.2 Recommendations for Preventing LAST

- Use the lowest effective dose of local anesthetic (dose = volume × concentration).
- Use the least toxic local anesthetic. Single-enantiomer local anesthetics such as levobupivacaine are claimed to be safer than their racemic counterparts such as racemic bupivacaine.
- Use slow, incremental injections of local anesthetics, administering 3–5 ml every 15–30 seconds.
- Aspirate the epidural catheter before each injection, recognizing that there is still a significant false-negative rate with this test.
- When injecting potentially toxic doses of local anesthetic, consider use of an intravascular marker: intravascular injection of epinephrine 10–15 µg/ml in adults produces an increase of >10 beats/min in heart rate or of >15 mmHg in systolic pressure. This test is not completely reliable and needs continuous ECG monitoring.
- Use of ultrasound has been advocated to help avoid intravascular placement and to minimize the required LA dose in some regional techniques, although its effectiveness in specific regard to epidural placement is unknown.
- Remain vigilant for the signs and symptoms of LAST.

Sources: Data from refs. 11 and 12.

Treatment of LAST

If LAST is suspected, prompt management is vital. Treatment should be systematic, following recognized guidelines for management.[13,14] This should be a team enterprise, with clear leadership. Local arrangements should ensure that wherever potentially toxic doses of LA are administered, relevant guidelines are immediately to hand, along with an adequate supply of the drugs required to treat LAST and the means to administer them. Prevention of hypercapnia, hypoxia, and acidosis is important because the presence of any of these will enhance LAST. As soon as LAST is suspected, stop the local anesthetic injection immediately, maintain the patient's airway, administer 100% oxygen, and secure IV access. Intubation of the trachea may be indicated. Seizures should be controlled immediately using benzodiazepines. Thiopental and propofol can also be used but must be administered with great care because they are associated with cardiovascular depression, which could be detrimental in this setting.[11]

Advanced life support should be started immediately in the case of cardiac arrest. LA-induced arrhythmias are difficult to control, especially when induced by bupivacaine. Dysrhythmias may be refractory to treatment, and prolonged cardiopulmonary resuscitation may be required. The preferred treatment of LA-induced arrhythmia is amiodarone, and unsurprisingly, lidocaine therapy is not indicated.[11]

213

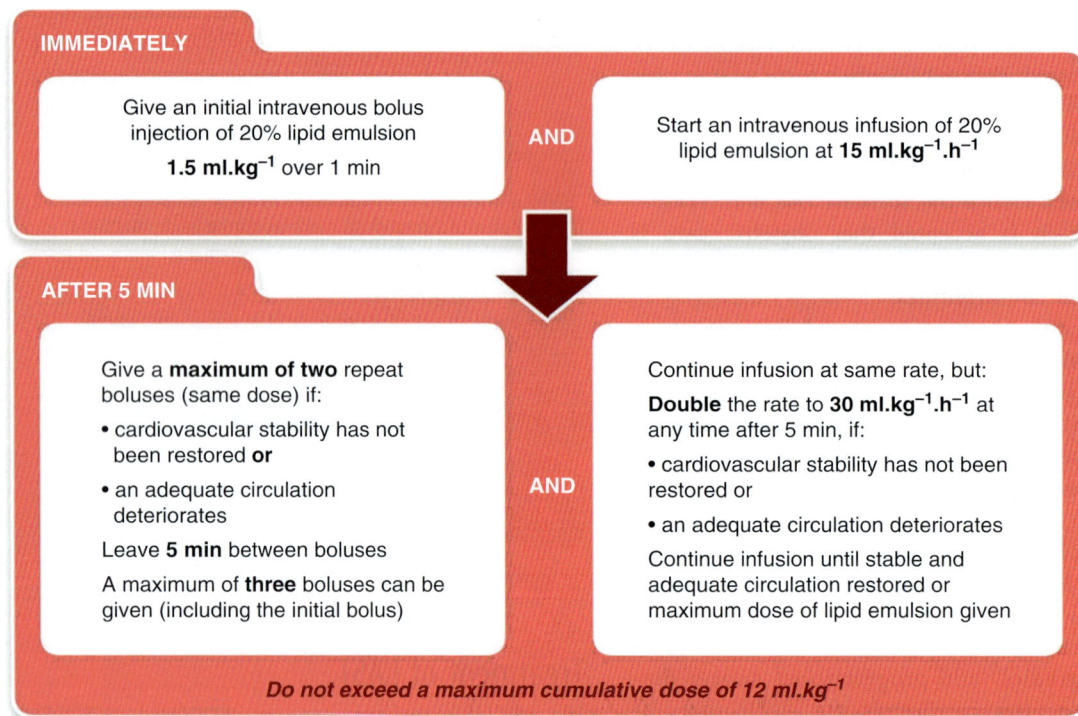

Figure 38.1 Lipid emulsion regimen
Source: Reproduced with permission from the Association of Anaesthetists of Great Britain and Ireland.[14]

Conventional treatments may be used for hypotension, bradycardia, and tachyarrhythmia in patients with circulatory arrest.

Lipid emulsion has been shown to be a potential antidote for LAST. Animal studies and clinical reports suggest that IV lipid emulsion is effective in the reversal of LAST and can contribute to successful resuscitation in the setting of cardiovascular collapse. Despite laboratory and clinical efficacy of lipid resuscitation, the exact mechanism has not been firmly established. At present, the "lipid sink" effect (whereby the lipid phase of the circulating volume acts as a partition removing free LA from the plasma) remains the dominant theory,[15] although other intracellular mechanisms are also postulated.[11] Treatment with lipid emulsion should be started simultaneously with other modalities of treatment.

Lipid Emulsion Regimen

Current treatment advice[13,14] is that lipid emulsion treatment should be started with an initial bolus of 20% lipid emulsion in a dose of 1.5 ml/kg over 1 minute, followed by an IV infusion of 20% lipid emulsion at 15 ml/kg per hour. Following the initial bolus dose, two repeat doses of lipid emulsion can be administered (5 minutes apart) if cardiovascular stability has not been restored or has deteriorated in the 5 minutes following the previous dose. The infusion dose may also be doubled after 5 minutes if required, and the infusion should be continued until stabilization of circulation or the maximum lipid emulsion dose has been given (12 ml/kg cumulative dose; see Figure 38.1).

Learning Points

- Pregnant women are at increased risk of local anesthetic systemic toxicity (LAST), and this demands extreme vigilance.
- Prevention is better than cure, but when cure is required, it is best provided promptly.
- The use of low doses of local anesthetics, with aspiration before injection, incremental injection,

and possibly intravascular markers, seems to reduce the likelihood of LAST.

- There is no single safety precaution that rules out LAST, so multiple precautions are mandated.
- All anesthetists and all facilities should be adequately prepared to treat LAST if it arises, with guidelines and drugs immediately to hand.
- Supportive measures, treatment with lipid emulsion, and prolonged resuscitation where necessary are central to treatment.

References

1. Di Gregorio G, Neal JM, Rosenquist RW, et al. Clinical presentation of local anesthetic systemic toxicity: a review of published cases, 1979 to 2009. *Reg Anesth Pain Med* 2010; **35**:181–87.

2. Dippenaar JM. Local anaesthetic toxicity. *SAJAA* 2007; **13**:23–28.

3. Barash PG, Cullen B, Stoelting RK. *Clinical Anesthesia*, 5th edn. Philadelphia,PA: Lippencott Williams & Wilkins; 2005, pp. 449–69.

4. Mather LE, Chang DH-T. Cardiotoxicity with modern local anesthetics: is there a safer choice? *Drugs* 2001; **61**:333–42.

5. Santos AC, Pedersen H, Harmon TW, et al. Does pregnancy alter the systemic toxicity of local anesthetics? *Anesthesiology* 1989; **70**:991–95.

6. Tsen LC, Tarshis J, Denson DD, et al. Measurements of maternal protein binding of bupivacaine throughout pregnancy. *Anesth Analg* 1999; **89**:965–68.

7. Moller RA, Datta S, Fox J, et al. Effects of progesterone on the cardiac electrophysiologic action of bupivacaine and lidocaine. *Anesthesiology* 1992; **76**:604–8.

8. Santos AC, DeArmas PI. Systemic toxicity of levobupivacaine, bupivacaine, and ropivacaine during continuous intravenous infusion to nonpregnant and pregnant ewes. *Anesthesiology* 2001; **95**:1256–64.

9. Auroy Y, Narchi P, Messiah A, et al. Serious complications related to regional anesthesia: results of a prospective survey in France. *Anesthesiology* 1997; **87**:479–86.

10. Brown DL, Ransom DM, Hall JA, et al. Regional anesthesia and local anesthetic-induced systemic toxicity: seizure frequency and accompanying cardiovascular changes. *Anesth Analg* 1995; **81**:321–28.

11. Brichant JF. Toxicity of Local Anaesthetics in Obstetric Anaesthesia and Lipid Rescue, European Society of Anaesthesiology Refresher Course, abstract, 2011. Available at www.esahq.org/~/media/ESA/Files/Refresher%20Courses/2011/Toxicity%20of%20local%20anaesthetics%20in%20obstetric%20anaesthesia%20and%20lipid%20rescue%20%282011%29.ashx (accessed December 23, 2014).

12. Mulroy MF, Hejmanek MR. Prevention of local anesthetic toxicity. *Reg Anesth Pain Med* 2010; **35**:177–80.

13. Neal JM, Bernards CM, Butterworth JF, et al. ASRA practice advisory on local anesthetic systemic toxicity. *Reg Anesth Pain Med* 2010; **35**:152–61.

14. Association of Anaesthetists of Great Britain and Ireland. AAGBI Safety Guideline: Management of Severe Local Anaesthetic Toxicity, 2010. Available at www.aagbi.org/sites/default/files/la_toxicity_2010_0.pdf (accessed January 6, 2015).

15. Bern S, Weinberg G. Local anesthetic toxicity and lipid resuscitation in pregnancy. *Curr Opin Anaesthesiol* 2011; **24**:262–67.

Addendum

Since this content was written, further studies have suggested alternate and additional mechanisms for the actions of lipid emulsion in the treatment of local anaesthetic toxicity. An editorial by Picard and Meek highlights these issues.

Reference

Picard J, Meek T. Lipid emulsion for intoxication by local anaesthetic: sunken sink? Anaesthesia 2016, 71, 879–882.

Medicolegal Issues

Alison Carter and Steve Yentis

Case Study

A 33-year-old woman presented at 40 weeks' gestation in spontaneous labor, requesting an epidural. She was low risk, with an uncomplicated vaginal delivery under epidural analgesia the year before. On assessment, the uterus was contracting well, the cardiotocogram (CTG) was normal, and her cervix was dilated 4 cm.

After a brief discussion of the risks and benefits of epidural analgesia with the patient (documented in the patient's notes), the trainee anesthetist (in the third year of anesthesia training and practising obstetric anesthesia independently) sited an epidural uneventfully at L3–L4 in the sitting position using a 16-gauge Tuohy epidural needle and loss of resistance to saline, with an initial dose of 15 ml low-dose epidural mixture (0.1% bupivacaine with 2 μg/ml fentanyl). After 20 minutes, the patient reported good pain relief, and a bilateral sensory block above T10 to cold using ethyl chloride spray was documented.

As labor progressed, the CTG became abnormal and necessitated a Category II cesarean delivery (fetal or maternal compromise that is not immediately life threatening[1]) 6 hours after the epidural was sited. The epidural was reportedly working well, and the block height on arrival in the OR was T10 to cold on the left and T12 on the right. An epidural bolus of 20 ml 2% lidocaine with epinephrine 1:200,000 was given 12 minutes after the decision for delivery was made. After 10 minutes, the block was documented as T5 to first sensation of cold and T6 to first sensation of touch bilaterally. Surgery proceeded, and a baby girl was delivered 6 minutes after skin incision with Apgar scores of 7 and 9 at 1 and 5 minutes, respectively.

The patient seemed to be comfortable until the uterus was incised but complained of right-sided abdominal pain during delivery. This worsened after delivery. IV acetaminophen and epidural diamorphine were administered with some benefit. Entonox

and general anesthesia were offered but refused. The epidural catheter was removed before transfer to the recovery area following completion of surgery. Later that evening, the patient was seen by the on-call trainee, who documented a full discussion explaining the sequence of events and including an offer of further follow-up.

The following afternoon, the patient complained of severe postural headache with no other associated symptoms. An explanation was given, with advice for initial conservative management with oral analgesics and caffeine, and an epidural blood patch if required. The patient was seen by consultant anesthetists daily, the headache diminished over the next 4 days without a blood patch, and the patient remained headache free at the outpatient anesthetic follow-up clinic 6 weeks later.

A year later, the hospital received a letter from a solicitor indicating a claim of negligence on the basis that incorrect epidural insertion and top-up had resulted in both pain during surgery, which should have been predicted before starting the operation and should have been managed better when it occurred, and additional suffering due to headache.

Key Points

- After receiving effective pain relief during her first delivery, this patient had epidural-associated complications (intraoperative pain and headache) with her second birth.
- Despite apparently successful management and a good outcome, she clearly felt strongly enough that the anesthetist was at fault to initiate a claim against the hospital 1 year later.

Discussion

Although anesthesia-related claims account for only 2.5 percent of all medicolegal claims in England, approximately 29 percent of these pertain to obstetric anesthesia.[2] It is important to note that patients sue the provider of care. Within the National Health Service (NHS) in the United Kingdom, although allegations may be made about a specific clinician, a claim of negligence would be directed against the hospital trust (in the United Kingdom, hospitals are usually managed by a body called an NHS Trust), not the trainee, who would be seen as an agent of the trust through vicarious liability. For a claim of negligence to succeed, the claimant must prove in court "on the balance of probabilities" that

1. The NHS Trust owed her a duty of care – this would not be in dispute because she was a patient of the Trust.
2. There was a failure ("breach") in that duty – this would hinge around whether the care she received was of an acceptable standard. There are two important principles that apply to this decision:

   a. *Bolam principle:* whether what was done (or not done) would be supported by a "significant body" of medical opinion, even a minority,[3] and
   b. *Bolitho principle:* whether this opinion is "reasonable" and "logical."[4]

3. Harm occurred – this would be in terms of pain and suffering in the case described plus any further harm she were to suffer (e.g., posttraumatic stress syndrome or a physical complication).
4. The harm occurred as a result of that failure ("causation").

From an anesthetic point of view, the main issues in this case were around breach of duty (i.e., standard of care) and causation. In the NHS, claims of negligence are managed by the NHS Resolution (formerly called the NHS Litigation Authority).[2] After local investigation and discussion between NHS Resolution and the Trust, the opinion of an expert witness, an independent obstetric anesthetist, was sought to consider these issues.

Appropriateness of Epidural

The patient was low risk, in established labor, and requested an epidural. With no contraindications, it was considered an entirely appropriate procedure for the anesthetist to perform.

Consent

In order to respect patient autonomy, informed consent should be obtained before epidural insertion. This requires provision of adequate information to a patient with the capacity and time to make a balanced decision, free from coercion.[5] The nature of the information given and whether a woman can have adequate capacity during painful labor are discussed further in Chapter 10. In this case, the documented discussion in the patient notes provided good evidence of the discussion that preceded the epidural, and care was considered acceptable. Such record-keeping is crucial to defend against an accusation of an inadequate consenting process, especially in cases where the woman's capacity is in doubt.

Standard of Epidural Insertion and Subsequent Management

The patient notes supported a good standard of care by the trainee, who had carefully documented the patient's position, the aseptic technique, the level of needle insertion, the method of loss of resistance, the depth of catheter insertion, the effect of the first dose, and the lack of complications. During the subsequent labor, the trainee had been too busy elsewhere to check the epidural regularly, but the midwife had carefully recorded on the chart that the patient was comfortable throughout (see Chapter 2). Management of the epidural was therefore considered acceptable.

Use of the Epidural for Cesarean Delivery

It would be preferable to use regional anesthesia for cesarean delivery when possible in order to avoid the complications of general anesthesia, such as difficult/failed intubation and aspiration of gastric contents. In this case, the obstetricians did not communicate to the anesthetist that the baby needed immediate delivery, and it was reasonable to top up the epidural with an appropriate solution of local anesthetic. The proposed standard or target for best practice indicated by the Royal College of Anaesthetists suggests that more than 85 percent of Category I–III cesarean deliveries and more than 50 percent of Category I cesarean sections should be carried out under regional anesthesia.[6] The trainee could perhaps be criticized for giving a 20-ml bolus of lidocaine without a test dose, but it could be argued that (1) a well-working epidural has only a very small chance of being intrathecal or intravenous, (2) a test dose would have risked delay, and (3) no apparent harm resulted (see Chapter 24). The standard of care for topping up the epidural was therefore considered acceptable.

Block Assessment before the Start of Surgery

It is important to document an acceptable block before allowing surgery to start so as to minimize the risk of intraoperative pain. There are a number of aspects of the block that should be specified in the notes: the sensory modality(ies) tested, the extent of the block (including whether the perineum is blocked), and the degree of lower limb motor block – and all of these on both sides of the mother's body. Further, the precise nature of the sensation should also be recorded because there may be a considerable difference between the level where, e.g., cold is first felt and where it feels "normal,"[7] so just recording, e.g., "T5 to cold" isn't very informative. In this case, the trainee was specific about the nature of the cold and touch sensation tested for but did not record the motor block, although subsequent witness statements confirmed that the patient was unable to move her legs after the top-up.

With regard to the minimal block required for pain-free surgery, a level of block to light touch to T5 has been shown to be the most reliable predictor of pain-free surgery,[7,8] although a significant proportion of anesthetists continues to use cold.[9] In the case described, the trainee could be criticized for allowing surgery to start when the block was at or around the lower end of the acceptable range (T5 to first sensation of cold and T6 to first sensation of touch, bilaterally), but with complete motor block and a rising sensory block 10 minutes after the top-up, together with a degree of urgency for delivery, allowing the surgeon to start could be defended on the basis that the block was likely to rise further beyond that point of testing (and indeed the patient didn't complain of pain until approximately 5–6 minutes after incision).

Overall, the expert considered the standard of care here to be acceptable, albeit with the above-mentioned caveats.

Intraoperative Pain and Its Management

"Pulling and pushing" are common during cesarean delivery under epidural anesthesia, so the first question is whether or not the patient actually felt pain. However, in this case, it was agreed by those present that she did complain of, and experience, pain just before and during/after delivery of the baby.

Appropriate intraoperative management once the patient complains of pain consists of asking the surgeons to stop, if possible; offering further analgesia; and, if all else fails, offering general anesthesia (see Chapter 30). In this case, there was no documentation that surgery was stopped although it would not have been possible to delay delivery after uterine incision because that may have compromised the baby's condition further. However, surgery could have paused after delivery if there was no major bleeding. The analgesics given (IV acetaminophen and epidural diamorphine) were reasonable choices, but many anesthetists might have considered further epidural local anesthetic and a more potent systemic analgesic such as alfentanil, fentanyl, or even ketamine. Nitrous oxide and general anesthesia were offered but declined. It is important when offering general anesthesia to be aware that mothers may decline because they are frightened – especially after a preoperative explanation of why it is generally avoided – and their refusal may not necessarily be a defense against a claim that it should have been administered. Therefore, if a patient is in extreme pain, the anesthetist should consider "strongly recommending" general anesthesia rather than just "offering" it.

The expert witness's view was that, overall, the anesthetic management once the patient complained of pain could be criticized for being less than ideal, but whether it fell below an *acceptable* standard (which is the key question) was debatable; further evidence from witness statements (including the claimant and the staff present) would help to illuminate this further (e.g., in terms of the timing and nature of the discussion between the anesthetist and the patient and whether surgery did pause at all). As to causation, if the court decided that care *was* substandard, then it would also be likely to decide that the patient's pain could have been lessened had the care been better and that it was the failure to provide better analgesia (the breach) that caused pain and suffering (the harm).

Follow-Up and Management of Headache

Prompt follow-up by the trainee, with early involvement of senior anesthetists, was highlighted by the expert witness as an example of good care, not only showing concern and empathy for the patient but also reinforcing good communication. There was no suggestion of substandard technique when the epidural was sited, as noted earlier, and no evidence that the catheter was intrathecal at any time. The expert considered therefore that the headache – which was carefully documented as being typical of a post–dural puncture headache – was likely to have arisen through a small and undetected breach in the dura, something that is known to occur in a minority of cases (see Chapter 42). The care given, including involvement of seniors, counseling, and follow-up, was felt to be exemplary and in accordance with the department's guidelines. The very good overall standard of documentation was also noted as, first, making it clearer to identify what happened and, second, suggesting an overall detailed and conscientious approach to care, thus assisting a medicolegal defense.

Subsequent Events

Further witness statements were gathered from the staff, and these supported the account given by the trainee anesthetist. NHS Resolution and The Trust agreed that the case should be defended, and a robust rebuttal of the points raised in the solicitor's letter was sent to the claimant. The Trust did not receive any further communication from the claimant or her solicitors.

Conclusion

This scenario illustrates two complications of epidural analgesia deemed to be the fault of the anesthetist. However, by demonstrating appropriate actions, along with careful documentation and clear communication, the trust was able to present a strong defense of the case such that the claimant did not pursue it.

Learning Points

- In the NHS, it is the provider of care (i.e., the Trust) that is sued, not its individual employees.
- A successful claim of negligence requires there to be a duty of care, a failure in that duty, and harm to occur as a result of that failure.

- Good documentation is essential for every case.
- Good communication, empathy, and regular follow-up, with involvement of senior staff if complications occur, always helps – in general, patients do not sue people they like.
- Compliance with departmental and/or national guidelines is extremely useful. Any reason for deviation should be meticulously documented.

References

1. Lucas DN, Yentis SM, Kinsella SM, et al. Urgency of caesarean section: a new classification. *J R Soc Med* 2000; **93**:346–50.

2. Cook TM, Bland L, Mihai R, Scott S. Litigation related to anaesthesia: an analysis of claims against the NHS in England 1995–2007. *Anaesthesia* 2009; **64**:706–18.

3. *Bolam* v. *Friern Hospital Management Committee* [1957] 2 All ER 118 at 122.

4. *Bolitho* v. *City and Hackney Health Authority* [1997] 4 All ER 771.

5. Yentis SM, Hartle AJ, Barker IR, et al. AAGBI: Consent for anaesthesia 2017. *Anaesthesia* 2017; **72**:93–105. Available at https://www.aagbi.org/sites/default/files/A AGBI_Consent_for_anaesthesia_2017_0.pdf.

6. Royal College of Anaesthetists. *Raising the Standard: A Compendium of Audit Recipes*, 3rd edn. London: Royal College of Anaesthetists; 2012. Available at www .rcoa.ac.uk/system/files/CSQ-ARB2012-SEC8.pdf.

7. Yentis SM. Height of confusion: assessing regional blocks before cesarean section. *Int J Obstet Anesth* 2006; **15**(1):2–6.

8. Russell IF. Levels of anesthesia and intraoperative pain at cesarean section under regional block. *Int J Obstet Anesth* 1995; **4**(2):71–77.

9. Husain T, Liu YM, Fernando R, et al. How UK obstetric anesthetists assess neuraxial anesthesia for cesarean delivery: national surveys of practice conducted in 2004 and 2010. *Int J Obstet Anesth* 2013; **22**(4):298–302.

Chronic Pain after Pregnancy

Ruth Landau and Carlos Delgado

Case Study

A 38-year-old woman with a history of chronic back pain, for which she was not taking any medications except for occasional ibuprofen, and one previous cesarean delivery was scheduled for an anesthetic consultation at 35 weeks' gestation because she was extremely concerned and somewhat traumatized with her previous delivery experience 2 years ago.

She reported that while her epidural placed for labor analgesia had worked fine, when the obstetrician decided to proceed with a cesarean delivery for failure to progress, the epidural didn't work that well, and while the anesthesiologist kept telling her that "feeling some pressure is normal during a cesarean delivery," she felt tremendous pain throughout the surgery and was sure the epidural wasn't working. She was afraid the anesthesiologist would decide to put to her to sleep and remembered vaguely receiving something intravenously. She also remembered having severe pain, mostly at the level of the incision, for several days after delivery and felt that the medication – IV patient-controlled analgesia (PCA) with morphine – did not help and just made her very nauseous. She reported having persistent pain around the incision for many weeks, with residual numbness and unpleasant "pins and needles" consistent with paresthesia and was extremely worried that she might again experience severe pain during this cesarean delivery and chronic pain after.

On reviewing the medical records from the previous cesarean delivery, it appeared that the epidural catheter had been topped up with 2% lidocaine with epinephrine 1:200,000 in 5-ml incremental boluses, up to a total of 20 ml, along with fentanyl 100 μg, and the reported sensory level to pinprick was T4 bilaterally. IV midazolam 2 mg was given after the baby was born, along with epidural preservative-free morphine 3 mg. Multimodal analgesia with a nonsteroidal anti-inflammatory drug (IV ketorolac followed by oral ibuprofen) and oral acetaminophen

was given in the recovery room, and because the patient reported severe pain, IV PCA morphine had also been started.

Key Points

- Women may present for obstetric surgery with a history of chronic pain related to a previous delivery with features of persistent neuropathic pain causing significant anxiety and fear of pain.
- It is important to reassure such women that all anesthetic and analgesic modalities will be tailored to their needs and to explain the different options for anesthesia and postcesarean analgesia.
- Strategies should include a dense neuraxial anesthetic block, with consideration of adjuvants to ensure anxiolysis and antihyperalgesia, such as intrathecal clonidine.
- IV ketamine and oral gabapentin may be considered for a prolonged period of time after delivery in an attempt to prevent hypersensitization and worsening of any preexisting neuropathic symptoms.

Discussion

Characteristics of Pain during and after Cesarean Delivery

Most women reporting pain during cesarean delivery complain of "intense pulling and tugging" along with nausea and vomiting, which can be exacerbated by uterine exteriorization[1] (which is a common practice in the United States to facilitate uterine exposure and closure) or if bilateral tubal ligation[2] is performed during the cesarean delivery; these unpleasant sensations reflect the intense visceral stimuli that accompany manipulation of the peritoneum. Ways to alleviate these sensations are to ensure an adequate dense surgical block up to T4, to be confirmed with pinprick testing, which can be easier to achieve with a spinal anesthetic than with an epidural anesthetic. Short-acting opioids are essential and can be given with the spinal local anesthetic or via an indwelling epidural catheter.[3–5] As an additional adjuvant, spinal or epidural clonidine may be used.[5] Clonidine has been shown to be extremely effective in reducing intraoperative pain.

Acute pain during cesarean delivery is an important event to identify and acknowledge because it has been consistently associated with an increased risk of developing *persistent postoperative pain* (pain that goes beyond the expected time of healing, typically up to 8–12 weeks after surgery, in this case after cesarean delivery).[6–11]

Chronic postcesarean pain, or pain that has developed in relation to the cesarean delivery and persists beyond 3 months after delivery, has been established to be quite rare,[12] particularly in comparison with other types of surgery, including hysterectomy.[13] The proposed mechanism for protection from chronic postcesarean pain is a putative effect of endogenous central oxytocin,[14] which was recently investigated in animal models of pain.[15,16] While chronic pain per se is uncommon after cesarean delivery, postoperative symptoms and specifically neuropathic characteristics of pain have been found to be common after cesarean deliveries.[11,17]

Neuropathic pain refers to pain after neural injury (peripheral or central), and a key feature is the combination of sensory loss with paradoxical hypersensitivity, including *hypoesthesia* (a reduced or partial sensation to touch), *dysesthesia* (a painful sensation after superficial touch), *allodynia* (a painful response to a normally innocuous stimuli, often to cold), *hyperalgesia* (an increased response to noxious stimuli), *hyperpathia* (an increased and persistent response to noxious stimuli) and burning pain. Not all patients with nerve damage will experience neuropathic pain; the type of nerve injury may explain the increase in both acute and chronic pain, but the extent of pain is mediated by other factors, including genetic, psychological, and physiologic factors that heighten pain sensitivity and impair pain modulation.

Predicting Women at Risk for Pain after Cesarean Delivery

There have been several studies trying to identify which women will be more likely to suffer acute and

persistent pain after cesarean delivery. Some have used experimental pain modalities such as quantitative sensory tests (QSTs) to predict women's risk for intense postcesarean pain.[18–24] Problems with such experimental tests is that depending on the pain modality used, these tests may not necessarily accurately predict postpartum pain because of its complex nature (including uterine cramping and postoperative pain). In addition, most of these tests are not easy to perform in a clinical setting and will not be directly useful and applicable to guide clinicians caring for women during cesarean delivery. Questions to assess women's pain catastrophization,[18] level of anxiety, and anticipated pain[25] have been shown to predict acute postcesarean pain. Finally, testing women undergoing a repeat cesarean delivery to assess whether some degree of scar hyperalgesia, which reflects hypersensitization, is present prior to surgery has been shown to predict acute postcesarean pain and analgesic consumption in the first 48 hours following the repeated procedure.[11] This confirms the concept that central sensitization preceding surgery may impair pain modulation and result in the second surgical procedure, here a repeat cesarean delivery, to cause more severe pain and potentially hyperalgesia and chronic pain. Identifying women with predisposing factors such as preexisting chronic pain, neuropathic symptoms, or other contributors such as psychological or genetic factors will ensure that antihyperalgesic/neuropathic adjuvants be targeted to the subset of women who actually need these additional medications (Figure 40.1).

Anesthetic Options for a Repeat Cesarean Delivery to Reduce Acute Pain and Minimize the Risk for Persistent Postoperative Pain in Women at Risk

1. A single shot spinal (SSS) with
   - A standard spinal solution with or without *clonidine*

2. A combined spinal-epidural (CSE) with
   - A standard spinal solution
   - Option to top up the epidural catheter intraoperatively if necessary
   - Option to keep the epidural catheter for postcesarean analgesia

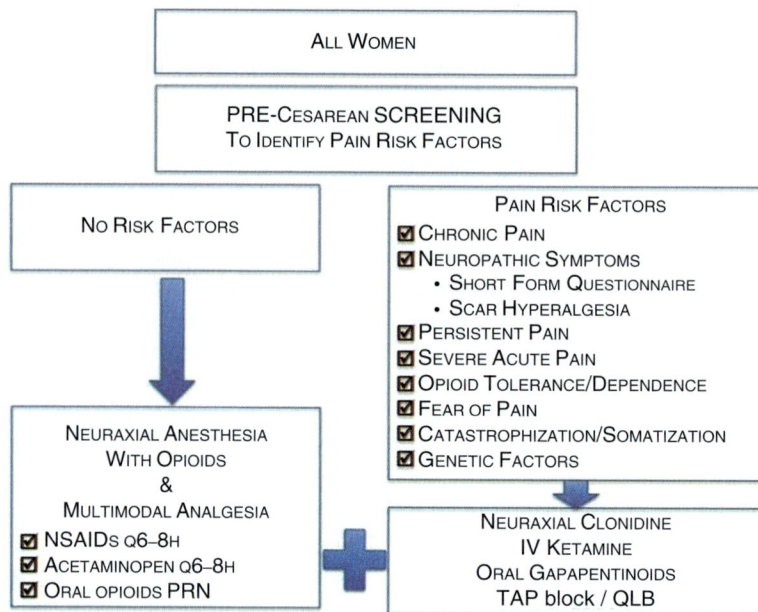

Figure 40.1 Proposed model for prescreening of pain risk factors to identify women likely to benefit from adjuvant modalities for postcesarean analgesia, in addition to standard multimodal analgesia. TAP, Transversus Abdominis Plane Block; QLB, Quadratus Lumborum Block.

- Intermittent dosing with long-acting opioids
- Continuous epidural infusion with PCEA
3. Intravenous *ketamine* intraoperatively
4. *Transversus abdominis plane (TAP) block* or *Quadratus Lumborum block (QLB)* for breakthrough pain
5. Prolonged oral *gabapentin* (see Table 40.1 for drug doses)

Neuraxial Clonidine

Clonidine is a potent α_2-adrenergic receptor agonist with antinociceptive effects acting via descending pathways to the dorsal horn of the spinal cord. It is effective for both somatic and visceral pain.[26] Intrathecal clonidine added to local anesthetics for surgery prolongs the surgical block time (sensory regression to L2 and duration of motor block) and the time to first analgesic request.[27] Multiple studies have evaluated the effect of intrathecal clonidine on intraoperative analgesia, onset and duration of surgical block, time to first analgesic request, morphine-sparing effect, shivering, and side-effect profile in women receiving varying doses of intrathecal clonidine for elective cesarean delivery.[5,28–35]

Taken together, all these studies suggest that adding an "intermediate" dose of clonidine (60–100 μg) prolongs the surgical block by up to 60 minutes, delays the time to first analgesic request for breakthrough pain, and has a beneficial effect on intraoperative shivering.[36] None of the studies reported severe hypotension with any of the studied doses, including relatively high doses (150 μg).[33,35] The proposed explanation is that hypotension occurs in almost 100 percent of women immediately after injection of the spinal solution; therefore, adding clonidine will not increase the incidence of hypotension and will be easily managed with the current practice of using a vasopressor infusion (typically phenylephrine) during cesarean delivery. However, because the effect of neuraxial clonidine may outlast the surgical time, maternal blood pressure may remain low in the post-anesthesia care unit (PACU), and maintaining a phenylephrine infusion for a few hours in the PACU may be required in some cases. While the sedative effect of clonidine has been evaluated, the anxiolytic effect of spinal clonidine has not been assessed. It is unclear whether spinal clonidine reduces the likelihood of suffering chronic postcesarean pain, most likely because this event is so uncommon, and much larger studies

Table 40.1 Anesthetic Options for a Repeat Cesarean Delivery to Reduce Acute Pain and Minimize the Risk for Persistent Postoperative Pain in Women at Risk

Option				Additional adjuvant
Single-shot spinal (standard spinal dose)				
Spinal	Hyperbaric Bupivacaine	Fentanyl	Morphine	Clonidine
	12 mg	10–15 µg	100–300 µg	60–100 µg
Combined spinal-epidural (CSE) (standard spinal dose followed by epidural dosing)				
Epidural	*Intraoperatively*			
	Lidocaine 2% + epinephrine 1:200,000 5-20 ml as needed			Clonidine 60–150 µg
	Postoperatively			
	Solution: Bupivacaine 0.0625% + fentanyl 2 µg/ml for 24–48 hours			
	Regimen:1: Continuous epidural infusion (CEI) (8–12 ml) with PCEA (bolus 5-8 ml)			
	Regimen 2: Programmed intermittent epidural bolus (PIEB) with PCEA			
	May be followed by a dose of epidural morphine 3 mg before epidural catheter is removed or epidural morphine 3 mg (every 18–24 hours) for 24–72 hours			
Transversus abdominis plane (TAP) block / Quadratus Lumborum Block (QLB)				
Single-shot TAP	*Postoperatively* (or on day 1–2 postpartum)			
	Ropivacaine 0.2% or bupivacaine / levobupivacaine 0.25%, 15–20 ml per side			
TAP catheters	*Postoperatively* (or on day 1–2 postpartum)			
	Repeat bolus (see Single-shot TAP) every 8 hours through catheters			
QLB	Postoperatively levobupivacaine 0.25% 20ml per side.			
Systemic medication				
Intravenous	Ketamine 0.15–0.5 mg/kg			
Oral	Gabapentin 300–600 mg two to three times a day			
	Start at least 2 hours (ideally 48 hours) before cesarean delivery			
	Duration may be up to 2–3 weeks for maximal effect in preventing neuropathic pain			

would be needed to explore this effect or studies that prescreen women to identify those most likely to benefit from the addition of an antihyperalgesic drug. Based on our vast clinical experience with spinal clonidine for cesarean deliveries, clonidine is best suited for women who either already suffer chronic pain, are opioid tolerant, have had a suboptimal experience with a previous cesarean delivery (anesthetic block not sufficiently dense, not lasting long enough, severe postcesarean pain) and/or are extremely anxious.

Intravenous Ketamine

Ketamine, an *N*-methyl-D-aspartate (NMDA) receptor antagonist, has been suggested as an intraoperative adjuvant to reduce acute postoperative pain,

reduce opioid-related side effects, and potentially prevent chronic postoperative pain. Systematic reviews have demonstrated a morphine-sparing effect postoperatively[37] but insufficient evidence to support its routine use to prevent chronic pain.[38] In a recent systematic review and meta-analysis of the effects of ketamine during cesarean delivery under spinal or general anesthesia,[39] ketamine significantly delayed time to first analgesic request and reduced pain scores 2 hours after cesarean delivery under spinal anesthesia.

To our knowledge, no academic center in the United States uses IV ketamine (as a bolus or per infusion) to prevent intraoperative pain at the beginning of the procedure. Current recommendations are not for its routine use, although doses of titrated IV

223

ketamine may be offered to women reporting significant intraoperative pain.

Oral Gabapentin

Preoperative administration of gabapentinoids (gabapentin or pregabalin) to prevent severe acute and chronic postoperative pain has been evaluated.[40] In the context of cesarean delivery, only three studies have evaluated the effect of a single preoperative dose of oral gabapentin, with mixed results.[41-43] Doses were either 300 mg[41,42] or 600 mg[42,43] taken 2 hours before cesarean delivery. It is possible that both the timing and duration were insufficient for both a morphine-sparing effect and the prevention of neuropathic pain. Starting gabapentinoids 48 hours prior to surgery and for a duration of at least 2–3 weeks to elicit a long-lasting effect has been proposed.[40] Women at low risk for severe acute postcesarean pain are unlikely to benefit from the administration of a single oral dose of gabapentin preoperatively, but for selected women at risk for neuropathic pain, prolonged gabapentin may be beneficial.

Regional Truncal Blocks

The transversus abdominis plane (TAP) block is a recently investigated regional technique that is effective and relatively simple to manage. The duration of a single-shot TAP block does not seem to exceed 15–18 hours. Multiple studies have evaluated the efficacy of TAP blocks regarding their opioid-sparing ability, and when compared with spinal morphine, studies have shown that they are *not* more effective than spinal morphine and that there are probably no advantages in giving them routinely to women already receiving a morphine-containing spinal anesthetic.[44-51] One study also reported the same lack of efficacy when morphine had been administered epidurally.[52] Reasons for this are that the analgesic effect of a single-shot TAP block does not last as long as the analgesia provided by a spinal dose of morphine and that uterine cramping is not relieved by a TAP block. It has therefore been suggested that TAP blocks should only be offered to selected women who cannot, or did not, receive spinal morphine or to those experiencing severe breakthrough pain despite multimodal analgesia,[53-57] particularly if abdominal wall pain is the dominant feature of the severe pain. Other studies on TAP block have confirmed its limited role in postoperative analgesia when spinal anaesthesia with a long acting opioid such as morphine is used as well as the use of TAP block for cesarean delivery under general anesthesia.[58-60] The benefit of adding antihyperalgesic adjuvants (i.e. clonidine) to TAP solutions remains to be further studied.[61] Threading bilateral catheters into the TAP for repeated boluses every 8 hours have been shown to provide successful analgesia for up to 72 hours after delivery.[62] Of note, local anesthetic toxicity has been reported within 30 minutes of injection,[63-65] and it is therefore important to adjust the local anesthetic dosing to women's weight, to monitor for possible signs of systemic toxicity, and to be prepared to manage seizures.

The Quadratus Lumborum block (QLB) has also been used for postoperative analgesia after cesarean delivery. The main advantage of QLB compared to the TAP block is the extension of local anesthetic agent beyond the transversus abdominis plane to the thoracic paravertebral space. Two studies on QLB for post-operative analgesia after caesarean section under spinal, have reported it significantly reduces morphine consumption in combination with a multimodal analgesic regimen.[66,67]

In summary, severe acute pain after cesarean delivery despite multimodal analgesia is not uncommon and requires early identification and management of severe pain to prevent persistent pain, surgery-related symptoms with neuropathic characteristics, and the very rare case of chronic postcesarean pain. In women with risk factors for postoperative pain or with allergies precluding the use of morphine and/or NSAIDs, additional modalities should be offered. In the future, more studies to identify preoperatively who may be at risk for pain are likely to propose tailored postcesarean analgesia.[68]

Learning Points

- Severe acute pain after cesarean delivery is relatively common, and multimodal analgesia including neuraxial opioids, acetaminophen, and NSAIDs is recommended as a minimum requirement.
- Severe acute pain has been associated with persistent pain and postpartum depression, which is why it is essential to offer appropriate management of acute postcesarean pain.
- Women at risk for severe postcesarean pain should be offered additional modalities because standard multimodal analgesia will likely not be sufficient; risk factors include a history of chronic pain,

opioid tolerance, severe acute postcesarean pain in a previous delivery, anxiety, and fear of pain.

- Neuraxial clonidine, IV ketamine, and/or oral gabapentin may each be beneficial (alone or in a combination) when standard multimodal analgesia is anticipated not to be sufficient. TAP or QLB blocks may be offered as a rescue for abdominal wall breakthrough pain postoperatively.

- Chronic pain after cesarean delivery is rare, but surgery-related neuropathic symptoms are quite common and could be precursors or markers for central sensitization and abnormal neuronal signaling that may result in chronic pain.

References

1. Nafisi S. Influence of uterine exteriorization versus in situ repair on post-cesarean maternal pain: a randomized trial. *Int J Obstet Anesth* 2007; **16**:135–38.

2. Sng BL, Lim Y, Sia AT. An observational prospective cohort study of incidence and characteristics of failed spinal anesthesia for cesarean section. *Int J Obstet Anesth* 2009; **18**:237–41.

3. Bogra J, Arora N, Srivastava P. Synergistic effect of intrathecal fentanyl and bupivacaine in spinal anesthesia for cesarean section. *BMC Anesthesiology* 2005; **5**:5.

4. Choi DH, Ahn HJ, Kim MH. Bupivacaine-sparing effect of fentanyl in spinal anesthesia for cesarean delivery. *Reg Anesth Pain Med* 2000; **25**:240–45.

5. Benhamou D, Thorin D, Brichant JF, et al. Intrathecal clonidine and fentanyl with hyperbaric bupivacaine improves analgesia during cesarean section. *Anesth Analg* 1998; **87**:609–13.

6. Kainu JP, Sarvela J, Tiippana E, Halmesmaki E, Korttila KT. Persistent pain after caesarean section and vaginal birth: a cohort study. *Int J Obstet Anesth* 2010; **19**:4–9.

7. Sng BL, Sia AT, Quek K, Woo D, Lim Y. Incidence and risk factors for chronic pain after caesarean section under spinal anaesthesia. *Anaesth intensive Care* 2009; **37**:748–52.

8. Eisenach JC, Pan PH, Smiley R, et al. Severity of acute pain after childbirth, but not type of delivery, predicts persistent pain and postpartum depression. *Pain* 2008; **140**:87–94.

9. Nardi N, Campillo-Gimenez B, Pong S, et al. Chronic pain after cesarean: impact and risk factors associated. *Ann Fran Anesth* 2013; **32**:772–78.

10. Liu TT, Raju A, Boesel T, Cyna AM, Tan SG. Chronic pain after caesarean delivery: an Australian cohort. *Anaesth Intensive Care* 2013; **41**:496–500.

11. Ortner CM, Turk DC, Theodore BR, et al. The Short-Form McGill Pain Questionnaire-Revised to evaluate persistent pain and surgery-related symptoms in healthy women undergoing a planned cesarean delivery. *Reg Anesth Pain Med* 2014; **39**: 478–86.

12. Eisenach JC, Pan P, Smiley RM, et al. Resolution of pain after childbirth. *Anesthesiology* 2013; **118**:143–51.

13. Brandsborg B, Nikolajsen L, Kehlet H, Jensen TS. Chronic pain after hysterectomy. *Acta Anaesthesiol Scand* 2008; **52**:327–31.

14. Yaksh TL, Hobo S, Peters C, et al. Preclinical toxicity screening of intrathecal oxytocin in rats and dogs. *Anesthesiology* 2014; **120**:951–61.

15. Gutierrez S, Liu B, Hayashida K, Houle TT, Eisenach JC. Reversal of peripheral nerve injury-induced hypersensitivity in the postpartum period: role of spinal oxytocin. *Anesthesiology* 2013; **118**:152–59.

16. Gutierrez S, Hayashida K, Eisenach JC. The puerperium alters spinal cord plasticity following peripheral nerve injury. *Neuroscience* 2013; **228**:301–8.

17. Loos MJ, Scheltinga MR, Mulders LG, Roumen RM. The Pfannenstiel incision as a source of chronic pain. *Obstet Gynecol* 2008; **111**:839–46.

18. Strulov L, Zimmer EZ, Granot M, et al. Pain catastrophizing, response to experimental heat stimuli, and post-cesarean section pain. *Journal of Pain* 2007; **8**: 273–79.

19. Nielsen PR, Norgaard L, Rasmussen LS, Kehlet H. Prediction of post-operative pain by an electrical pain stimulus. *Acta Anaesthesiol Scand* 2007; **51**:582–86.

20. Pan PH, Coghill R, Houle TT, et al. Multifactorial preoperative predictors for postcesarean section pain and analgesic requirement. *Anesthesiology* 2006; **104**:417–25.

21. Granot M, Lowenstein L, Yarnitsky D, Tamir A, Zimmer EZ. Postcesarean section pain prediction by preoperative experimental pain assessment. *Anesthesiology* 2003; **98**:1422–26.

22. Landau R, Kraft JC, Flint LY, et al. An experimental paradigm for the prediction of post-operative pain (PPOP). *J Vis Exp* 2010; **35**:1671.

23. Buhagiar LM, Cassar OA, Brincat MP, et al. Pre-operative pain sensitivity: a prediction of post-operative outcome in the obstetric population. *J Anaesthesiol Clin Pharmacol* 2013; **29**:465–71.

24. Ortner CM, Granot M, Richebe P, et al. Preoperative scar hyperalgesia is associated with post-operative pain in women undergoing a repeat caesarean delivery. *Eur J Pain* 2013; **17**:111–23.

25. Pan PH, Tonidandel AM, Aschenbrenner CA, et al. Predicting acute pain after cesarean delivery using

three simple questions. *Anesthesiology* 2013;
118:1170–79.

26. Eisenach JC, De Kock M, Klimscha W. Alpha(2)-
    adrenergic agonists for regional anesthesia: a clinical
    review of clonidine (1984–1995). *Anesthesiology* 1996;
    85:655–74.

27. Elia N, Culebras X, Mazza C, Schiffer E, Tramer MR.
    Clonidine as an adjuvant to intrathecal local
    anesthetics for surgery: systematic review of
    randomized trials. *Reg Anesth Pain Med* 2008; **33**:
    159–67.

28. Khezri MB, Rezaei M, Delkhosh Reihany M, Haji Seid
    Javadi E. Comparison of postoperative analgesic effect
    of intrathecal clonidine and fentanyl added to
    bupivacaine in patients undergoing cesarean section:
    a prospective randomized double-blind study. *Pain Res
    Treat* 2014; 2014:513–628.

29. Singh R, Gupta D, Jain A. The effect of addition of
    intrathecal clonidine to hyperbaric bupivacaine on
    postoperative pain after lower segment caesarean
    section: a randomized control trial. *Saudi J Anaesth*
    2013; **7**:283–90.

30. Braga Ade F, Frias JA, Braga FS, Pereira RI, Titotto SM.
    Spinal anesthesia for elective ceasarean section: use of
    different doses of hyperbaric bupivacaine associated
    with morphine and clonidine. *Acta Cir Brasil* 2013;
    28:26–32.

31. Bajwa SJ, Bajwa SK, Kaur J, et al. Prevention of
    hypotension and prolongation of postoperative
    analgesia in emergency cesarean sections:
    a randomized study with intrathecal clonidine.
    Int J Crit Illness Injury Sci 2012; **2**:63–69.

32. Kothari N, Bogra J, Chaudhary AK. Evaluation of
    analgesic effects of intrathecal clonidine along with
    bupivacaine in cesarean section. *Saudi J Anaesth* 2011;
    5:31–35.

33. Lavand'homme PM, Roelants F, Waterloos H,
    Collet V, De Kock MF. An evaluation of the
    postoperative antihyperalgesic and analgesic effects of
    intrathecal clonidine administered during elective
    cesarean delivery. *Anesth Analg* 2008; **107**:948–55.

34. van Tuijl I, van Klei WA, van der Werff DB,
    Kalkman CJ. The effect of addition of intrathecal
    clonidine to hyperbaric bupivacaine on postoperative
    pain and morphine requirements after caesarean
    section: a randomized controlled trial. *Br J Anaesth*
    2006; **97**:365–70.

35. Paech MJ, Pavy TJ, Orlikowski CE, et al.
    Postcesarean analgesia with spinal morphine,
    clonidine, or their combination. *Anesth Analg* 2004;
    98:1460–66.

36. Crespo S, Dangelser G, Haller G. Intrathecal clonidine
    as an adjuvant for neuraxial anaesthesia during

caesarean delivery: a systematic review and meta-
analysis of randomised trials. *Int J Obstet Anesth* 2017
Nov; **32**:64–76.

37. Ding X, Jin S, Niu X, et al. Morphine with adjuvant
    ketamine versus higher dose of morphine alone for
    acute pain: a meta-analysis. *Int J Clin Exp Med* 2014; 7:
    2504–10.

38. McNicol ED, Schumann R, Haroutounian S.
    A systematic review and meta-analysis of ketamine for
    the prevention of persistent post-surgical pain. *Acta
    Anaesthesiol Scand* 2014; **58**:1199–213.

39. Heesen M, Bohmer J, Brinck EC, et al. Intravenous
    ketamine during spinal and general anaesthesia for
    caesarean section: systematic review and
    meta-analysis. *Acta Anaesthesiol Scand* 2015; **59**:
    414–26.

40. Clarke H, Bonin RP, Orser BA, et al. The prevention of
    chronic postsurgical pain using gabapentin and
    pregabalin: a combined systematic review and
    meta-analysis. *Anesth Analg* 2012; **115**:428–42.

41. Najafi Anaraki A, Mirzaei K. The effect of gabapentin
    versus intrathecal fentanyl on postoperative pain and
    morphine consumption in cesarean delivery:
    a prospective, randomized, double-blind study. *Arch
    Gynecol Obstet* 2014; **290**:47–52.

42. Short J, Downey K, Bernstein P, Shah V, Carvalho JC.
    A single preoperative dose of gabapentin does not
    improve postcesarean delivery pain management:
    a randomized, double-blind, placebo-controlled
    dose-finding trial. *Anesth Analg* 2012; **115**:1336–42.

43. Moore A, Costello J, Wieczorek P, et al. Gabapentin
    improves postcesarean delivery pain management:
    a randomized, placebo-controlled trial. *Anesth Analg*
    2011; **112**:167–73.

44. McDonnell JG, Curley G, Carney J, et al. The analgesic
    efficacy of transversus abdominis plane block after
    cesarean delivery: a randomized controlled trial.
    Anesth Analg 2008; **106**:186–91.

45. Fusco P, Scimia P, Paladini G, et al. Transversus
    abdominis plane block for analgesia after cesarean
    delivery: a systematic review. *Minerva Anestesiol* 2015;
    81:195–204.

46. Mishriky BM, George RB, Habib AS. Transversus
    abdominis plane block for analgesia after cesarean
    delivery: a systematic review and meta-analysis. *Can
    J Anaesth* 2012; **59**:766–78.

47. Costello JF, Moore AR, Wieczorek PM, et al.
    The transversus abdominis plane block, when used as
    part of a multimodal regimen inclusive of intrathecal
    morphine, does not improve analgesia after cesarean
    delivery. *Reg Anesth Pain Med* 2009; **34**:586–89.

48. Kanazi GE, Aouad MT, Abdallah FW, et al. The analgesic
    efficacy of subarachnoid morphine in comparison with

ultrasound-guided transversus abdominis plane block after cesarean delivery: a randomized controlled trial. *Anesth Analg* 2010; **111**:475–81.

49. McMorrow RC, Ni Mhuircheartaigh RJ, Ahmed KA, et al. Comparison of transversus abdominis plane block vs spinal morphine for pain relief after caesarean section. *Br J Anaesth* 2011; **106**:706–12.

50. Singh S, Dhir S, Marmai K, et al. Efficacy of ultrasound-guided transversus abdominis plane blocks for post-cesarean delivery analgesia: a double-blind, dose-comparison, placebo-controlled randomized trial. *Int J Obstet Anesth* 2013; **22**:188–93.

51. McKeen DM, George RB, Boyd JC, Allen VM, Pink A. Transversus abdominis plane block does not improve early or late pain outcomes after caesarean delivery: a randomized controlled trial. *Can J Anaesth* 2014; **61**: 631–40.

52. Onishi Y, Kato R, Okutomi T, et al. Transversus abdominis plane block provides postoperative analgesic effects after cesarean section: additional analgesia to epidural morphine alone. *J Obstet Gynaecol Res* 2013; **39**:1397–405.

53. Sharkey A, Finnerty O, McDonnell JG. Role of transversus abdominis plane block after caesarean delivery. *Curr Opin Anaesthesiol* 2013; **26**:268–72.

54. Mirza F, Carvalho B. Transversus abdominis plane blocks for rescue analgesia following cesarean delivery: a case series. *Can J Anaesth* 2013; **60**:299–303.

55. Belavy D, Cowlishaw PJ, Howes M, Phillips F. Ultrasound-guided transversus abdominis plane block for analgesia after caesarean delivery. *Br J Anaesth* 2009; **103**:726–30.

56. Baaj JM, Alsatli RA, Majaj HA, Babay ZA, Thallaj AK. Efficacy of ultrasound-guided transversus abdominis plane (TAP) block for postcesarean section delivery analgesia–a double-blind, placebo-controlled, randomized study. *Middle East J Anaesthesiol* 2010; **20**: 821–26.

57. Loane H, Preston R, Douglas MJ, et al. A randomized controlled trial comparing intrathecal morphine with transversus abdominis plane block for post-cesarean delivery analgesia. *Int J Obstet Anesth* 2012; **21**: 112–18.

58. Tan TT, Teoh WH, Woo DC, et al. A randomised trial of the analgesic efficacy of ultrasound-guided transversus abdominis plane block after caesarean delivery under general anaesthesia. *Eur J Anaesthesiol* 2012; **29**:88–94.

59. Eslamian L, Jalili Z, Jamal A, Marsoosi V, Movafegh A. Transversus abdominis plane block reduces postoperative pain intensity and analgesic consumption in elective cesarean delivery under general anesthesia. *J Anesth* 2012; **26**:334–38.

60. Lee AJ, Palte HD, Chehade JM, et al. Ultrasound-guided bilateral transversus abdominis plane blocks in conjunction with intrathecal morphine for postcesarean analgesia. *J Clin Anesth* 2013; **25**:475–82.

61. Bollag L, Richebe P, Siaulys M, et al. Effect of transversus abdominis plane block with and without clonidine on post-cesarean delivery wound hyperalgesia and pain. *Reg Anesth Pain Med* 2012; **37**:508–14.

62. Bollag L, Richebe P, Ortner C, Landau R. Transversus abdominis plane catheters for post-cesarean delivery analgesia: a series of five cases. *Int J Obstet Anesth* 2012; **21**:176–80.

63. Weiss E, Jolly C, Dumoulin JL, et al. Convulsions in 2 patients after bilateral ultrasound-guided transversus abdominis plane blocks for cesarean analgesia. *Reg Anesth Pain Med* 2014; **39**:248–51.

64. Griffiths JD, Le NV, Grant S, et al. Symptomatic local anaesthetic toxicity and plasma ropivacaine concentrations after transversus abdominis plane block for Caesarean section. *Br J Anaesth* 2013; **110**:996–1000.

65. Chandon M, Bonnet A, Burg Y, et al. Ultrasound-guided transversus abdominis plane block versus continuous wound infusion for post-caesarean analgesia: a randomized trial. *PloS ONE* 2014; **9**:e103971.

66. Blanco R, Ansari T, Girgis E. Quadratus lumborum block for postoperative pain after caesarean section: A randomised controlled trial. *Eur J Anaesthesiol* 2015; **32**:812–8.

67. Blanco R, Ansari T, Riad W, Shetty N. Quadratus lumborum block versus transversus abdominis plane block for postoperative pain after cesarean delivery: A randomized controlled trial. *Reg Anesth Pain Med.* 2016; **41**:757–62.

68. Booth JL, Harris LC, Eisenach JC, Pan PH. A randomized, controlled trial comparing two multimodal analgesic techniques in patients predicted to have severe pain after cesarean delivery. *Anesth Analg* 2016; **122**(4):1114–19.

Neurologic Deficits Following a Primary Elective Cesarean Delivery under Spinal Anesthesia

Anthony Chau and Lawrence C. Tsen

Case Study

A 23 year-old gravida 1, para 0 woman at 39 weeks' gestation with a body mass index (BMI) of 28 kg/m^2 was admitted to the labor and delivery suite for a scheduled elective cesarean delivery due to a breech presentation. The patient was healthy with no past medical, surgical, or obstetric history and reported an uncomplicated pregnancy. A preoperative assessment revealed no concerning features for difficult airway management or neuraxial placement; informed consent was obtained for a single-shot spinal anesthetic technique.

Following aseptic preparation and patient positioning in the seated position, a spinal technique with a 25-gauge Whitacre needle was attempted at the presumed L3–L4 interspace, as determined by palpation. During the first attempt, the spinal needle hit bone. Despite repeated attempts with needle angle readjustment, passage of the spinal needle into the subarachnoid space was not successful. The anesthesiologist subsequently moved to the next higher interspace and reinserted the spinal needle to a depth of 4–5 cm when a sudden change in resistance was felt. At this point, the patient screamed and indicated the presence of a sharp pain radiating from her right hip to her foot. The pain gradually subsided without moving the needle; with removal of the spinal needle stylet, the anesthesiologist observed clear CSF return and administered an admixture containing hyperbaric 0.5% bupivacaine 12 mg, fentanyl 10 µg, and preservative-free morphine 100 µg. The injection occurred without patient discomfort and resulted in a bilateral T4 sensory level block to pinprick with a Bromage grade 3 motor block of the lower limbs. The operation proceeded uneventfully, and a healthy baby girl was born.

At 24 hours postoperatively, the patient complained of throbbing pain and paresthesias in her right thigh and buttock radiating down her right leg.

She also reported right-sided numbness over her lateral calf and the dorsum of her foot. She was able to stand and walk, but not without dragging her right foot and toes. An examination revealed preserved bilateral hip, knee, and ankle reflexes, with weak right-sided ankle dorsiflexion and plantar flexion, manifesting as a foot drop. The patient also reported difficulty passing urine, which required intermittent catheterization. A MRI scan of the lumbar/sacral spine revealed a high T2-weighted signal in the conus at the L1 vertebral level.

Key Points

- This patient experienced neurologic deficits after a routine single-shot spinal anesthetic technique.
- The anesthesiologist selected a lumbar interspace that was inadvertently one or more segments higher than intended and made direct needle contact with the spinal cord/conus.
- Although rare, lower extremity neurologic complications after neuraxial anesthesia techniques can occur, and this patient most likely suffered a conus medullaris injury.

Discussion

Neurologic Complication Following Central Neuraxial Anesthesia

Although the incidence of permanent neurologic dysfunction is extremely low, the consequences can be devastating.[1] The Royal College of Anaesthetists' Third National Audit Project (NAP3) estimated the incidence of permanent injury after central neuraxial blockade to be 4.2 per 100,000 (95% confidence interval [CI] 2.9–6.1) and the incidence of paraplegia or death to be 1.8 per 100,000 (95% CI 1.0–3.1).[2] Among the obstetric population, the risk for complications

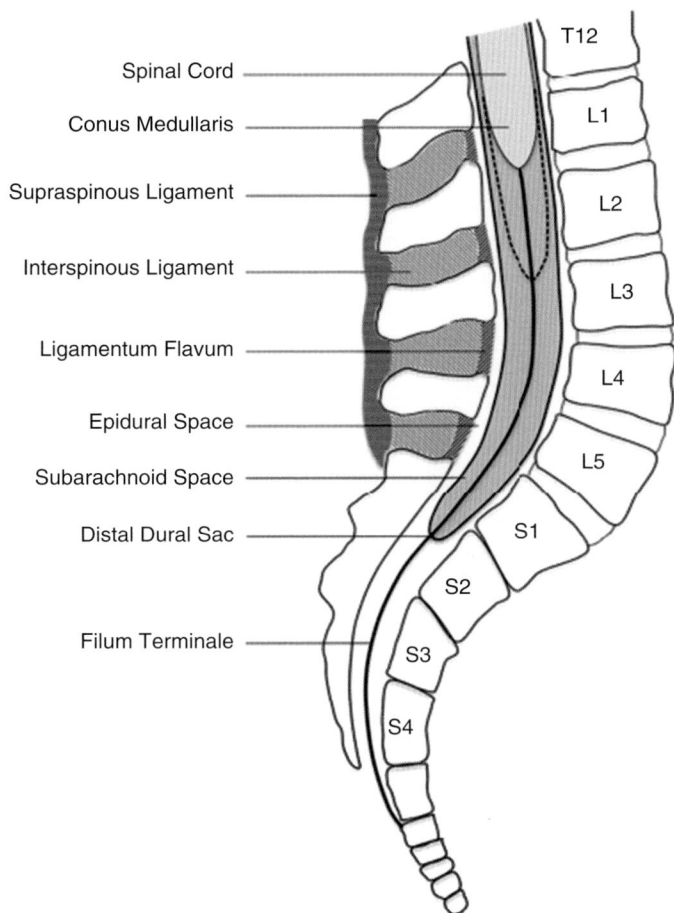

Figure 41.1 Adult spine illustrating the caudal spinal cord and conus medullaris. In some individuals, the lower ends of the conus medullaris may extend to L2–L3 (dotted lines). Spinal anesthesia placed at this level may potentially cause direct needle injury to the conus medullaris.

was greatest for the combined spinal-epidural technique, intermediate for the spinal technique, and lowest for the conventional epidural technique.[2]

Anatomic and Clinical Considerations of the Spinal Cord

Knowledge of normal and abnormal spinal cord anatomy and the limitations of external landmark palpation is essential for the safe administration of lumbar neuraxial techniques. The spinal cord terminates as the conus medullaris before dividing into nerve fibers known as the cauda equina, which includes the filum terminale and the lumbosacral nerve roots[3] (Figure 41.1). Functionally, the conus medullaris represents a major site of transition between the central and

peripheral nervous systems. As a consequence, injuries distal to the conus medullaris (e.g., the nerve roots and cauda equina) result in symptoms and signs consistent with cauda equina syndrome, lumbosacral radiculopathies, or peripheral nerve injuries.

The spinal cord typically terminates at the interspace between the first and second lumbar vertebral level (L1–L2), but this can vary widely (range T12 to L3–L4).[4] In 43 percent of women, the conus medullaris reaches the upper part of the L2 vertebral body, and in up to 10 percent of the population, the spinal cord may terminate caudal to L2.[5]

A spinal needle inserted at the level of the L2–L3 interspace may contact the conus medullaris in 4–20 percent of patients[6] (Figure 41.2). As a consequence, instruction for neuraxial techniques emphasizes

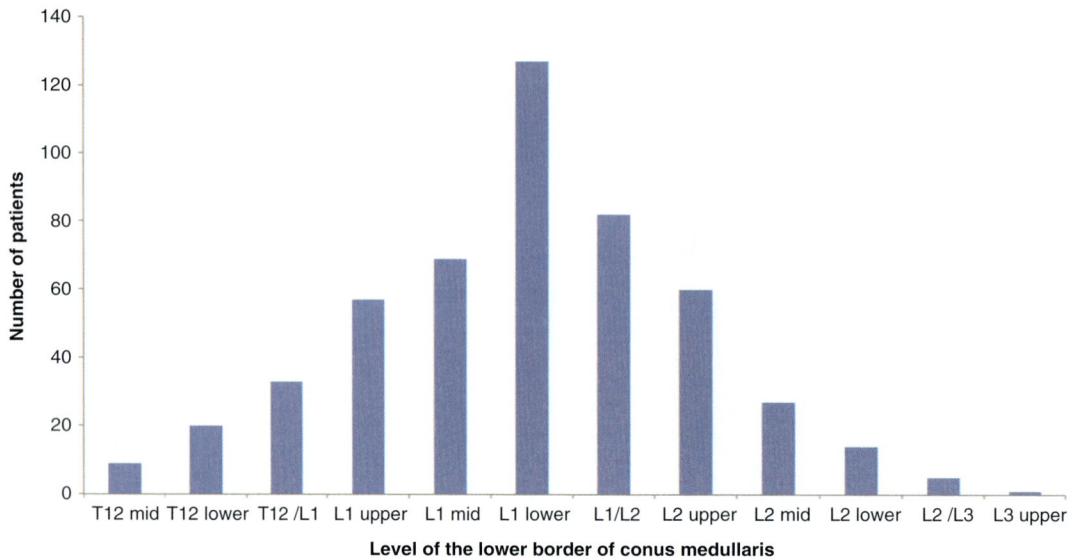

Figure 41.2 Normal distribution of the lower border of the conus medullaris, illustrating the inherent variability in the healthy adult population without spinal deformity
Source: Data derived from Saifuddin et al.[18]

insertion below Tuffier's line, an imaginary line between the posterosuperior iliac crests that is believed to intersect the L4 vertebral body or the L4–L5 interspace.[4] Radiologic studies indicate that the anatomic location identified by Tuffier's line can range from L1 to L5.[7,8] Even experienced anesthesiologists identify lumbar intervertebral spaces correctly in only 29 percent of patients.[9]

Conus Medullaris Injury

Injury to the conus medullaris has been reported in parturients receiving neuraxial anesthesia using 25- and 27-gauge pencil-point spinal needles; these needles have a tip that is at least 1 mm beyond the opening and require deeper insertion into the subarachnoid space to obtain CSF return than a beveled, open-tip needle.[6] Most patients who have experienced this outcome recall having pain on needle insertion but not on medication injection; CSF flow through the needle and the resulting spinal anesthesia block pattern or spread characteristics were described as being normal.[6]

The conus medullaris gives origin to the lumbar sympathetic, sacral parasympathetic, and sacral nerve roots; provides important lower extremity sensory, motor, and autonomic functions[3]; and when injured, results in disabilities related to sacral outflow (S2–S4).

In the largest case series of seven conus medullaris injury patients following spinal anesthesia (six obstetric, one surgical; all placed at the L2–L3 level), unilateral sensory and motor deficits occurred, and a syrinx was demonstrated on MRI (T2 weighted).[6] Symptoms experienced by these patients included numbness in the lower extremities and saddle area along L4–S2, weakness manifesting as foot drop, and urinary dysfunction.[6]

Bladder dysfunction related to conus medullaris injuries is variable depending on the neuroanatomic structures involved, but typically weak or flaccid detrusor activity results in urinary retention and overflow incontinence.[3] Treatment consists of intermittent catheterization to prevent bladder overdistension and kidney retrograde flow injuries and infections.[3]

Management and Prognosis of Neurologic Injury

When a neurologic injury is suspected, and particularly when symptoms or signs are worsening, prompt diagnosis and management may prevent the possibility of permanent damage.[10] The neurosurgical team should be consulted immediately to determine whether an operative intervention is required. Meanwhile, arrangements should be made for a spine MRI or, if not available, CT scan.[10]

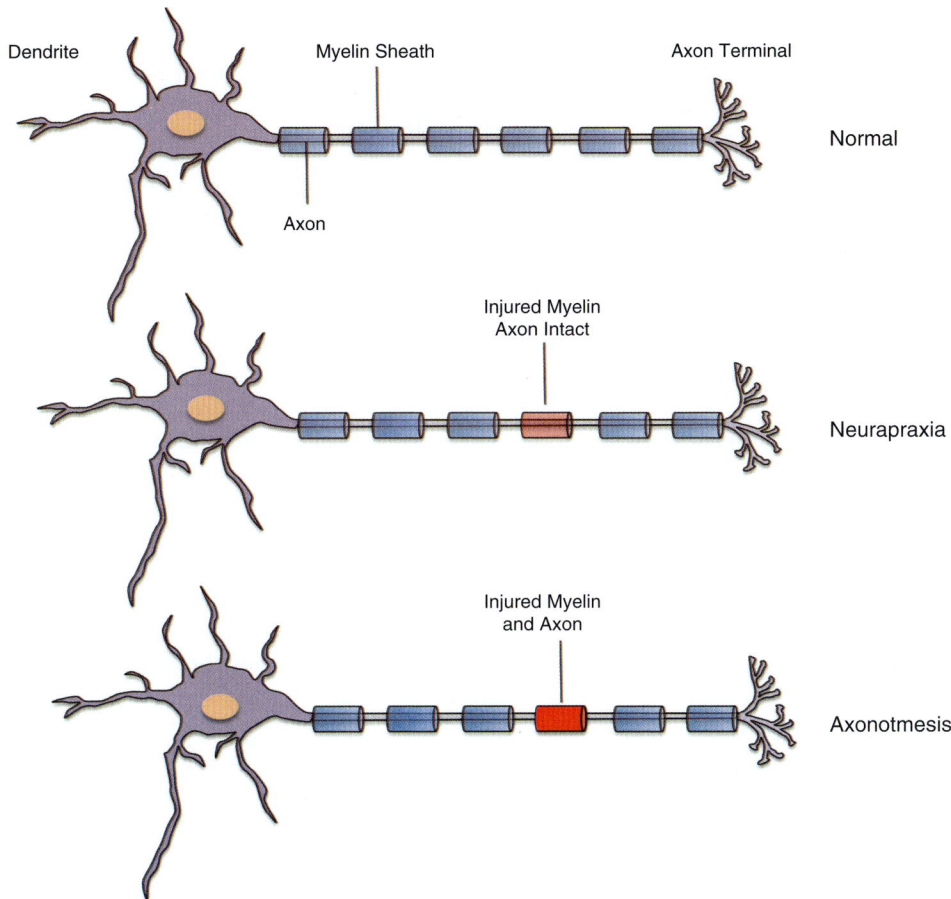

Figure 41.3 Schematic drawing of normal and injured nerve fibers. Neurapraxia is the mildest type of nerve injury resulting in segmental demyelination and reversible loss of nerve function. Axonotmesis occurs when injury to a nerve is sufficient to cause damage to both myelin and axon. When there is damage to the myelin sheath, axon, and connective tissue components, complete recovery is unlikely.

In general, the prognosis of neurologic injuries depends on the degree of nerve damage. After a nerve injury, damage to the myelin sheath or axonal loss may follow.[11] When damage is limited to the myelin sheath, neurapraxia (not neuropraxia, as it is commonly misspelled) ensues.[12] In neurapraxia, the nerve cannot conduct action potentials, resulting in motor and sensory loss; however, once the myelin sheath heals, the nerve typically regains its original function.[11] Neurapraxia generally recovers without medical or surgical interventions over the course of several hours to months, with full function often restored within 12 weeks, assuming no further injuries or compression.[13,14] Neurapraxia has also been used to describe a transient conduction block that lasts only minutes, a phenomenon that cannot be attributed to structural myelination damage but likely due to focal ischemia (e.g., when one's foot is "falling asleep"). If nerve injury is accompanied by axonal loss, but most of the connective tissues remain intact, axonotmesis results (Figure 41.3). Axonotmesis is typically seen in crush or stretch injuries rather than direct needle trauma. Recovery after axonotmesis depends on the rate of axonal regeneration, a slow process (0.25–2 mm/day) that may take many months.[13,14]

Compared with spinal cord injury patients, the prognosis of conus medullaris injury patients is generally good; symptoms may improve partially or completely within the first 2 years following injury.[15] Most cases of major complications in the NAP3 report following central neuraxial blockade resolved within

6 months,[2] although persistent neurologic deficits have been described.[6]

Preventing Direct Spinal Cord Injury during Neuraxial Blockade

If the insertion of a spinal needle results in significant, often radiating pain, injection should be avoided; unfortunately, the injury may already have occurred.[6] Prevention of direct contact with the spinal cord and conus medullaris is one of the most important ways to reduce the risk of injury.

The avoidance of neuraxial needle placement above the L2–L3 interspace is critical.[16]

Although ultrasonography has allowed anesthesiologists to visualize neuraxial anatomy and objectively determine vertebral levels with minimal training,[17] the technology is not uniformly available and takes time to set up and use. Palpation techniques, such as counting vertebra from C7 or finding the vertebra attached to the twelfth rib, have not been validated and may be impractical in patients with high body mass index (BMI). However, improving the knowledge and responses to the conventional palpation of the superior iliac crest can potentially increase the safety margin.

In a recent study,[8] 110 women undergoing elective cesarean delivery via spinal anesthesia were randomized into two groups based on Tuffier's line: (1) group A, in which the intervertebral space identified by the line was marked or, if a spinous process was intersected, the space immediately above was marked, and (2) group B, in which the intervertebral space immediately below the identified space or spinous process was marked. When the marked interspace was compared with an ultrasound-determined actual vertebral level, 45.5 percent versus 7.3 percent were at or above the L2–L3 interspace in groups A and B, respectively.[8] In the accompanying editorial, a maxim based on Tuffier's line palpation was suggested: "Feel a space, down one place: bone pokes through, go down two."[17]

Anesthesia providers should always strive to use the lowest possible lumbar interspace when inserting a neuraxial anesthetic, particularly via a subarachnoid technique, and to be mindful of the range of anatomic locations identified by palpation of Tuffier's line. Additionally, providers should consider ways, including the application of preprocedure ultrasonography, maintenance of close attention to patient symptoms or signs during needle and medication insertion, and active postprocedure management, to improve the safety of neuraxial anesthetic techniques.

Learning Points

- Direct spinal cord injury following central neuraxial placement is rare but can result from inadvertently higher lumbar interspace placement.
- Tuffier's line cannot accurately identify intervertebral levels but should serve as a landmark to stay below.
- Lumbar ultrasonography, awareness of the inaccuracy of vertebral level estimation by palpation, and knowledge of risk factors that contribute to altered patient anatomy may minimize injury to the conus medullaris.
- Conus medullaris injuries may result in unilateral lower extremity sensory and motor deficit with or without bladder and bowel dysfunction. In most cases, prognosis is good, but chronic neurologic deficits may persist.

References

1. Brull R, McCartney CJL, Chan VWS, El-Beheiry H. Neurological complications after regional anesthesia: contemporary estimates of risk. *Anesth Analg* 2007; **104**:965–74.

2. Cook TM, Counsell D, Wildsmith JAW, Royal College of Anaesthetists. Major complications of central neuraxial block: report on the Third National Audit Project of the Royal College of Anaesthetists. *Br J Anaesth* 2009; **102**:179–90.

3. Kingwell SP, Curt A, Dvorak MF. Factors affecting neurological outcome in traumatic conus medullaris and cauda equina injuries. *Neurosurg Focus* 2008; **25**:e7.

4. Boon JM, Abrahams PH, Meiring JH, Welch T. Lumbar puncture: anatomical review of a clinical skill. *Clin Anat* 2004; **17**:544–53.

5. Thomson A. Fifth annual report of the Committee of Collective Investigation of the Anatomical Society of Great Britain and Ireland for the year 1893–94. *J Anat Physiol* 1894; **29**:35–60.

6. Reynolds F. Damage to the conus medullaris following spinal anaesthesia. *Anaesthesia* 2001; **56**:238–47.

7. Pysyk CL, Persaud D, Bryson GL, Lui A. Ultrasound assessment of the vertebral level of the palpated intercristal (Tuffier's) line. *Can J Anaesth* 2010; **57**:46–49.

8. Srinivasan KK, Deighan M, Crowley L, McKeating K. Spinal anesthesia for cesarean section: an ultrasound comparison of two different landmark techniques. *Int J Obstet Anesth* 2014; **23**:206–12.

9. Broadbent CR, Maxwell WB, Ferrie R, et al. Ability of anaesthetists to identify a marked lumbar interspace. *Anaesthesia* 2000; **55**:1122–26.

10. Neal JM, Bernards CM, Hadzic A, et al. ASRA practice advisory on neurologic complications in regional anesthesia and pain medicine. *Reg Anesth Pain Med* 2008; **33**:404–15.

11. Sorenson EJ. Neurological injuries associated with regional anesthesia. *Reg Anesth Pain Med* 2008; **33**:442–48.

12. Huntley JS. Neurapraxia and not neuropraxia. *J Plast Reconstr Aesthet Surg* 2014; **67**:430–31.

13. Campbell WW. Evaluation and management of peripheral nerve injury. *Clin Neurophysiol* 2008; **119**:1951–65.

14. Tsen LC. Neurologic complications of labor analgesia and anesthesia. *Int Anesthesiol Clin* 2002; **40**:67–88.

15. Podnar S. Epidemiology of cauda equina and conus medullaris lesions. *Muscle Nerve* 2007; **35**:529–31.

16. Reynolds F. Logic in the safe practice of spinal anaesthesia. *Anaesthesia* 2000; **55**:1045–46.

17. Bogod D. Keeping in the Reynolds zone. *Int J Obstet Anesth* 2014; **23**:201–3.

18. Saifuddin A, Burnett SJ, White J. The variation of position of the conus medullaris in an adult population: a magnetic resonance imaging study. *Spine* 1998; **23**:1452–56.

Management of Post–Dural Puncture Headache

Michael J. Paech and Han T. Truong

Case Study

A 28-year-old nulliparous woman had labor induced for prolonged preterm rupture of membranes at 35 weeks' gestation. Apart from obesity, her prebooking body mass index (BMI) being 34 kg/m^2, she had no other medical comorbidities. That morning, the insertion of an epidural catheter via a 16-gauge Tuohy needle at the L3–L4 interspace was complicated by an accidental dural puncture (ADP). The epidural catheter was successfully inserted 3 cm into the subarachnoid space, aspiration of cerebrospinal fluid (CSF) was confirmed, and the catheter secured. An initial intrathecal injection of 2 ml of 0.125% plain bupivacaine with fentanyl 5 µg/ml provided good analgesia. This was maintained using a patient-controlled spinal analgesia method of the same drug doses by bolus with a 45 minute lockout interval via an electronic pump. No change was made to her labor management plan, and the patient had a spontaneous vaginal delivery 7 hours later. The epidural catheter was removed within 1 hour. The woman was advised of the complication that had occurred and the risk of headache. She was reassured that she would be reviewed by the pain service next morning but was asked to inform hospital staff prior to this should she develop a headache.

On review the following morning, approximately 24 hours after the ADP, the patient reported having mild nausea and a moderate frontal headache that had developed shortly after sitting up in bed but that resolved when lying flat. After discussing the options of either an epidural blood patch (EBP) or expectant management, a conservative symptomatic treatment approach of bed rest and regular acetaminophen and ibuprofen was started. However, the patient's headache worsened considerably over the day such that she was unable to sit upright without the onset of severe frontal and occipital headache and neck stiffness. She was confined to bed, making nursing of her baby very difficult, and she requested further review.

In the absence of fever or other relative contraindications, the woman agreed to and provided written consent for an EBP that evening, 36 hours after the ADP. The procedure was performed in the operating room (OR) by two anesthesiologists. An intravenous (IV) cannula was inserted, and the antecubital fossa of the other arm prepped with antiseptic. With the patient in the left lateral position with lumbar flexion and under full aseptic conditions, the epidural space was located without difficulty at L4–L5. The second anesthesiologist, using sterile gloves and an aseptic technique, obtained 20 ml of venous blood that was then injected slowly over 60 seconds via the epidural needle by the other anesthesiologist. The patient complained of lower back pain radiating to the legs after injection of 15 ml, and this limited total injected volume of blood to 18 mL. However, the patient commented on an immediate reduction in the severity of her headache.

After a short period of time in the recovery area to monitor her vital signs, the patient was returned to the postnatal ward, where she was instructed to remain flat in bed for 2 hours. Thereafter, she started ambulatory care of her infant, and on review the following morning, she reported that she had been headache-free since the EBP. She was discharged that day, with written instructions, including contact information, should the headache recur or other concerning symptoms arise. At telephone contact a week later, she remained symptom free.

Key Points

- Post–dural puncture headache (PDPH) is one of the most common complications of neuraxial anesthesia. It adversely affects the ability of mothers to self-care and care for their newborns and prolongs hospital stay.
- PDPH is uncommon, of mild to severe intensity, and lasts up to several days. It varies in incidence

with spinal needle gauge and point design from 0.5 to 2 percent.

- ADP in an obstetric patient confers a 50–80 percent risk of subsequent postural headache that is most commonly moderate to severe, of onset within 48 hours, and persistent for at least a week. Pharmacologic therapies are largely ineffective.

- Although invasive, a therapeutic EBP is the best way to immediately and completely relieve PDPH. Although very effective against postspinal headache, after ADP most of the obstetric population obtains benefit, but only a third gets complete and sustained relief from a single EBP due to headache recurrence.

- Repeat EBP may be appropriate, but other diagnoses need to be considered and possibly excluded through appropriate investigation. Regular care and follow-up should be routine regardless of whether an expectant or interventional approach is taken.

Discussion

Accidental dural puncture is a not uncommon complication of a labor epidural, the reported incidence varying from 0.5 to 2 percent.[1–3] The leak of CSF through the arachnoid and dura mater (meninges) is the precipitating event for PDPH, which is characterized by its postural nature – being worse when erect and relieved by lying flat. Low intracranial pressure in the upright position is thought to cause traction on the meninges, meningeal veins, and cranial nerves. Intracranial hypotension due to caudad redistribution of CSF when upright results in compensatory cerebral vasodilation, similar to that of migrainous headache, and this may also contribute.[3,4]

PDPH is typically described as a frontal-occipital headache associated with neck stiffness, nausea, tinnitus, and occasionally hearing loss or visual disturbance.[2] Rarely, cranial nerve palsies, seizures, or other neurologic pathologies and events are associated, so if symptoms are atypical or neurologic evaluation is suggestive, it is essential to exclude other serious pathologies (see Table 42.1).[2]

Following an ADP in pregnancy, the incidence of PDPH varies between 50 and 80 percent depending mainly on the size and type of epidural needle used as well as various patient factors.[1–3,5] The obstetric population appears particularly susceptible, with observational studies identifying adults younger than age 40 and female gender as independent risk

Table 42.1 Causes of Postpartum Headache

- Preeclampsia
- Tension headache
- Migraine
- Sinusitis
- Myofascial neck pain
- Caffeine withdrawal
- Cerebral vein thrombosis
- Subdural hematoma
- Meningitis/encephalitis
- Intracranial hemorrhage
- Cerebral tumor

factors for PDPH.[3,6] Obesity may have an impact on the incidence of PDPH, with lower rates of headache observed among morbidly obese women.[1] Compared with an incidence of PDPH of less than 2 percent when using atraumatic spinal needles, the larger size of an epidural needle is a major factor contributing to morbidity.[2,3,5] Accidental dural puncture with a 16-gauge epidural needle appears almost twice as likely to result in PDPH as ADP with an 18-gauge needle.[7,8] With conservative management, the median duration of PDPH from large spinal needles may be longer than 7 days,[9] and 10 percent of women who experience ADP are still symptomatic after 1 month.[1,2] It is possible that those who develop PDPH will be more likely to suffer from chronic headaches subsequently.[10]

The onset of headache within 5 days of dural puncture is required to meet the diagnostic criteria for PDPH set forth in the *International Classification of Headache Disorders* (3rd edn; ICHD-3), but 90 percent of women with an ADP are likely to be symptomatic within 48 hours.[1] Debilitating headache can prolong hospital stay due to compromise of a mother's ability to care for both herself and her newborn baby. Daily follow-up should be instituted because the diagnosis of PDPH is clinical. Although typical changes occur in the presence of low intracranial pressure (Figure 42.1), neuroimaging is normally reserved for when other pathologies are suspected or headache fails to respond to multiple blood patches. The woman needs to be monitored to ensure that she does not develop a rare but serious complication, for example, a subdural hematoma, cranial nerve palsy, or cerebral vein thrombosis.

Following an ADP, women are often advised to limit ambulation, maintain hydration, and drink coffee or take caffeine (caffeine is a cerebral vasoconstrictor) and are prescribed regular oral analgesia (opioid and nonopioid) in an attempt to prevent PDPH or minimize its severity. Unfortunately, the drug

235

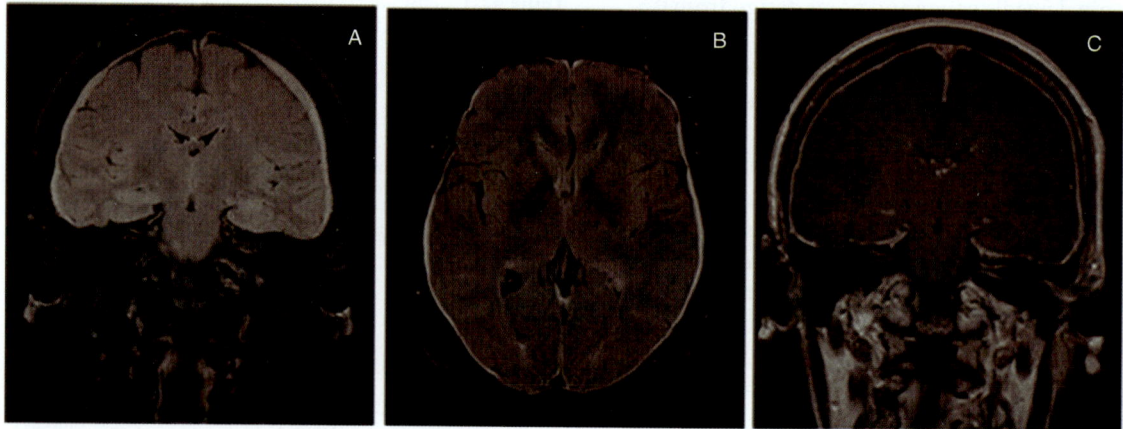

Figure 42.1 Brain MRI scans showing typical findings in intracranial hypotension with coronal and axial fluid attenuated inversion recover-weighted images. A, B Thickening of the pachymeninges. C. Coronal gadolinium-enhanced T1-weighted image.
Source: Reproduced from Ferraro et al.[22] with permission from the Australian Society of Anaesthetists.

therapies lack good supporting evidence and are at best of limited efficacy. Restricting ambulation and providing supplemental fluid are of no benefit.[11] Evidence that oral or IV caffeine and other cerebral vasoconstrictors are of benefit is equivocal and compliance problematic due to the high incidence of side effects and insomnia.[1,5,12] Low levels of evidence suggest a possible therapeutic benefit from analgesia with IV cosyntropin (a synthetic adrenocorticotropic hormone analogue), epidural morphine, occipital nerve blocks, or oral gabapentin or pregabalin, but without further validation, neither these nor other pharmacologic therapies can be recommended for routine use.[11]

The invasive procedure of EBP is the best supported treatment of PDPH.[11,13] Expansion of the epidural space with blood usually produces an immediate and sustained increase in epidural and subarachnoid space pressure, with shift of CSF relieving intracranial hypotension and inducing cerebral vasoconstriction. This may rapidly relieve headache. Additionally, further CSF loss may be prevented by sealing the meningeal hole with a hemostatic plug that also stimulates collagen repair of the defect.[4] A therapeutic EBP provides complete or partial relief in up to 95 percent of women with PDPH, but recurrence of headache is common, especially when the CSF leak is greater through a larger meningeal perforation after an ADP.[14] Given the poor initial efficacy or recurrence of PDPH (usually within 48 hours), 15–30 percent of these women may request a repeat EBP.[5,14,15]

Hence, only a third of women receiving a single EBP obtain complete and sustained relief from headache after ADP.[6,14,15] This contrasts with the efficacy of EBP for PDPH subsequent to use of an atraumatic or small-gauge spinal needle, where permanent resolution of PDPH is much more likely.[11]

A prophylactic EBP, in which blood is administered through a reinserted epidural catheter before the onset of PDPH, has been used to try to reduce the incidence, severity, and/or duration of symptoms. Research has been limited by small sample sizes and bias due to the inability to blind study subjects, and the two largest randomized trials have produced conflicting results.[16,17] One reported excellent outcomes,[16] but the other study, which included a sham procedure, found no difference in the incidence of PDPH or need for therapeutic EBP.[17] Concern about bacteremia immediately postpartum and the risk of injecting a growth medium such as blood, possibly through a colonized catheter, have led to a major decline in the popularity of this approach.[18] A consensus recommendation to defer the conduct of a therapeutic EBP until at least 24–48 hours after ADP is based on observational studies indicating a higher success rate, although this may be attributable in part to selection bias, given that the natural history of PDPH is to improve with time.[6,14] On balance, EBP tends to be offered early for women with severe headache (one that prevents normal ambulation and care of the neonate) and late for those with persisting moderate headache.

Prior to performing an EBP, it is important to ensure that the timing falls within a recommended "safe" window with respect to any anticoagulant therapy (e.g., low-molecular-weight heparin thromboprophylaxis) and that there are no relative contraindications, for example, systemic or local infection. Maintenance of procedural sterility is best achieved by two physicians – one performing venesection and the other the epidural needle placement. The postural nature of PDPH means that most women are more comfortable in the lateral position, but the anesthesiologist should select his or her preferred patient position for insertion to minimize the risk of a repeat ADP. Performing the EBP at the same vertebral level or a nearby interspace is recommended, although success may still occur after distant injection because magnetic resonance imaging (MRI) has shown blood to spread at least three to five vertebral levels within the epidural space, and spontaneous low-intracranial-pressure headache can be relieved irrespective of the location of the dural leak. The optimal volume of autologous blood for EBP is unclear. Two randomized trials have compared 7.5 ml versus 15 ml or 15 ml versus 20 ml versus 30 ml, and an attempt to slowly inject at least 20 ml appears a reasonable strategy, recognizing that back pain during the procedure may limit the total volume able to be administered.[6,19]

Best practice after an EBP is also uncertain, with weak evidence supporting the advice to remain lying supine for 2 hours.[20] It is postulated that remaining supine allows time for CSF production and cerebral vasoconstriction, which correct intracranial hypotension and allow a more stable hemostatic plug of the meningeal perforation to form. Valsalva maneuvers have been linked to recurrence of headache, presumably through disruption of the hemostatic plug, so attempts to prevent sudden increases in lumbar subarachnoid pressure include advice against heavy lifting or coughing and prescription of stool softeners. In the event that PDPH does recur, a repeat EBP can be offered, but again, the optimal timing is unknown – the authors suggest delaying for at least 24 hours after recurrence. A third EBP should not be performed without considering alternative causes for symptoms, seeking neurologic advice, and considering neuroimaging to exclude other causes of postpartum headache.

Back pain can occur during the administration of blood and is also the most common subsequent complication of an EBP. It typically lasts up to 5 days but is not usually distressing.[6] Pain is thought

Table 42.2 Red Flag Symptoms Following an Epidural Blood Patch

- Fever
- Drowsiness
- Worsening headache
- Worsening back pain
- Urinary retention
- Fecal incontinence
- Leg weakness or numbness

to be due to a direct irritant effect of blood on the nerve roots or nerve root compression caused by the substantial increase in spinal canal pressure.[6] Daily review of women with PDPH is important to monitor symptoms and for early detection of potentially serious complications such as epidural abscess or lumbovertebral syndrome, in which back pain occurs in association with neurologic deficits of the lower limbs. Other rare neurologic complications include arachnoiditis, subdural hematoma, seizures, cranial nerve palsies, and worsening headache due to raised intracranial pressure following the EBP.

Strategies to minimize the incidence and/or severity of PDPH are difficult to investigate because of the infrequency and unpredictability of ADP. Promising results are often not confirmed in larger and better-controlled studies. The insertion of an epidural catheter intrathecally to prevent PDPH following ADP is one such approach that became popular because of encouraging observational studies. However, meta-analysis shows limited efficacy, with the requirement for EBP reduced but no significant difference in the incidence of PDPH.[21]

Regardless of whether an expectant or interventional approach is taken to the management of PDPH, mothers should be reviewed daily while in hospital, with phone follow-up and notification of their general practitioner after discharge. Providing written information about "red flag" symptoms (see Table 42.2) is recommended, as well as contact instructions for questions or concerns. Local protocols should be in place, ideally offering ongoing counseling and the opportunity for anesthetic outpatient review during a subsequent pregnancy.

Learning Points

- PDPH has a characteristic postural component in almost all cases – this assists with the clinical diagnosis, but other serious causes of postpartum headache must always be considered.

237

- Conservative measures to treat PDPH have proven disappointing. Recent therapies, such as epidural morphine or oral gabapentin or pregabalin, require validation before they can be recommended routinely.
- An epidural blood patch is the most effective treatment for PDPH, but only a third of obstetric patients with PDPH after an ADP will obtain complete and sustained relief, mainly due to headache recurrence.
- Regardless of whether an expectant or interventional management approach is taken, patient follow-up should continue until there has been satisfactory resolution of symptoms.

References

1. Paech M, Banks S, Gurrin L. An audit of accidental dural puncture during epidural insertion of a Tuohy needle in obstetric patients. *Int J Obstet Anesth* 2001; **10**:162–67.

2. Sprigge JS, Harper SJ. Accidental dural puncture and post dural puncture headache in obstetric anaesthesia: presentation and management: a 23-year survey in a district general hospital. *Anaesthesia* 2008; **63**:36–43.

3. Choi PT, Galinski SE, Takeuchi L, et al. PDPH is a common complication of neuraxial blockade in parturients: a meta-analysis of obstetrical studies. *Can J Anesth* 2003; **50**:460–69.

4. Kroin JS, Nagalla SK, Buvanendran A, et al. The mechanisms of intracranial pressure modulation by epidural blood and other injectates in a postdural puncture rat model. *Anesth Analg* 2002; **95**:423–29.

5. Van de Velde M, Schepers R, Berends N, Vandermeersch E, De Buck F. Ten years of experience with accidental dural puncture and post-dural puncture headache in a tertiary obstetric anesthesia department. *Int J Obstet Anesth* 2008; **17**:329–35.

6. Paech MJ, Doherty DA, Christmas T, Wong CA. The volume of blood for epidural blood patch in obstetrics: a randomized, blinded clinical trial. *Anesth Analg* 2011; **113**:126–33.

7. Morley-Forster PK, Singh S, Angle P, et al. The effect of epidural needle type on postdural puncture headache: a randomized trial. *Can J Anesth* 2006; **53**:572–78.

8. Russell IF. A prospective controlled study of continuous spinal analgesia versus repeat epidural analgesia after accidental dural puncture in labour. *Int J Obstet Anesth* 2012; **21**:7–16.

9. van Kooten F, Oedit R, Bakker SL, Dippel DW. Epidural blood patch in post dural puncture headache: a randomised, observer-blind, controlled clinical trial. *J Neurol Neurosurg Psychiatry* 2008; **79**:553–58.

10. Webb CA, Weyker PD, Zhang L, et al. Unintentional dural puncture with a Tuohy needle increases risk of chronic headache. *Anesth Analg* 2012; **115**:124–32.

11. Paech MJ. Iatrogenic headaches: giving everyone a sore head. *Int J Obstet Anesth* 2012; **21**:1–3.

12. Halker RB, Demaerschalk BM, Wellik KE, et al. Caffeine for the prevention and treatment of postdural puncture headache: debunking the myth. *Neurologist* 2007; **13**:323–27.

13. Boonmak P, Boonmak S. Epidural blood patching for preventing and treating post-dural puncture headache. *Cochrane Database Syst Rev* 2010; (1):CD001791.

14. Banks S, Paech M, Gurrin L. An audit of epidural blood patch after accidental dural puncture with a Tuohy needle in obstetric patients. *Int J Obstet Anesth* 2001; **10**:172–76.

15. Williams EJ, Beaulieu P, Fawcett WJ, Jenkins JG. Efficacy of epidural blood patch in the obstetric population. *Int J Obstet Anesth* 1999; **8**:105–9.

16. Stein MH, Cohen S, Mohiuddin MA, Dombrovskiy V, Lowenwirt I. Prophylactic vs therapeutic blood patch for obstetric patients with accidental dural puncture: a randomized, controlled trial. *Anaesthesia* 2014; **69**:320–26.

17. Scavone BM, Wong CA, Sullivan JT, et al. Efficacy of a prophylactic epidural blood patch in preventing post dural puncture headache in parturients after inadvertent dural puncture. *Anesthesiology* 2004; **101**:1422–27.

18. Agerson AN, Scavone BM. Prophylactic epidural blood patch after unintentional dural puncture for the prevention of postdural puncture headache in parturients. *Anesth Analg* 2012; **115**:133–36.

19. Chen LK, Huang CH, Jean WH, et al. Effective epidural blood patch volumes for postdural puncture headache in Taiwanese women. *J Formosan Med Assoc* 2007; **106**:134–40.

20. Martin R, Jourdain S, Clairoux M, Tetrault JP. Duration of decubitus position after epidural blood patch. *Can J Anesth* 1994; **41**:23–25.

21. Heesen M, Klohr S, Rossaint R, et al. Insertion of an intrathecal catheter following accidental dural puncture: a meta-analysis. *Int J Obstet Anesth* 2013; **22**:26–30.

Nonobstetric Surgery during Pregnancy

Neeti Sadana

Case Study

A 22-year-old gravida 2, para 1 woman at 28 weeks' gestation presented to the triage area for evaluation with a 24-hour history of worsening abdominal pain, nausea, anorexia, and fever. Her medical history was unremarkable. She previously had a vaginal delivery of a healthy baby at term. On admission, her vital signs were stable. The Emergency Department team immediately contacted the surgical team to investigate a potential surgical diagnosis, such as acute appendicitis. The junior surgeon performing the initial assessment was hesitant to recommend any form of imaging because of the pregnancy. The patient subsequently spent several hours in the Emergency Department without any investigations or interventions. Her condition worsened over the next few hours. Finally, the obstetric team was consulted, and a presumptive diagnosis of appendicitis was made. The fetal condition was evaluated by the obstetric team at the same time and found to be stable. The patient was then prepared for open surgery, with the attending surgeon adamant that laparoscopy was contraindicated in pregnancy. Unfortunately, during this period, the patient became severely septic, with fetal compromise. This resulted in a joint obstetric/surgical procedure that included an urgent cesarean delivery together with an open appendectomy. Following a protracted period in the high-dependency unit, the patient made a full recovery and was discharged 10 days later with her healthy baby.

Key Points

- Essential to an understanding of the risks of nonobstetric surgery during pregnancy is an awareness of the physiologic changes during pregnancy.
- The available evidence-based literature suggests that surgery during pregnancy is much safer than previously thought.

- There is no strong evidence as to the preferred way to perform an appendectomy (open or laparoscopic) during pregnancy from a fetal or maternal safety viewpoint.
- Delay in the diagnosis and treatment of conditions such as acute appendicitis dramatically increases maternal and fetal morbidity and mortality.
- The perioperative team should aim to minimize the operative time and use the most appropriate anesthesia technique with the safest anesthetic drugs.
- Preterm delivery and fetal loss remain the most prevalent concerns for nonobstetric surgery during pregnancy. Some surgeons are hesitant to perform laparoscopic surgery during the third trimester due to the risk of greater fetal loss and potentially increased surgical complication rates.
- In cases of appendectomy in pregnancy, the most experienced surgical team should be used to minimize complications, and the decision to perform a laparoscopy versus open procedure should depend on the expertise of the surgical team.

Discussion

It is generally estimated that up to 2 percent of parturients undergo nonobstetric surgery during pregnancy. The most common nonobstetrical surgical emergencies complicating pregnancy are acute appendicitis, cholecystitis, and intestinal obstruction.[1] Nonobstetric surgery during pregnancy must initiate a discussion about how the physiologic changes of pregnancy affect the mother while also being highly sensitive to the effects of surgery and anesthesia on the unborn fetus. Ideally, elective surgery should be postponed until the postpartum period, and if possible, it also should be avoided during the organogenesis phase of the first trimester.

The multidisciplinary team must be cognizant of the physiologic changes of pregnancy, especially those involving the cardiovascular, respiratory, and gastrointestinal systems. Major cardiovascular changes include an increase in cardiac output by 30–40 percent during the first trimester and up to 50 percent at term.[2] Blood pressure decreases secondary to reduced systemic vascular resistance and can result in the supine hypotensive syndrome. In cases of trauma or infection, this syndrome can alter uteroplacental perfusion significantly, as well as maternal hemodynamic stability. Changes in cardiac output can speed up the rate of intravenous (IV) drug induction and alter rates of uptake and removal of drugs from the maternal circulation, altering the depth of anesthesia. Significant respiratory changes secondary to increased progesterone levels lead to increases in minute ventilation. The growing fetus causes anatomic changes in the location of the diaphragm, resulting in a significant 20 percent reduction in functional residual capacity (FRC). These changes, together with increases in alveolar ventilation, result in an increased risk of hypoxemia during periods of apnea as well as rapid uptake and distribution of inhaled anesthetics. In addition, airway changes include laryngeal and pharyngeal edema as well as capillary engorgement of the mucosal lining of the airway. These changes may make securing the airway a potential challenge.[3]

While almost every system in the parturient undergoes some alteration, the gastrointestinal system is also very relevant. Recently, Wong et al.[4] found no change in gastric emptying in obese and nonobese pregnant women compared with nonpregnant patients. While gastric emptying may not be delayed, there certainly are changes such as a reduction in lower esophageal sphincter tone and increases in intragastric pressure due to the gravid uterus. An increase in gastric acid secretion has been seen in parturients as well, although the finding is not consistent. It is not clear whether these gastrointestinal changes increase the risk of parturients developing acute appendicitis and other abdominal pathology. Of course, in acute abdominal pathology, as seen in the Case Study, "full stomach" considerations are valid irrespective of the patient's pregnancy.

During pregnancy, the well-being of the fetus is paramount. Teratogens are drug and environmental agents that increase the incidence of non-chance-related defects. Fetal organs develop throughout gestation, but days 15–60 are essential for organogenesis in humans. For the fetus, the greatest risk involves spontaneous abortion, premature labor, and preterm delivery, which can result in significant morbidity and mortality to the newborn. And while no anesthetic agent or technique is superior, each agent and technique carries risks that must be evaluated. Finally, it is not certain whether the underlying medical condition requiring surgery, surgery itself, or the anesthetic agents used poses the greatest risk to the fetus, but all should be minimized during pregnancy. The most current evidence suggests that no anesthetic agents, including the previously suspect nitrous oxide and benzodiazepines, are teratogenic in humans.

The Case Study illustrates the difficulty that imaging and diagnosis pose for both maternal and fetal outcome. In the case of acute appendicitis, a 24-hour delay of surgery after presentation can lead to a 66 percent increase in the perforation rate as well as a 20 percent rate of fetal loss compared with a 5 percent rate of fetal loss with uncomplicated acute appendicitis.[5] Radiation to the fetus from x-rays and CT scans has been a major factor in delays in diagnosis. Most physicians are concerned about the potential negative effects on the developing fetus. Radiation comes in two types: ionizing and nonionizing. Examples of nonionizing radiation include ultrasound and MRI. Examples of ionizing radiation include x-rays and gamma rays. Ionizing radiation originates from space and natural resources and exists everywhere, including soil, water, and air. On average, a person is exposed to some discreet level of background radiation every year.[6] The precise amount of background radiation exposure varies in different parts of the world depending on the altitude and the quality of the atmosphere. When looking specifically at the effects of radiation on a fetus, it is important to first note that the radiation dose that a pregnant woman is exposed to or absorbs may not directly transfer to the fetus. A fetus is partly protected from radiation injury by a pregnant woman's surrounding soft tissues and uterus, both of which generally stop alpha and beta particles from penetration if they are not ingested, injected, or inhaled.[7] However, gamma and x-rays directed toward the abdomen of a pregnant woman who is not appropriately shielded can reach and harm a fetus. The effects of ionizing radiation on an embryo and fetus can include pregnancy loss, malformations, neurobehavioral abnormalities, fetal growth restriction, and cancer.[8] The American College of Obstetricians and Gynecologists (ACOG) has indicated that the threshold for medical concern, particularly regarding congenital malformations, should be lowered to 50 mGy (5 rad).[9] It is important to remember that there is a less than 0.001 rad exposure per chest x-ray. According to these statistics, it would take thousands of x-rays to cause significant risk. However abdominal shields should be placed when possible, and time to exposure should be minimized.

Now, with the presence of ultrasonography and MRI scanning that provide minimal radiation exposure to the unborn fetus and a knowledgeable multidisciplinary team with an obstetric anesthesiologist to facilitate imaging and surgery, delays should not occur.

The long term effects of surgery and anesthesia on the fetus are highly controversial. Animal models have shown that exposure to anesthetic agents during a period of synaptogenesis in rats results in neuronal apoptosis and can infer later-in-life learning defects. These data are difficult to extrapolate to human models. Several provocative studies have recently shown an association of surgery and anesthesia with both learning disabilities and deviant behavior.[10] In addition, in 2017 the U.S. Food and Drug Administration (FDA) issued a warning that repeated or lengthy use of general anesthesia and sedation during surgery or procedures in children younger than 3 years old or pregnant women during the 3rd trimester or lasting greater than 3 hours may affect fetal brain development and cognitive behavior.[11]

Once a decision is made to proceed with surgery, an anesthetic technique is selected. If at all possible, regional and neuraxial techniques should be used because they confer minimal transfer of drugs and agents to the fetus. If general anesthesia is used, animal models suggest that fetal skeletal abnormalities or death may followed repeated or prolonged exposure of mice to anesthetic concentrations of volatile agents, but no evidence has suggested reproductive toxicity with either sevoflurane or desflurane in clinical concentrations.[12] Nitrous oxide use has been studied extensively in rat models, and the literature suggests that the teratogenicity is complex and involves the inhibition of methionine synthase. Teratogenesis has been associated with the use of any of the commonly employed induction agents, including the barbiturates, ketamine, and the benzodiazepines, as well as opioids, when given in clinical doses.[13] It is common to see fetal heart rate variability with opioids and induction agents, but these changes may indicate an anesthetized fetus and are not of concern in the presence of maternal stability. Toxicity is not associated with small doses of muscle relaxants, and no evidence supports teratogenicity associated with any local anesthetic used clinically in humans.[14]

Continuous fetal heart rate monitoring during surgery certainly can be performed if the surgical site allows, and someone who can interpret the cardiotocography (CTG) monitor should be present. A plan also must be in place when faced with persistent nonreassuring or pathologic CTG tracings. The ACOG has stated that "the decision to use fetal monitoring should be individualized and, if used, should be based on gestational age, type of surgery, and facilities available."[15]

The decision to perform open versus laparoscopic surgery is a controversial one and should be based on the skill level of the surgical team for optimal safety of the mother and fetus. When laparoscopic surgery was in its infancy, some argued that laparoscopy was contraindicated during pregnancy owing to concerns for uterine injury and fetal perfusion. As surgeons have gained more experience with laparoscopy, it has become the preferred treatment for many surgical diseases in pregnant patients. Concerns for the fetus during laparoscopy include fetal trauma, fetal acidosis from absorbed carbon dioxide, and decreased maternal cardiac output and resulting decrease in uteroplacental perfusion from iatrogenic increases in intraabdominal pressure.

Benefits of laparoscopy during pregnancy appear similar to those in nonpregnant patients, including less postoperative pain, less postoperative ileus, decreased length of hospital stay and faster return to work. There are many advantages of laparoscopy in pregnant patients as well, including decreased fetal respiratory depression due to diminished postoperative narcotic requirements, lower risk of wound complications, diminished postoperative maternal hypoventilation, and decreased risk of thromboembolic events.[16] Laparoscopic treatment of acute abdominal disease has the same indications in pregnant and nonpregnant patients and may even confer some benefit. The improved visualization in laparoscopy may reduce the risk of uterine irritability by decreasing the need for uterine manipulation. Decreased uterine irritability results in lower rates of spontaneous abortion and preterm delivery.[17] Laparoscopic appendectomy may be performed safely in pregnant patients with appendicitis, and laparoscopic cholecystectomy is the treatment of choice in

241

the pregnant patient with gallbladder disease regardless of trimester.[18]

Learning Points

- Nonobstetric surgery during pregnancy is more common than once thought.
- Delays in proper imaging and diagnosis can lead to worsened outcome for mother and newborn.
- No anesthetic technique is superior, but exposure time should be minimized.
- Multidisciplinary teams should discuss anesthetic technique, surgical approach, radiation risk, and plan for potential complications.

References

1. Kort B, Katz VL, Watson WJ. The effect of nonobstetric operation during pregnancy. *Surg Gynecol Obstets* 1993; **177**:371–76.

2. Capeless EL, Clapp JF. Cardiovascular changes in the early phase of pregnancy. *Am J Obstet Gynecol* 1989; **161**:1449–53.

3. Lewis G, ed. Confidential inquiry into maternal and child health, saving mother's lives: reviewing maternal deaths to make motherhood safer: 2003–2005. *The Seventh Report of the Confidential Inquiries into Maternal Death in the United Kingdom*. London: CEMACH; 2007.

4. Brock-Utne JG, Dow TGB, Dimopoulos GE, et al. Gastric and lower esophageal sphincter pressures early in pregnancy. *Br J Anaesth* 1981; **53**:381–84.

5. Park SH, Park MI, Choi JS, et al. Laparoscopic appendectomy performed during pregnancy by gynecological laparoscopists. *Eur J Obstet Gynecol Reprod Biol* 2010; **148**:44–48.

6. United Nations Scientific Committee on the Effects of Atomic Radiation (UNSCEAR). *Sources and Effects of Ionizing Radiation*. New York: UNSCEAR; 2010.

7. Harrison J, Stather J. The assessment of doses and effects from intakes of radioactive particles. *J Anat* 1996; **189**:521.

8. Fattibene P, Mazzei F, Nuccetelli C, Risica S. Prenatal exposure to ionizing radiation: sources, effects and regulatory aspects. *Acta Paediatr* 1999; **88**:693–702.

9. Donnelly EH, Smith JM, Farfan EB, Ozcan I. Prenatal radiation exposure: background material for counseling pregnant patients following exposure to radiation. *Disaster Med Public Health Prep* 2011; **5**:62–68.

10. Palanisamy A, Baxter MG, Keel PK, et al. Rats exposed to isoflurane in utero during early gestation are behaviorally abnormal as adults. *Anesthesiology* 2011; **114**(3):521–28.

11. United States Food and Drug Administration. FDA Safety Communication:FDA review results in a new warning about using general anesthesia and sedation drugs in young children and pregnant women. Available at http://wwwfda.gov/Drugs/DrugSafety/ucm.532356.htm.

12. Mazze RI, Wilson AI, Rice SA, et al. Fetal development in mice exposed to isoflurane. *Teratology* 1985; **32**:339–45.

13. Briggs GC, Freeman Rk, Yaffe Sj. *Drugs Used in Pregnancy and Lactation*, 3rd edn. Baltimore, MD: Williams & Wilkins; 1990.

14. Shepard TH. *Catalog of Teratogenic Agents*, 7th edn. Baltimore: Johns Hopkins University Press; 1973, pp. 1–82.

15. American College of Obstetricians and Gynecologists Committee on Obstetric Practice. ACOG Committee Opinion No. 474: Nonobstetric surgery in pregnancy. *Obstet Gynecol* 2011; **117**:420–21.

16. Pucci RO, Seed RW. Case report of laparoscopic cholecystectomy in the third trimester of pregnancy. *Am J Obstet Gynecol* 1991; **165**:401–2.

17. Curet MJ. Special problems in laparoscopic surgery: previous abdominal surgery, obesity, and pregnancy. *Surg Clin North Am* 2000; **80**:1093–110.

18. Pearl J, Price R, Richardson W, Fanelli R, Society of American Gastrointestinal and Endoscopic Surgeons. Guidelines for diagnosis, treatment, and use of laparoscopy for surgical problems during pregnancy. *Surg Endosc* 2011; **25**(11):3479–92.

Trauma in Pregnancy

Tom Hurst and Andre Vercueil

Case Study

A 27-year-old primiparous woman at 31 weeks gestation was involved in a road traffic collision (RTC). She was the front seat passenger in a car that came off the road and hit a tree at 40–50 mph. She required extrication by the fire service and received oxygen, spinal immobilization, femoral traction, morphine, and ketamine in the prehospital phase. She was secured to a scoop stretcher tilted to 30 degrees to the left to avoid aortocaval compression and triaged to a major trauma center. On arrival, her vital signs were heart rate 116 beats/min, blood pressure 105/84 mmHg, SpO_2 100% on 15 liter/min oxygen, and a Glasgow Coma Score (GCS) of 13 (E3 V4 M6). She was complaining of some tenderness over the left chest wall, and there was clinical evidence of a closed fracture of the right femur.

The patient was received by the trauma team and, following a primary survey, was taken to the CT scanner, where she underwent CT scanning of her head, neck, chest, abdomen, and pelvis. This revealed a simple pneumothorax on the left and a grade 3 splenic laceration with extravasation of contrast material into surrounding hematoma. Tranexamic acid 1 g was administered as a bolus, followed by an infusion of 1 g over 8 hours.

The patient was transferred to the interventional radiology suite for angioembolization of her spleen. On arrival, her blood pressure was 88/60 mmHg, and a massive transfusion protocol was activated. Preparations were made for emergency cesarean delivery, and in the absence of an appropriate wedge, manual uterine displacement was performed. The patient received 2 units of O-negative blood and 2 units of AB fresh frozen plasma (FFP) through a fluid warmer, following which her blood pressure increased to 124/80 mmHg. Angioembolization proceeded uneventfully, and the patient received a further 2 units of FFP and blood. She was transferred to the ICU following her stabilization for ongoing monitoring. A senior midwife and obstetrician were consulted to monitor the fetus using cardiotocographic monitoring. Fortunately, the fetal heart rate remained normal, and there was no clinical evidence of placental abruption. The mother was questioned regarding antenatal anti-Rhesus D (RhD) immunization, and because she had already received the 28-week dose, she was given the 34-week dose prior to her transfer to the labor ward

Key Points

- This patient had a significant mechanism of injury and sustained polytrauma. Clinicians need to have a high incidence of suspicion in such cases, and occult injuries should be anticipated.
- The patient required rapid comprehensive imaging to identify all her injuries based on the fact that she was tachycardic and had a reduced GCS. High-quality CT imaging of all organs was appropriate, regardless of the fact that the woman was pregnant.
- Following deterioration, she was resuscitated with blood and blood products, while preparing for emergency surgical delivery of the fetus.
- Thankfully, there was a good response to resuscitation and maneuvers aimed at reducing aortocaval compression, making emergency cesarean delivery unnecessary.
- Two potential patients mean that the multidisciplinary team should include senior obstetric and midwife support and monitoring.

Discussion

It is difficult to know the true incidence and epidemiology of trauma during pregnancy, and a recent meta-analysis has noted the many shortcomings of the published literature. These include publication bias, the retrospective nature of all the studies, and wide variations in the outcomes reported.

243

Nevertheless, it has been reported that trauma is now the most common cause of non-obstetric maternal death in the United States, and complicates approximately 6 percent of pregnancies worldwide. Unlike many other causes of death, it is increasing in frequency. Motor vehicle accidents and non-accidental injury due to domestic violence are the most common reported causes, with falls also common.[1] As pregnancy progresses, patterns of injury change, with predominantly blunt abdominal injuries becoming increasingly common, whereas the incidence of head injury falls.[2]

Transport of seriously injured patients to a major trauma center is associated with a reduction in mortality.[3] Most trauma systems select patients for direct transport to a major trauma center on grounds of altered physiology, apparent injuries, mechanism of injury, and patient factors such as age, pregnancy, and comorbidities. The exact inclusion criteria vary both nationally and internationally. The current London Major Trauma decision tool states that ambulance crews should assess special patient or system considerations following trauma. If the woman is more than 20 weeks' pregnant, she will be taken to a major trauma center for assessment, even if the rest of the decision tree suggest that the patient could be managed locally.[4]

The initial approach to the severely injured pregnant patient is almost identical to that in the non-pregnant patient. A structured primary survey should be performed and immediately life-threatening injuries identified and treated, but CT imaging should proceed if indicated because the treatment of the mother takes priority over radiation risk to the fetus. Comprehensive early CT imaging of polytrauma patients is associated with lower mortality.[5]

Physiology of Pregnancy and Hemorrhage

The physiologic changes of pregnancy are adaptive for surviving hemorrhage but may make detection of hypovolemia more difficult. Increases in both blood volume and erythrocyte count of 50 and 30 percent, respectively, mean that pregnant women have a physiologic anemia due to hemodilution, both of which may provide a degree of protection from blood loss. This may mean that by the time of decompensation due to blood loss, the intravascular volume and red cell deficit may be very substantial. Cardiac output is increased by up to 50 percent by the beginning of

the first trimester, and this is coupled with a reduction in systemic vascular resistance and increased uterine blood flow. The uterine blood flow is not autoregulated, and is thus entirely dependent on maternal blood pressure. Aortocaval compression, which can occur from the twentieth week of pregnancy, can impair venous return to the right side of the heart, significantly reducing both cardiac output and blood pressure in the mother, with obvious deleterious effects on the fetus. These factors, coupled with the increase in metabolic rate of up to 20 percent in the pregnant mother, mean that by the time the blood pressure begins to fall, shock is advanced, with both limited reserves and increased oxygen consumption. Speedy and effective resuscitation, including uterine displacement and consideration of operative delivery, is required to save the life of the mother.

In the non-pregnant patient, it should be noted that the likelihood of requiring blood transfusion following injury increases progressively as systolic blood pressure falls below 110 mmHg, this being a more logical definition of hypotension in trauma.[6] However, fluid resuscitation prior to hemorrhage control is associated with increased hemorrhage, and many clinicians would advocate resuscitation that aims for a systolic blood pressure of less than 100 mmHg until definitive surgical or radiologic control of bleeding has been achieved. The relatively low number of traumatically injured pregnant women seen in both emergency and radiology departments means that staff may be unfamiliar with the need to correctly position the patient to avoid aortocaval compression, and this may precipitate hemodynamic deterioration and even cardiac arrest. Should this occur, the cause should be addressed. Chest compressions may be easier to perform in the supine position, with lateral manual displacement of the uterus.[7]

Coagulation and Trauma

Following major trauma, a subset of patients develop a coagulopathy early in their clinical course related to the magnitude of their shock and tissue damage. This coagulopathy is distinct from disseminated intravascular coagulopathy and the coagulopathy that arises secondary to hypothermia and dilution, although these may all coexist. The exact mechanism remains to be elucidated, although a mismatch between the coagulation cascade and the thrombolytic pathway, resulting in overproduction of activated protein C, has been implicated.[8] The increasing appreciation of this clinical entity has meant recent alterations in transfusion strategies. There is an increase in fixed-ratio transfusion protocols of blood to FFP and platelets. There remains debate over the ideal ratios, with a recent trial reporting similar mortality outcomes for a 1:1:1 ratio versus a 2:1:1 ratio for blood, FFP, and platelets, respectively.[9] There were, however, fewer deaths due to exsanguination in less than 24 hours in the 1:1:1 group, and more patients achieved hemostasis. While there are no data to guide transfusion in traumatically injured pregnant women, there is increasing interest in optimizing transfusion both in trauma and during obstetric hemorrhage. Trauma may also result in placental abruption in anything from 2 to 4 percent following minor injury, to as much as 50 percent following major injury and is also associated with significant coagulopathy. Near-patient testing using rotational thromboelastography may offer a way of ensuring that optimal transfusion ratios are used, limiting unnecessary transfusions while ensuring clot strength. Specific fibrinogen replacement using fibrinogen concentrate, rather than depending on the relatively modest levels present in FFP, has shown promise in the treatment of obstetric hemorrhage, with prompt correction of coagulopathy, and a reduction in blood product requirements.[10]

Tranexamic acid is an antifibrinolytic agent that has been shown in the CRASH-2 trial to reduce mortality in trauma patients with or at risk of severe bleeding. Adult patients with a heart rate greater than 110 beats/min or a systolic BP of less than 90 mmHg or who were considered to be at significant risk of bleeding were included within 8 hours of injury. Over 20,000 patients were enrolled, and the relative risk of death in the tranexamic acid group was 0.91 (95% confidence interval [CI] 0.85–0.97, $p = 0.0035$).[11] Subsequent analysis indicates that treatment should be initiated within 3 hours of injury.[12]

An additional risk associated with trauma in pregnancy, particularly blunt trauma to the abdomen, is fetomaternal hemorrhage. This presents the potential for rhesus sensitization if the fetus is rhesus positive and the mother's blood type is rhesus negative. There remains a lack of awareness of the requirement for anti-RhD following blunt abdominal trauma in pregnant women,[13] although it forms part of NICE guidance,[14] with potentially devastating consequences in subsequent pregnancies.

Emergency cesarean delivery is indicated *to save the life of the mother* in situations where there is hemodynamic instability unresponsive to initial therapy. Resuscitation of the trauma patient increasingly happens in a dynamic and mobile fashion, and key members of the trauma team should accompany the patient during their initial assessment and treatment. In the case of obstetric patients, this should include an obstetrician of sufficient seniority to perform an emergent cesarean delivery.

Learning Points

- Traumatically injured pregnant women present unique challenges. There are two patients for the multidisciplinary team to consider, and the physiologic changes of pregnancy may mean that hypovolemic shock is detected late.
- Aortocaval compression may reduce venous return, with serious consequences related to reduced cardiac output and hypotension, and should always be considered and avoided by left lateral tilt or uterine displacement.
- The focus of the team should be on saving the life of the mother. All necessary imaging should be performed. Refractory hypotension or cardiac arrest of the mother may require emergency cesarean delivery to save her life.
- Blunt abdominal trauma is more common in pregnancy and may result in Rhesus immunization or placental abruption.
- Coagulopathy is common following major trauma and obstetric hemorrhage and should be managed with either fixed-ratio transfusion or near-patient testing and appropriate use of tranexamic acid.

References

1. Mendez-Figueroa H, Dahlke JD, Vrees RA, Rouse DJ. Trauma in pregnancy: an updated systematic review. *Am J Obstet Gynecol* 2013; **209**(1):1–10.

2. Shah KH, Simons RK, Holbrook T, et al. Trauma in pregnancy: maternal and fetal outcomes. *J Trauma* 1998; **45**(1):83–86.

3. Celso B, Tepas J, Langland-Orban B, et al. A systematic review and meta-analysis comparing outcome of severely injured patients treated in trauma centers following the establishment of trauma systems. *J Trauma* 2006; **60**(2):371–78.

4. Adult Major Trauma Decision Tree. 2015. Available at www.google.co.uk/search?q=London+Trauma+Office+and+London+Ambulance+Service+NHS+Trust+Major+Decision+Tree&client=safari&rls=en&biw=1289&bih=787&source=lnms&sa=X&ved=0CAYQ_AUoAGoVChMImsChveLnxwIV0xfbCh35WQ8S&dpr=2 (accessed August 2015).

5. Huber-Wagner S, Lefering R, Qvick LM, et al. Effect of whole-body CT during trauma resuscitation on survival: a retrospective, multicentre study. *Lancet* 2009; **373**: 1455–61.

6. Eastridge BJ, Salinas J, McManus JG, et al. Hypotension begins at 110 mmHg: redefining "hypotension" with data. *J Trauma* 2007; **63**:291–99.

7. Butcher M, Ip J, Bushby D, Yentis SM. Efficacy of cardiopulmonary resuscitation in the supine position with manual displacement of the uterus vs lateral tilt using a firm wedge: a manikin study. *Anaesthesia* 2014; **69**:868–71.

8. Frith D, Goslings JC, Gaardner C, et al. Definition and drivers of acute traumatic coagulopathy: clinical and experimental investigations. *J Thromb Haemost* 2010; **8**(9):1919–25.

9. Holcolmb JB, Tilley BC, Baraniuk S, et al. Transfusion of plasma, platelets, and red blood cells in a 1:1:1 vs a 1:1:2 ratio and mortality in patients with severe trauma. The PROPPR Randomized Clinical Trial. *JAMA* 2015; **313**(5):471–82.

10. Mallaiah S, Barclay P, Harrod I, Chevannes C, Bhalla A. Introduction of an algorithm for ROTEM-guided fibrinogen concentrate administration in major obstetric haemorrhage. *Anaesthesia* 2015; **70**:166–75.

11. CRASH-2 Trial Collaborators. Effects of tranexamic acid on death, vascular occlusive events, and blood transfusion in trauma patients with significant haemorrhage (CRASH-2): a randomised, placebo-controlled trial. *Lancet* 2010; **376**:23–32.

12. CRASH-2 Trial Collaborators. The importance of early treatment with tranexamic acid in bleeding trauma patients: an exploratory analysis of the CRASH-2 randomised controlled trial. *Lancet* 2011; **377**: 1096–101.

13. Eager R, Sutton J, Spedding R, et al. Use of anti-D immunoglobulin in maternal trauma. *Emerg Med J* 2003; **20**:498.

14. National Institute for Health and Clinical Excellence. Pregnancy: routine anti-D prophylaxis for RhD-negative women, 2008. Available at www.nice.org.uk/guidance/ta156/resources/guidance-routine-antenatal-antid-prophylaxis-for-women-who-are-rhesus-d-negative-pdf (accessed August 2015).

Ischemic Heart Disease and Myocardial Infarction in Pregnancy

Rachel Hignett and Lindzi Peacock

Case Study

A 42-year-old primigravida woman at 34 weeks' gestation presented to her local Emergency Department. She gave a history of severe central chest pain radiating to her left arm at rest for 1 hour requiring IV morphine analgesia. Significantly, she reported smoking 20 cigarettes per day since age 18, and her body mass index (BMI) at booking of antenatal care was 39 kg/m^2. There was a strong family history of ischemic heart disease (IHD). A 12-lead ECG demonstrated an acute ST-segment elevation myocardial infarction (STEMI) in the inferoposterior territory (Figure 45.1). Shortly after arrival, the patient suffered a ventricular fibrillation cardiac arrest. Cardiopulmonary resuscitation was commenced according to European Advanced Life Support guidelines. Two biphasic DC shocks at 150 J two minutes apart resulted in return of spontaneous circulation within 3 minutes. She recovered to a Glasgow Coma Scale score of 15 and was given 300 mg aspirin and 600 mg clopidogrel orally before being transferred unintubated with an anesthetic escort by ambulance to a tertiary interventional cardiology unit. She underwent percutaneous coronary intervention (PCI) through a radial artery approach. IV unfractionated heparin was given by infusion during the PCI. Occlusion of the proximal circumflex coronary artery was demonstrated: excellent flow was restored with balloon angioplasty and the use of a bare metal stent. Continuous fetal heart rate was monitored by cardiotocography (CTG) prior to transfer and was recommenced on arrival in the cardiac catheterization area. The CTG was reassuring, and the patient herself remained stable cardiovascularly throughout the procedure. Her chest pain and ST-segment elevation both resolved with coronary reperfusion, and she was transferred to the coronary care unit. Cardiac enzymes peaked at 29.2 µg/liter for troponin-I and 1340 units/liter for creatinine kinase. The patient was discharged home on day 5 on dual antiplatelet medication and twice-daily 25 mg metoprolol.

The remainder of her pregnancy was closely monitored by a multidisciplinary team of obstetricians, cardiologists, anesthetists, and midwives, who met to discuss her care every 1–2 weeks. ECG demonstrated good left ventricular function. However, concerns regarding fetal growth restriction based on abnormal umbilical artery Doppler flows prompted a Category III cesarean delivery at 37/40 weeks' gestation.

Cesarean delivery was carried out uneventfully under general anesthesia (GA) due to concerns about safety of regional anesthesia with clopidogrel, with invasive arterial blood pressure (IABP) monitoring. A 2.9-kg male baby was delivered in good condition. The patient was observed on the labor ward high-dependency unit (HDU) for 24 hours after delivery. Both mother and baby were discharged home on day 4 postnatally.

Key Points

- Myocardial infarction (MI) in women of childbearing age is a rare event.
- A woman presenting with severe chest pain needing potent IV opioid analgesia, such as morphine, should be investigated to rule out acute MI or other serious pathology.[1]
- Risk factors for MI and ischemic heart disease (IHD) in pregnancy include the typical risk factors for nonpregnant patients with IHD,[2] but pregnancy itself increases the risk of MI three- to fourfold.[3]
- The treatment of choice for coronary reperfusion is percutaneous coronary intervention.[4]
- A pregnant woman who has a history of IHD should be reviewed on a frequent basis by a multidisciplinary team.[3,4]
- A care plan should be agreed on in the third trimester to cover all aspects of perinatal care, including choice of anesthesia, if required.[3]

247

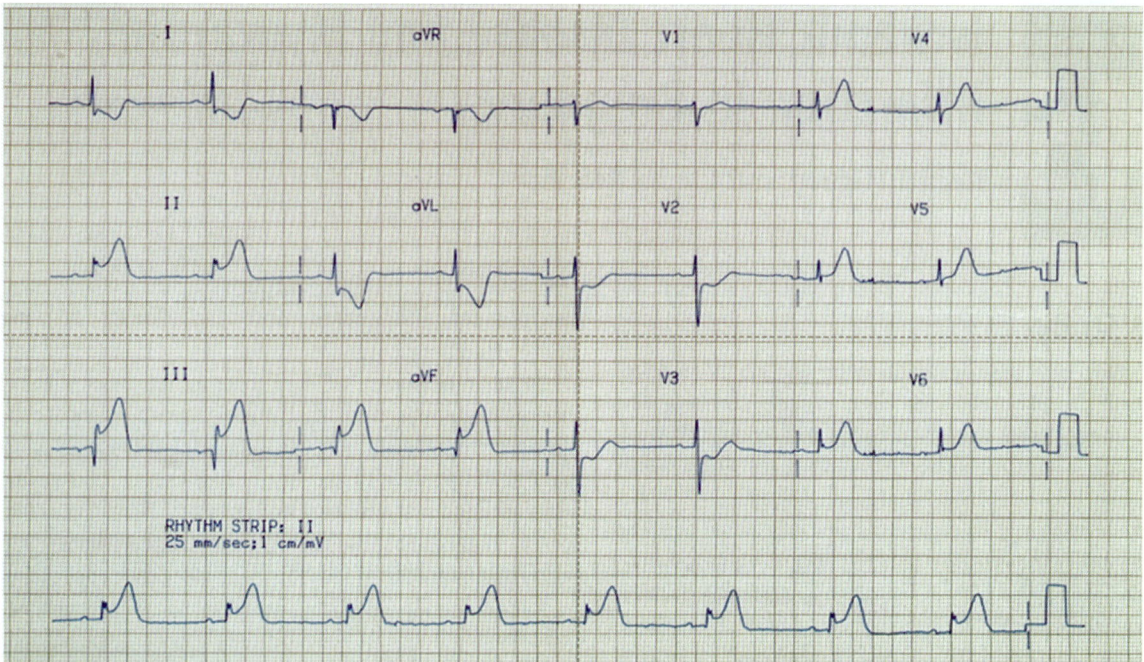

Figure 45.1 Twelve-lead ECG demonstrating acute inferoposterior STEMI

Discussion

Background

Worldwide, cardiac disease is a leading cause of death in many resource-rich countries.[3] In the United Kingdom, the most common cause of maternal death is cardiac disease, of which acquired conditions account for the majority.[5] In the recent UK Confidential Enquiry into Maternal Deaths, Saving Lives, Improving Mothers' Care,[5] there were 49 deaths from cardiac disease, with ischemic heart disease (IHD) accounting for 20 percent. These deaths were due to either an acute myocardial infarction (MI) or preexisting IHD, where death was presumed to be due to an arrhythmia or heart failure.

IHD is rare in women of childbearing age.[6] In the UK Obstetric Surveillance System (UKOSS) study of MI in pregnancy (2005–10), the incidence of MI complicating pregnancy or the first week postpartum was 0.7 per 100,000 maternities.[2] The rate of maternal and fetal demise is high following MI in pregnancy: maternal mortality rates between 5 and 11 percent have been reported, with most deaths occurring peri-infarct or in the peripartum period.[7–9] Fetal mortality is around 9–13 percent,[9] with most deaths occurring

in association with maternal death. The outcome of pregnancy in women who have suffered an MI before pregnancy may be better. In 2007, the European Registry on Pregnancy and Heart Disease was initiated by the European Society of Cardiology (ESC) to collect data on women with structural heart disease or IHD.[10] Between 2007 and 2011, pregnancy occurred in 20 women who had suffered an MI previously, with only one woman suffering a new acute coronary syndrome (ACS). Overall, a total of six women had ACS during pregnancy, and all of them survived.

Risk Factors

The risk factors for ACS in pregnancy are the same as those for the general population:[2]

- Diabetes mellitus
- Hypertension
- Obesity
- Smoking
- Family history
- Hypercholesterolemia

Advanced maternal age is a significant risk factor for MI. In the UKOSS study of MI in pregnancy, the mean age of women suffering an MI was 37 years compared with 29 years in the control group.[2] The risk of MI is 30 times greater in women over age 40 compared with those under 20 years of age.[3,7] This is a concerning observation in view of the increasing tendency of women in developed countries to delay having children.

Pregnancy itself increases the risk of ACS three- to fourfold.[3] Increased circulating blood volume and increased cardiac output in pregnancy result in an increase in myocardial oxygen demand. At the same time, the physiologic anemia and reduction in diastolic blood pressure reduce myocardial oxygen supply.[11] Blood vessel walls are more vulnerable to damage during pregnancy: shearing forces are increased, and blood vessel walls are weakened by elevated levels of estrogen and progesterone.[4] When these factors are combined with the prothrombotic state of pregnancy, clot formation and subsequent ischemia are more likely. Other pregnancy-specific risk factors identified by UKOSS include twin pregnancy and preeclampsia.[2]

Pathophysiology

ACS is usually the result of atherosclerotic plaque rupture or instability. When complicated by overlying thrombus formation, complete occlusion to blood flow may result, producing an MI. However, in pregnancy, this mechanism accounts for only 40–50 percent of cases of MI.[2,9,12] The other mechanisms contributing to MI are coronary dissection (16–27 percent), which is a rare event in the nonpregnant population at 1 percent or less, and coronary thrombus occurring in normal coronary arteries (6–21 percent), which is thought to occur from paradoxical embolism through a patent foramen ovale. Normal coronary arteries at angiography have been found in up to 29 percent of patients.[2,9,12]

Diagnosis

IHD may present as stable angina or as an acute coronary syndrome (ACS). ACS consists of three different clinical entities: unstable angina, non-ST-segment elevation MI (NSTEMI), and ST-segment elevation MI (STEMI). Patients with unstable angina may present with chest pain at rest or on minimal exertion but have no rise in cardiac enzymes or 12-lead ECG changes. NSTEMI patients have chest pain associated with raised cardiac enzymes, and the ECG may show ST-segment depression or T-wave changes.

Patients with STEMI typically have severe chest pain associated with elevated ST segments or new left bundle-branch block and raised cardiac enzymes.

In pregnant women, the diagnosis of ACS is the same as in nonpregnant patients, consisting of a triad of history and examination, 12-lead ECG, and troponin levels. STEMI is a clinical diagnosis and does not rely on waiting for cardiac enzyme results because this would delay prompt treatment. ACS may present atypically in pregnant women, making the diagnosis more challenging. Classic central crushing chest pain may be absent, and atypical symptoms such as abdominal or epigastric pain, vomiting, and dizziness may be attributed to pregnancy per se rather than ACS.[1] Previous recommendations from the Confidential Enquiries into Maternal Deaths in the UK recommend that any women who is suffering chest or epigastric pain severe enough to warrant opioid analgesia should have appropriate investigations to rule out cardiac disease.[1] The 12-lead ECG in pregnant women may also be more difficult to interpret because nonspecific ST-segment and T-wave changes may occur due to pregnancy.

The differential diagnoses for ACS in pregnancy are acute pulmonary embolism, preeclampsia, and aortic dissection. Echocardiography may be a useful tool to identify wall motion abnormalities suggestive of ischemia, and exercise treadmill testing can be performed in pregnancy, although this test has a high false-positive rate.[13] There have been no reported adverse effects from dobutamine stress echocardiography, and more recently cardiac MRI has been used in the second and third trimesters of pregnancy.[13] Coronary angiography can be both diagnostic and therapeutic (see below).

Management

The immediate management of ACS in pregnancy is the same as in the nonpregnant state, that is, high-flow oxygen, morphine analgesia with an antiemetic, and loading doses of aspirin 300 mg and clopidogrel 600 mg.[13]

Primary Percutaneous Coronary Intervention (PCI)

Patients presenting with STEMI require urgent coronary artery reperfusion.[4] PCI is preferred to thrombolysis with recombinant tissue plasminogen activator (rtPA) because it will differentiate between occluded, dissected, and normal coronary arteries.[4] PCI also has reduced bleeding complications compared with thrombolysis. However, there appears to be a general reluctance to perform angiography in pregnant women because in the UKOSS study only 60 percent of women presenting with MI underwent coronary angiography.[2] This appears to be due to concerns regarding radiation exposure to the fetus. However, this can be minimized by lead shielding, reducing the duration of screening, and using a radial or brachial approach. The risks to the fetus from radiation exposure are greatest in the first trimester because this is the peak time of organogenesis. After 20 weeks' gestation, the mother should have a left lateral tilt performed during the procedure to minimize aortocaval compression. Most reports of coronary artery stenting in pregnant women have used a bare metal stent (BMS) rather than drug-eluting stents (DESs).[4] The use of BMSs in pregnancy is preferred because dual antiplatelet therapy is required for a minimum of 1 month versus 12 months for DESs. BMSs undergo rapid endothelialization within this time frame. The cessation of antiplatelet drugs will reduce the risk of peripartum bleeding.

Thrombolysis

Thrombolysis has been used successfully for MI and should be considered if there is likely to be a significant delay to PCI.[4] Thrombolysis can result in subplacental hemorrhage. It is best avoided in the first few weeks postnatally due to the risk of hemorrhage. There are no data to support one thrombolytic agent over another in pregnancy, and the choice of agent should be based on local policy. Streptokinase is associated with a higher risk of allergic reactions and hypotension, whereas rtPA such as alteplase and reteplase is associated with marginally higher survival in nonpregnant patients but carries a greater risk of hemorrhage.[14]

In women presenting with NSTEMI, use of a risk scoring system such as TIMI (Thrombolysis in Myocardial Infarction) or GRACE (Global Registry of Acute Coronary Events), can help to identify women at higher risk who may benefit from early coronary angiography. Those at lower risk should be managed medically.

Medical Management

The medical management of IHD in pregnant women is limited compared with nonpregnant patients because some drugs are contraindicated.[13] Low-dose aspirin and beta-blockers are considered to be relatively safe for use in pregnancy and breastfeeding. Low-molecular-weight heparin should be given until at least 48 hours after the last episode of chest pain or dynamic ECG changes.[14] There is very little information relating to the safety of thienopyridines during pregnancy, and as a consequence, clopidogrel usage should be for a minimal duration in women who have undergone coronary stenting. Due to a lack of safety data and concerns about bleeding, glycoprotein IIb/IIIa antagonists (such as abciximab and tirofiban) are contraindicated. Calcium channel antagonists, nitrates, and nicorandil appear to be safe, but ACE inhibitors, angiotensin receptor blockers, renin antagonists, and statins are contraindicated during pregnancy due to their teratogenic effects.[4]

There is only limited evidence from case studies of emergency coronary artery bypass grafting during pregnancy, and these suggest that mortality rates for mother and fetus are high.[7,9]

Care during Pregnancy

Women with a history of IHD should receive preconceptual counseling from a cardiologist and an obstetrician.[3] The ESC advocates that pregnancy may be considered in women with no ongoing evidence of ischemia or left ventricular dysfunction.[4] General opinion recommends allowing 1 year following an ACS to allow for full recovery and repair of the myocardium.[14]

During pregnancy, women should be reviewed regularly by a multidisciplinary team (MDT).[3,4] The ESC recommends that women are risk assessed early in pregnancy against the Modified WHO Classification of Maternal Cardiovascular Risk, which includes the type of heart disease and functional status. Women who fall into low- to medium-risk categories (classes 1–2) may be seen infrequently during pregnancy; those falling into high- (class 3) and very-high-risk categories (in whom pregnancy is not recommended; class 4) should be seen once or twice per month by the MDT. A care plan to cover all aspects of labor and delivery should be decided on by the MDT and the patient in the third trimester.[3]

Management of Labor and Delivery

General goals in managing women with IHD during labor and delivery include

1. Minimizing the cardiovascular (CVS) work of labor and delivery by limiting surges in cardiac output and heart rate.
2. Monitoring fluid balance.
3. Avoiding aortocaval compression.
4. A low threshold for the use of invasive monitoring, most commonly IABP.
5. Reducing the risk of venous thromboembolism (VTE).

In general, vaginal delivery with epidural analgesia and an assisted second stage is the preferred mode of delivery.[3] Cesarean delivery (CD) is planned for women who have obstetric indications or women with severe heart disease who are thought to be unable to withstand the CVS stress of labor.

Compared with CD, assisted vaginal delivery (AVD) is associated with reduced blood loss, stress response, postpartum pulmonary complications, sepsis, and VTE.[4] Avoidance of pushing by the mother in the second stage by assisting the delivery with low-cavity forceps limits further increases in cardiac output. Slow, incremental epidural analgesia is advantageous because good analgesia limits surges in cardiac output due to pain. Other advantages include reduction of preload and afterload, titration of block height to limit sympathetic blockade, and ability to provide surgical anesthesia if required. Blood pressure, continuous ECG, and pulse oximetry should be monitored throughout labor, and supplemental oxygen should be given. Cardiac medications such as beta-blockers and aspirin should be continued. To reduce the risk of postpartum hemorrhage (PPH), active third-stage management should be used; an initial dose of 2–5 IU syntocinon infused slowly over 15–30 minutes avoids hemodynamic instability. This can be followed by 40 IU syntocinon infused over 4 hours if there are concerns regarding uterine tone or bleeding.

For CD, both risks and benefits of GA versus regional anesthesia (RA) need to be considered, and wishes and preferences of the mother and anesthetist should be taken into consideration. RA can be achieved using an epidural or a low-dose spinal component (e.g., 1.5 ml 0.5% heavy bupivacaine and 300 μg diamorphine) combined spinal-epidural (CSE). These regional techniques allow for slow titration of anesthesia aiming for cardiovascular stability. A single-shot spinal anesthetic is relatively contraindicated due to the rapid onset of sympathetic block. Additional advantages of RA are avoidance of complications of GA (i.e., failed

intubation, aspiration), reduced blood loss, and reduced risk of VTE. The cardiac depressant effect of GA drugs and the hemodynamic stress of intubation and extubation are also avoided. By contrast, a GA can also provide a hemodynamically stable anesthetic and will reduce perioperative anxiety in the mother, thereby attenuating catecholamine surges. GA will be required where anticoagulation or dual antiplatelet therapy precludes RA and where the mother is unable to lie flat.

The conduct of GA will require a modified rapid-sequence induction. This is commonly performed using either thiopentone or propofol as induction agents, suxamethonium or rocuronium 1 mg/kg to provide rapid paralysis, and an opioid such as 1 mg IV alfentanil to attenuate the hemodynamic response to intubation. Invasive monitoring, most commonly arterial monitoring, is advocated. Myocardial function, ventricular filling, and regional wall motion abnormalities can be directly observed by transesophageal echocardiography. Volatile anesthesia is usually used for maintenance of anesthesia. Again, 2–5 IU syntocinon given as third-stage management should be infused slowly over 15–30 minutes.

Good postoperative analgesia is required. This can be achieved by use of intrathecal or epidural opioids with or without continuation of the epidural for a period postoperatively. For women who have had GA, analgesia should be achieved with IV patient-controlled morphine or fentanyl in conjunction with transversus abdominis plane blocks. Some patients with heart disease having GA will benefit from having an epidural sited preinduction to provide analgesia postoperatively due to the beneficial reduction in preload and afterload.

Drug Protocol for Atonic Postpartum Hemorrhage

Drugs used in the management of atonic postpartum hemorrhage (PPH) may have profound CVS effects.[4] Where drug treatment options are limited, early recourse to obstetric interventions, such as Bakri balloons for uterine tamponade and B-Lynch uterine compression sutures, may be needed.

1. Oxytocin analogues (such as syntocinon) cause rapid reduction in systemic vascular resistance and myocardial contractility with reflex tachycardia. Bolus injection should be avoided: 2–5 IU can be slowly infused over 15–30 minutes.

3. Ergometrine causes coronary vasoconstriction and hypertension. It is generally contraindicated in significant cardiac disease.
4. Prostaglandin F_2 alpha-analogues (such as carboprost) cause smooth muscle contraction, bronchospasm, intrapulmonary shunting, hypoxemia, pulmonary and systemic hypertension, and pulmonary edema. They are generally contraindicated in significant cardiac disease.
5. Misoprostol commonly causes shivering and rarely causes hyperpyrexia.

Postnatal Care

The immediate postpartum period is a high-risk time for women with IHD due to rapid fluid redistribution, which can occur during delivery (e.g., up to 500 ml auto transfusion from the placenta) and the initial postnatal days. High-dependency-unit (HDU) or level 2 care for 1–2 days after delivery[4] will provide a safe environment in which to monitor the mother's cardiac status and fluid balance, optimize analgesia, observe vital signs. and encourage mobilization.

Learning Points

- Cardiac disease is a leading cause of maternal death worldwide.[3]
- Women presenting with severe chest pain requiring strong opioid analgesia should be fully investigated for MI.[1]
- PCI is the treatment of choice for STEMI in pregnant women.[4]
- Pregnant women with IHD should be cared for by a MDT (RCOG).
- A care plan for labor and delivery should be agreed on during the third trimester.[3]
- AVD with incremental epidural analgesia is the preferred mode of delivery.[3,4]
- The relative risks and benefits of GA versus RA for CD need to be considered on an individual basis.

References

1. Centre for Maternal and Child Enquiries (CMACE). Saving mothers' lives: reviewing maternal deaths to make motherhood safer: 2006–2008. The Eighth Report on Confidential Enquiries into Maternal Deaths in the United Kingdom. *BJOG* 2011; **118**:1–203.

2. Bush N, Nelson-Piercy C, Spark P, et al. Myocardial infarction in pregnancy and postpartum in the UK. *Eur J Prevent Cardiol* 2013; **20**:12–20.

3. Royal College of Obstetricians and Gynaecologists. *Cardiac Disease and Pregnancy* (Good Practice No. 13). London: RCOG; June 2011.

4. Regitz-Zagrosek V, Lundquist CB, Borghi C, et al. ESC guidelines on the management of cardiovascular diseases during pregnancy. *Eur Heart J* 2011; **32**:3147–97.

5. Knight M, Tuffnell D, Kenyon S, et al. on behalf of MBRRACE-UK, eds. Saving lives, improving mother's care: surveillance of maternal death in the UK 2011–13 and lessons learned to inform maternity care from the UK and Ireland Confidential Enquiries into Maternal Deaths and Morbidity 2009–13, National Perinatal Epidemiology Unit, University of Oxford, Oxford.

6. Centers for Disease Control and Prevention. Prevalence of coronary heart disease US, Morb*id* Mortal Weekly Rep, October 14, 2011. Available at www.cdc.gov/mmwr/preview/mmwrhtml/mm6040a1.htm (accessed May 7, 2015).

7. James AH, Jamison MG, Biswas MS, et al. Acute myocardial infarction in pregnancy: a United States population-based study. *Circulation* 2006; **113**:1564–71.

8. Ladner HE, Danielson B, Gilbert WM. Acute myocardial infarction in pregnancy and the puerperium: a population-based study. *Obstet Gynecol* 2005; **105**:480–84.

9. Roth A, Elkayam U. Acute myocardial infarction associated with pregnancy. *J Am Coll Cardiol* 2008; **52**:171–80.

10. Roos-Hesselink JW, Ruys TP, Stein JI, et al. Outcome of pregnancy in patients with structural or ischaemic heart disease: results of a registry of the European Society of Cardiology. *Eur Heart J* 2013; **34**:657–65.

11. Kealey AJ. Coronary artery disease and myocardial infarction in pregnancy: a review of epidemiology, diagnosis and medical and surgical management. *Can J Cardiol* 2010; **26**:e185–89.

12. Roth A, Elkayam U. Acute myocardial infarction associated with pregnancy. *Ann Intern Med* 1996; **125**:751–62.

13. Fryearson J, Adamson DL. Heart disease in pregnancy: ischaemic heart disease. *Best Pract Res Clin Obstet Gynaecol* 2014; **28**:551–62.

14. Adamson DL, Dhanjal MK, Nelson-Piercy C. Ischaemic heart disease, in Adamson D, Dhanjal M, Nelson-Piercy C, eds., *Heart Disease in Pregnancy*. Oxford: Oxford University Press; 2011, pp. 57–76.

Intracranial Lesions in Pregnancy

Roulhac D. Toledano and Lisa Leffert

Case Study

A 31-year-old gravida 1, para 0 woman with a recently diagnosed intracranial mass presented for planned cesarean delivery at 37 weeks' gestation. On admission, she denied headache, nausea, vomiting, seizure activity, visual changes, and altered level of consciousness. A recent MRI confirmed a 2 × 3 cm lesion consistent with low-grade glioma in the anterior frontal lobe without mass effect. The patient's medical history was otherwise unremarkable.

The patient requested to be "awake" during the procedure, and a spinal anesthetic was administered on first attempt with a small-gauge atraumatic needle at the L3–L4 interspace after consultation with her neurosurgeon. A T4 surgical level was attained, and a healthy boy was delivered without incident. The patient underwent surgical resection of the glioma (WHO grade II) under general anesthesia 3 weeks later, followed by radiation therapy and chemotherapy.

Key Points

- This patient with a known intracranial lesion requested regional anesthesia for her planned cesarean delivery.
- Concern for herniation after deliberate or accidental dural puncture (ADP) is often cited as a reason to avoid neuraxial techniques in parturients with intracranial tumors or vascular lesions, even in the absence of clinical and radiographic evidence of increased intracranial pressure.[1]

This patient had an uneventful spinal anesthetic after a multidisciplinary discussion about her care.

Discussion

Neuraxial anesthesia is considered the technique of choice for cesarean delivery, when feasible, for several reasons, including improved pain management and maternal satisfaction, avoidance of volatile agent–induced uterine relaxation and fetal depression, prevention of intraoperative recall in a high-risk patient population, reduced fetal exposure to the potentially toxic effects of general anesthetics,[2] and avoidance of instrumentation of the parturient's airway. It also allows the patient and her partner to experience the birth of their child. More broadly, the increased use of neuraxial techniques for labor and delivery has been associated with a reduction in airway and aspiration-related morbidity and mortality in serial obstetric safety audits.[3]

However, the use of spinal or epidural anesthesia for cesarean delivery is not without risks, including the possibility of block failure with subsequent conversion to general anesthesia, high or total spinal, postdural puncture headache (PDPH) in a population at increased risk for this untoward complication, and the less common risks of nerve damage, epidural hematoma, and infection. In patients with clinically significant intracranial pathology, the initiation of neuraxial anesthesia may also carry the risk of significant brain tissue shifts (i.e., herniation) after dural puncture.

Case-by-case assessment by the obstetric anesthesiologist and neurologist or neurosurgeon of the risk of neurologic deterioration with spinal or epidural anesthesia and analgesia in parturients with intracranial lesions is strongly recommended. Although many factors should be taken into consideration, appropriate neuroimaging and knowledge of the following lesion characteristics are paramount: the type of intracranial lesion; its size, location, and growth rate; whether it obstructs CSF flow at or above the foramen magnum; and whether it causes intracranial tissue shifts. This information is required to properly assess the risks of neuraxial or general anesthesia in these patients and to plan accordingly.

Lesion Size, Location, and Growth Rate

Not all intracranial lesions place the patient at risk for complications from neuraxial analgesia and

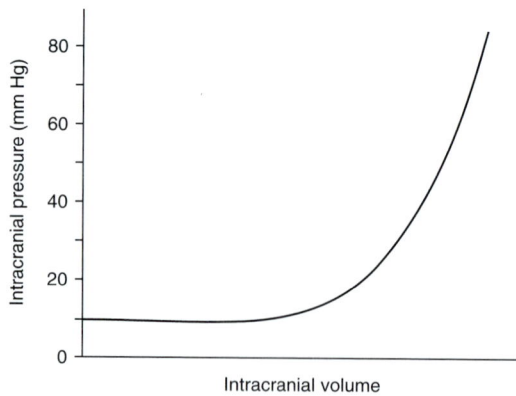

Figure 46.1 Intracranial compliance curve

anesthesia. In this Case Study, the tumor is small, without significant mass effect. Its location in an area remote from the foramen magnum and CSF pathways reduces the risks of partial or complete foramen magnum obstruction or ventricular compression, permitting translocation of the CSF from the cranium to the spinal part of the neuraxis after dural puncture. By contrast, intracranial lesions that impede the free flow of CSF and cause obstructive (or noncommunicating) hydrocephalus, such as those located in the posterior fossa, near the third ventricle or cerebral aqueduct, or at the foramen magnum, can place a patient at significant risk of herniation. Similarly, large or fast-growing intracranial lesions exert mass effect and displace the intracranial contents around them; brain tissue rather than CSF will be displaced caudally if there is a sudden loss of CSF from a lumbar dural puncture.

The Monro-Kellie doctrine provides the explanation for these assertions: the total intracranial volume (comprised of brain tissue, CSF, and cerebral blood volume) remains constant within the noncompliant bony skull. This means that an increase in the volume of one element causes a compensatory decrease in the volume of another. If the intracranial volume increases because of a small, remotely located intracranial lesion, the intracranial pressure remains relatively unchanged as long as CSF can be displaced caudally (Figure 46.1). However, once this compensatory mechanism is exhausted or can no longer function because of obstruction, even a small increase in volume from peritumoral edema or bleeding or from a transient increase in intracranial blood or

Table 46.1 Signs and Symptoms of Elevated Intracranial Pressure

- Headache
- Drowsiness
- Nausea and vomiting
- New-onset seizures
- Decreased level of consciousness
- Papilledema
- Pupillary changes
- Focal neurologic signs

CSF (with physiologic maneuvers such as coughing, vomiting, gagging, or Valsalva) will cause an increase in ICP.

In this patient's case, the small, slow-growing tumor in the frontal lobe without clinical or radiographic evidence of CSF obstruction or significant mass effect presents a low likelihood of herniation after dural puncture. Therefore, it may be reasonable to proceed with spinal anesthesia with a small-gauge needle, preferably after consultation with a neurologic expert. Even a dural puncture with a large-gauge epidural needle would most likely result in normal flow of CSF rather than herniation of brain tissue in this setting. Similarly, the transient increase in ICP associated with epidural catheter dosing should also be well tolerated (see below).

Role of Elevated Intracranial Pressure

This patient is unlikely to have elevated ICP because she lacks suggestive clinical signs and symptoms (Table 46.1) and radiologic findings. Nonetheless, elevated ICP is not necessarily associated with increased risk of herniation after deliberate or unintentional dural puncture. Increased ICP is seen in the pathologic condition pseudotumor cerebri, which, by definition, is characterized by the absence of an intracranial lesion. Because there is no obstruction to CSF flow and no baseline intracranial-intraspinal pressure gradient, repeated lumbar punctures are not only safe but also therapeutic. There are also several examples of physiologic and pathologic increases in ICP that are well tolerated. Both the cardiac and respiratory cycles, for example, are marked by a transient increase in ICP, followed by rapid reequilibration.[4] During pregnancy, transient increases in ICP have been documented during the second stage of labor, in particular when the parturient is bearing down. A similar phenomenon has been observed during injection of medication into the lumbar epidural space, when CSF is displaced upward into the intracranial compartment.[5]

Conversely, normal ICP does not necessarily ensure the safety of neuraxial techniques. Some patients with normal ICP may have underlying conditions that can predispose them to herniation after dural puncture. Parturients with Arnold-Chiari malformation, for example, pose a particular challenge to the obstetric anesthesiologist. Patients with the most common form, type I, may be asymptomatic, have normal ICP, or even be undiagnosed at the time of presentation despite low-lying cerebellar tonsils. By contrast, there may be a component of obstruction or severe crowding at the foramen magnum. In patients without these severe features or who have been surgically corrected, it can be safe to proceed with neuraxial techniques after appropriate neurologic consultation. However, if they develop a PDPH, expert consultation and early blood patch should be strongly considered because a persistent CSF leak can result in further cerebellar descent and neurologic deterioration.

Is There a Preferred Neuraxial Technique?

A common misconception about neuraxial anesthesia in parturients with intracranial pathology is that a small dural puncture with a spinal needle is acceptable if there are concerns about herniation in the setting of an ADP with a large-gauge epidural needle. While CSF loss may be of shorter duration through smaller dural puncture sites[6] and with the use of pencil-point versus cutting needles, studies have demonstrated that persistent CSF leakage can occur after spinal anesthetics in both these scenarios.[7] Another misconception is that an epidural technique is a safe alternative when an intentional dural puncture with a small-gauge spinal needle is considered to be too risky. Unfortunately, even in experienced hands, the incidence of ADP may be as high as 1 percent. In addition, epidural dosing itself can increase ICP, particularly in patients with baseline elevated ICP.

In summary, if a spinal technique is considered to be too dangerous in a patient with clinically significant intracranial pathology, then an epidural technique is also likely not advisable. If a general anesthetic is selected, then care must be taken to avoid increases in ICP (see below).

Risks and Benefits of General Anesthesia

Performing a general anesthetic in a parturient with a clinically significant intracranial lesion is not without risks. In addition to the usual challenges of the parturient (e.g., weight gain, airway swelling, reduced functional residual capacity, and increased oxygen consumption), these patients can develop an acute deterioration in neurologic status from increases in ICP during tracheal intubation and extubation and during episodes of hypoxia, hypercarbia, coughing, and valsalva. The preservation of adequate maternal cerebral perfusion pressure is vital in this setting; the use of adjuncts to induction agents (e.g., remifentanil), modest hyperventilation, and osmotic agents (e.g., furosemide and mannitol) is generally considered to be safe if needed.

Intracranial Vascular Pathology

The anesthetic management of parturients with intracranial arterial or venous pathology requires a precise understanding of the type of vascular abnormality (e.g., arterial malformation, aneurysm, venous thrombosis, moyamoya syndrome) and its likelihood of peripartum rupture. Multidisciplinary consultation with the obstetrician and the neurologic or neurosurgical expert is needed to determine the mode of delivery (vaginal or cesarean) and anesthetic management. Although, historically, pregnant patients with unruptured brain aneurysms have been counseled against vaginal delivery, a recent retrospective study found that the expulsive efforts associated with labor did not increase the risk of aneurysmal subarachnoid hemorrhage.[8]

Anesthetic considerations for cesarean delivery in parturients with intracranial vascular malformations (e.g., arteriovenous malformations, brain aneurysms) include whether the lesion is stable, the type and timing of additional surgical intervention, and whether the patient has experienced a recent intracranial hemorrhage. For stable patients who do not require simultaneous aneurysm repair, a neuraxial technique is appropriate, provided that extreme fluctuations in blood pressure are avoided. General anesthesia, often with a total IV technique, is commonly performed for combination procedures (craniotomy, embolization, and cesarean delivery). In cases of recent intracranial hemorrhage from either an aneurysm or an arteriovenous malformation, maintenance of strict hemodynamic stability is paramount, as is ascertaining the likelihood of the lesion creating a mass effect or obstruction to CSF flow. Overall, a case-by-case approach to the anesthetic management of patients with intracranial vascular lesions is recommended, with input from obstetric, neonatal, neurosurgical, and neurologic team members.

Learning Points

- Newly diagnosed brain tumors or other intracranial lesions are relatively rare during pregnancy but, when present, provide challenges for anesthesia providers.
- Case-by-case assessment by the obstetric anesthesiologist in consultation with a neurologist or neurosurgeon of the risk of neurologic deterioration with neuraxial procedures in parturients with intracranial lesions is strongly recommended.
- The presence of an intracranial lesion does not necessarily mean (a) increased ICP and (b) high risk of herniation after deliberate or unintentional dural puncture.
- Neuraxial anesthesia and analgesia may be appropriate in the presence of an intracranial lesion that is not associated with mass effect or CSF obstruction at or above the foramen magnum.
- An epidural technique *should not be considered a safe alternative* if a spinal technique is considered too risky.
- If a general anesthetic is indicated, adjuncts to induction medications, osmotic agents, and mild to moderate hyperventilation can be used safely during cesarean delivery.

References

1. Leffert LR, Schwamm LH. Neuraxial anesthesia in parturients with intracranial pathology: a comprehensive review and reassessment of risk. *Anesthesiology* 2013; **119**: 703–18.

2. Jevtovic-Todorovic V. Functional implications of an early exposure to general anesthesia: are we changing the behavior of our children? *Mol Neurobiol* 2013; **48**:288–93.

3. Ngan Kee WD. Confidential enquiries into maternal death: 50 years of closing the loop. *Br J Anaesth* 2005; **94**: 413–16.

4. Heiss JD, Patronas N, DeVroom HL, et al. Elucidating the pathophysiology of syringomyelia. *J Neurosurg* 1999; **91**:553–62.

5. Hilt H, Gramm HJ, Link J. Changes in intracranial pressure associated with extradural anaesthesia. *Br J Anaesth* 1986; **58**:676–80.

6. Cruickshank RH, Hopkinson JM. Fluid flow though dural puncture sites: an in vitro comparison of needle point types. *Anaesthesia* 1989; **44**:415–18.

7. Ready LB, Cuplin S, RH. Haschke, et al. Spinal needle determinants of rate of transdural fluid leak. *Anesth Analg* 1989; **69**:457–60.

8. Tiel Groenestege AT, Rinkel GJ, van der Bom JG, et al. The risk of aneurysmal subarachnoid hemorrhage during pregnancy, delivery, and the puerperium in the Utrecht population: case-crossover study and standardized incidence ratio estimation. *Stroke* 2009; **40**:1148–51.

Sepsis in Obstetrics

Gabriela Frunza and Nuala Lucas

Case Study

A multiparous woman at 37 weeks' gestation was admitted to the delivery suite for induction of labor. She had ruptured her membranes 24 hours previously, but labor had not begun. She was induced with a syntocinon infusion and received an epidural for labor analgesia.

Two hours after the onset of labor, she developed a pyrexia and low-grade tachycardia. Her labor progressed uneventfully, and she delivered vaginally but suffered a postpartum hemorrhage of 1000 ml secondary to uterine atony.

The day after delivery, the patient complained of feeling tired and had abdominal pain but was keen to be discharged because she had another child at home.

The community midwife reviewed her the day after discharge (day 2 postpartum). She was noted to have a tachycardia of 110 beats/min, a temperature of 37.9°C (100.2°F), and her abdominal pain had worsened. She was advised to return to the maternity unit immediately.

On admission to the labor ward, clinical examination noted that in addition to the tachycardia and pyrexia, the patient was also tachypnea, with a respiratory rate of 22 breaths/min. The medical team assessed her urgently. A diagnosis of sepsis was made, and an abdominal ultrasound scan confirmed the presence of retained products of conception in her uterus. IV antibiotics and fluid resuscitation were started immediately. She underwent surgical removal of the retained products of conception, and she made a full recovery.

Key Points

- This patient had documented risk factors for sepsis (premature rupture of membranes, pyrexia in labor).
- The diagnosis of sepsis was initially delayed.

- When the diagnosis was made, prompt treatment including antibiotics and removal of the septic focus lead to a good outcome.

Discussion

Sepsis in obstetrics is an important cause of maternal mortality and morbidity worldwide and accounts for 11 percent of all maternal deaths.[1] The UK maternal mortality rate from sepsis almost tripled between 1980 and 2008.[2] In the United States, a retrospective analysis of almost 45 million hospitalizations for delivery between 1998 and 2008 demonstrated that sepsis complicated 1 per 3,333 deliveries, with severe sepsis complicating approximately 1 per 11,000 deliveries.[3] Sepsis in obstetrics is associated with significant morbidity, including fetal demise, organ failure, chronic pelvic inflammatory disease, bilateral tubal occlusion, and infertility. Early recognition and timely response are keys to ensuring a good outcome.

Risk Factors

A number of risk factors are associated with an increased risk of developing sepsis in obstetrics (Table 47.1). These may be broadly divided into intrinsic patient factors and obstetric factors. Obese women are twice as likely to develop obstetric sepsis as normal weight women.[4] Although relatively infrequent in pregnancy, chronic comorbid conditions such as congestive heart failure, chronic liver disease, and chronic renal disease are risk factors for sepsis in the general population, and these associations have been demonstrated in pregnancy as well.[3] Women with systemic lupus erythematosus are also at risk of developing sepsis, likely as a result of the immunologic effects of the disease itself but also secondary to the use of steroids and immunosuppressive medications. Although women with these conditions are a relatively small proportion of obstetric patients, the magnitude of risk associated with these conditions

Table 47.1 Risk Factors for Sepsis in Obstetrics

Obstetric factors
• Invasive intrauterine procedures (e.g., amniocentesis)
• Cervical suture
• Prolonged rupture of membranes (rupture prior to labor at or after 37 weeks' gestation)
• Prolonged labor with multiple (>5) vaginal examinations
• Vaginal trauma
• Cesarean delivery or operative vaginal delivery
• Retained products of conception after miscarriage or delivery

Patient factors
• Obesity
• Impaired glucose tolerance/diabetes
• Impaired immunity (e.g., immunosuppressive therapy)
• Anemia
• Chronic comorbid conditions (e.g., renal/hepatic/cardiac disease)
• History of pelvic infection

Table 47.2 Causes of Sepsis in Obstetrics

Obstetric causes	
Genital tract causes	**Non-genital tract causes**
Chorioamnionitis	Renal tract infection
Endometritis	Mastitis/breast abscess
Septic abortion	Septic pelvic thrombophlebitis
Wound infection following cesarean delivery/ episiotomy/vaginal tear	

Nonobstetric causes
Pneumonia
Human immunodeficiency virus
Tuberculosis
Malaria

prompts early consideration of the diagnosis and treatment of sepsis in patients with these conditions.

Causes of Sepsis in Obstetrics

The causes of sepsis in obstetrics may be divided into obstetric and other causes (Table 47.2). Sepsis can arise at any time during pregnancy, labor, and the postpartum period, and the cause may vary depending on the stage of pregnancy. In early pregnancy, the most common causes of sepsis are septic abortion and termination of pregnancy.

Surgical intervention, in particular cesarean delivery, is one of the most important risk factors for the development of sepsis in obstetrics. Women undergoing cesarean delivery have a 5- to 20-fold greater risk for infection and infectious morbidity compared with a vaginal birth.[5] It has been shown that the risk of postpartum infection within 30 days of delivery for women delivered by cesarean delivery (elective and emergency) was 7.6 percent versus 1.6 percent for women who had a vaginal delivery.[6] Following emergency cesarean delivery, there is a nearly 50 percent higher risk of postpartum wound infection compared with elective cesarean delivery. The use of prophylactic antibiotics before surgical incision is therefore recommended.[7,8] A Cochrane review found that prophylactic antibiotics in women undergoing cesarean delivery substantially reduced the incidence of febrile morbidity, wound infection, endometritis, and serious maternal infectious complications.[5] However, even with prophylactic antibiotics, infection remains a significant risk in women who deliver by cesarean delivery.

Pregnant women are more vulnerable to urinary tract infection, which can lead to sepsis. In pregnancy, there is decreased peristalsis of the ureters, increased bladder capacity, and urinary stasis caused by progesterone-induced smooth muscle relaxation. In addition, as a result of the mechanical effects of the gravid uterus, there may be renal pelvic and ureteric dilatation.[9,10]

Mastitis affects up to 20 percent of postpartum women but is comparatively rare as a cause of postpartum sepsis. It has been estimated that up to a third of women admitted with mastitis develop breast abscess that requires surgical drainage.[11]

Pneumonia is one of the leading causes of sepsis arising in the antepartum period and is associated with significant morbidity and mortality. In the United Kingdom, it is the most common reason for admission to intensive care for pregnant women.[12] Comorbidities in pregnancy including asthma, cardiac disease and obesity increase the risk of developing pneumonia. In pregnant women who develop pneumonia, there is a higher rate of maternal and fetal complications such as respiratory failure and pneumothorax, intrauterine growth retardation and in utero death; preterm delivery may be required to improve maternal respiratory function.[13,14]

The specific physiologic respiratory changes of pregnancy predispose the parturient with pneumonia to rapid desaturation and a reduced ability to compensate for the development of a metabolic acidosis. The differential diagnosis of pneumonia in pregnancy includes pulmonary embolus and pulmonary edema. Pregnancy does not exclude the use of chest radiography, which can assist with diagnosis. The consequences of viral pneumonia in pregnancy have been particularly topical in recent years as a result of the H1N1 flu pandemic. Women in pregnancy and the post-partum period are known to be at higher risk of complications of seasonal flu than the non-pregnant population. In previous flu pandemics, pregnant women had significantly higher mortality and morbidity rates, and this effect was seen in the 2009 pandemic.[15] Although the use of neuraminidase inhibitors has not been demonstrated to be beneficial in the non-obstetric population, there is good observational evidence that pregnant women may benefit from these drugs. A pregnant woman in whom influenza is suspected should be started on these drugs without delay, and pregnant women should be encouraged to receive seasonal influenza vaccination.[16]

Microbiology

The genitourinary tract is colonized with a wide variety of organisms, but not all of these will cause infection and sepsis. One of the most important organisms associated with obstetric sepsis in recent years has been Group A streptococcus. It has been estimated that in the developed world, between 5–30 percent of the community are asymptomatic carriers of Group A streptococci, usually on the skin or in the throat. In the UK Confidential Maternal Death Enquries of 2006–8, several of the women who died had a history of a recent upper respiratory tract infection and/or contact with young children.[2] It is thought that following contact with Group A streptococcus, these women autoinoculate themselves through contamination of the perineum, and the organism then ascends leading to systemic infection. The presence of upper respiratory tract symptoms should alert the clinician to the possibility of Group A streptococcus or influenza as a possible diagnosis. If a woman has a sore throat, the Centor criteria are useful to predict bacterial infection.[17] The presence of three or four of the following signs suggests that a woman may have a bacterial infection and would benefit from antibiotics:

- Tonsillar exudate
- Tender anterior cervical lymphadenopathy or lymphadenitis

- Fever
- An absence of cough

Other important microorganisms include *Escherichia coli, Meningococcus, Staphylococcus, Streptococcus pneumonia*, and *Pseudomonas*. Of particular concern is sepsis arising as a result of Extended-Spectrum-Beta-Lactamase-producing organisms.[18] Extended-Spectrum-Beta-Lactamases (ESBLs) are enzymes that can be produced by bacteria that make them resistant to third-generation cephalosporins commonly used for the treatment of serious infections. ESBL-producing organisms occur principally in *Enterobacter* species, *E. coli, Klebsiella pneumoniae*, and *Proteus mirabilis* (all recognized causes of obstetric sepsis).

One of the most important factors in obstetric sepsis, particularly in the undeveloped world, is the HIV/AIDS pandemic.[19] Pregnant women with HIV/AIDS are more susceptible to sepsis and postoperative complications. Many opportunistic infections associated with HIV/AIDS may complicate pregnancy and cause maternal mortality. Pregnant women with HIV/AIDS are more susceptible to infection, and in addition, infections such as *Pneumocystis jirovecii* (previously *carinii*) pneumonia have a more aggressive course during pregnancy, with an increase in both morbidity and mortality. The most significant infection contributing to maternal mortality in HIV-infected women is tuberculosis (which is the most common opportunistic infection associated with HIV in the undeveloped world). It has been estimated that maternal mortality in HIV-infected women is 6.2 times greater than in HIV-negative women.

Clinical Presentation and Diagnosis

Sepsis is initially a clinical diagnosis, and microbiologic investigations may be negative. There is overlap between the clinical features of sepsis (Table 47.3) and the physiologic changes of pregnancy (particularly around the time of delivery), and therefore diagnosis can be difficult. Sepsis can develop and progress rapidly, but it also can develop more slowly with nonspecific features. The clinician must rely on a high index of clinical suspicion. Early warning scores (physiologic track and trigger systems) are widely used in non-obstetric patients, and their use is recommended in obstetrics. There is currently no widely accepted validated early warning system for use in obstetrics. There is difficulty identifying appropriate physiologic triggers because of the altered physiology of pregnancy, and there is a high false-positive

Table 47.3 Clinical Features of Obstetric Sepsis

General	Specific
Fever	Premature contractions
Upper respiratory tract symptoms	Abdominal pain
Diarrhea and vomiting	Mastitis
Shortness of breath	Uterine atony associated with hemorrhage
Mottled skin	Wound infection
Confusion, mental changes	Vaginal discharge
Signs and laboratory findings	
Pyrexia or hypothermia, <36°C	
Tachycardia	
Tachypnea	
Decreased urine output	
Elevated white cell count or low white cell count/neutropenia	
Rising C-reactive protein (CRP)	
Lactic acidosis	

Table 47.4 Hour-1 Surviving Sepsis Campaign Bundle of Care

- Measure lactate level; remeasure if initial lactate ≥ 2 mmol/L
- Take blood cultures before giving antibiotics
- Give broad spectrum IV antibiotics
- Rapidly give 30ml/kg crystalloid for hypotension (or lactate ≥ 4mmol/L)
- Give vasopressors (during or after fluid resuscitation) to keep MAP ≥ 65mmHg

Surviving Sepsis Campaign guidelines.[21] The Hour-1 Surviving Sepsis Campaign Bundle of Care (Table 47.4) is a recently updated initial resuscitation bundle designed to offer basic intervention within the first hour.[22] In a prospective observational study, it has been demonstrated to reduce sepsis-associated mortality by as much as 50 percent.[23] The principles of management for the septic obstetric patient follow the same principles as for any septic patient: initial resuscitation, identification and treatment/removal of the source of sepsis, and management of complications such as hypotension and tissue hypoxia.

The objective of fluid resuscitation is to restore adequate oxygen delivery to peripheral tissues. Hemodynamic optimization before the development of secondary organ failure reduces morbidity and mortality. Even in early sepsis, some degree of fluid resuscitation is likely to be required. Obstetric patients are generally young with robust cardiovascular physiology, but it is of concern that deaths secondary to the effects of fluid overload have been reported in the obstetric population. There are various reasons why the obstetric patient may be vulnerable to fluid overload: the physiologic changes of pregnancy can predispose to volume overload because the parturient is already in a relatively volume overloaded state; she may have comorbidity such as preeclampsia and have received uterotonic drugs (e.g., oxytocin or carboprost) that can further predispose to fluid retention or pulmonary edema. It may be appropriate to use additional monitoring when fluid resuscitating a septic obstetric patient.

There is overwhelming evidence about the importance of starting antibiotic therapy as soon as possible after diagnosis, ideally within 1 hour of diagnosis (the "golden hour"). Delay in the initiation of antibiotic therapy is associated with increased mortality and has consistently been cited as an area of substandard care in successive UK Confidential Maternal Death Enquiries. Causes of delay include errors in administration, prescription errors, patients awaiting senior review, and patients being transferred between departments;

rate. However, work in this area is ongoing, and these systems are likely to be important in the detection of obstetric critical illness in the future.

A careful history should aim to elicit features of localized symptoms and clarify the possible source of infection; the presenting features vary depending on the source of infection. The uteroplacental circulation does not exhibit autoregulation, so fetal perfusion and oxygenation depend on the well-being of the maternal cardiovascular system; any disturbance can lead to compromised fetal perfusion, and a septic woman may present with an abnormal fetal heart rate pattern or intrauterine fetal death. Investigations should include laboratory analysis of hematologic indices (full blood count and clotting screen), renal and hepatic assessment (urea and electrolytes and liver function tests) and C-reactive protein and lactate measurement (as an indicator of organ dysfunction). Blood should be sent for culture and other samples sent for culture as guided by the clinical history. Recent publications on the definition of sepsis may lead to further changes in management in the future.[20]

Management

Recommendations from the Royal College of Obstetricians and Gynaecologists (RCOG) are that sepsis should be managed in accordance with the

Table 47.5 Antibiotic Dos and Don'ts

- Start urgently.
- Use adequate doses given intravenously, not via the oral route.
- Seek senior microbiologic advice as soon as possible.
- Daily clinical review to check response.
- Don't delay starting antibiotics while waiting for microbiology results.
- Don't stop antibiotics too soon; pelvic infection may require several days of treatment.

strenuous efforts must be made to avoid such delays. Broad-spectrum antibiotics should be used initially and because of the polymicrobial nature of the genitourinary tract, two or more agents may be needed, at least until a pathogen has been identified. Urgent microbiologic advice should be sought as soon as possible, but this should not delay starting antibiotics. A list of antibiotic dos and don'ts is provided in Table 47.5.

The management of sepsis arising in the antenatal period is complicated by the presence of the fetus; in this situation, maternal resuscitation is the key to ensuring fetal well-being. Attempting early delivery in women with cardiovascular compromise due to sepsis may increase maternal and fetal mortality and can be extremely technically challenging if the woman is in the Intensive Care unit (ICU). The only exception is when intrauterine infection is suspected as the source of sepsis; then delivery must be expedited. Other features that may indicate that delivery is appropriate include rapid maternal deterioration, difficulty with mechanical ventilation due to the gravid uterus, multiorgan failure, and fetal compromise.[24]

Learning Points

- The diagnosis of sepsis in obstetrics may be difficult as the physiological changes of pregnancy can mask the pathophysiology of sepsis. A high index of suspicion is required
- There is good evidence that the use of sepsis bundles can improve outcomes in the management of sepsis
- A key component of the sepsis bundle is the timely administration of antibiotics, which should be given within 1 hour of diagnosis.

References

1. www.who.int/mediacentre/factsheets/fs348/en/ (accessed June 2015).

2. Centre for Maternal and Child Enquiries (CMACE). Saving mothers' lives: reviewing maternal deaths to make motherhood safer: 2006–2008. The Eighth Report on Confidential Enquiries into Maternal Deaths in the United Kingdom. *BJOG* 2011; **118**(suppl. 1):1–203.

3. Bauer ME, Bateman BT, Bauer ST, Shanks AM, Mhyre JM. Maternal sepsis mortality and morbidity during hospitalization for delivery: temporal trends and independent associations for severe sepsis. *Anesth Analg* 2013; **117**:944–50.

4. Acosta CD, Bhattacharya S, Tuffnell D, Kurinczuk JJ, Knight M. Maternal sepsis: a Scottish population-based case–control study *BJOG* 2012; **119**:474–83.

5. Smaill FM, Gyte GML. Antibiotic prophylaxis versus no prophylaxis for preventing infection after cesarean section. *Cochrane Database Syst Rev* 2010; (**10**):CD007452.

6. Leth RA, Moller JK, Thomsen RW, Uldbjerg N, Norgaard M. Risk of selected postpartum infections after cesarean section compared with vaginal birth: a five-year cohort study of 32,468 women. *Acta Obstet Gynaecol Scand* 2009; **88**: 976–83.

7. American College of Obstetricians and Gynecologists (ACOG). Antimicrobial prophylaxis for cesarean delivery: timing of administration (ACOG Committee Opinion No. 465). *Obstet Gynecol* 2010; **116**:791–92.

8. National Institute for Health and Care Excellence. Caesarean section. Clinical guideline. update, 2011. Available at www.nice.org.uk/guidance/cg132/resources/caesarean-section-pdf-35109507009733 (accessed June 2015).

9. Macejko AM, Schaeffer AJ. Asymptomatic bacteriuria and symptomatic urinary tract infections during pregnancy. *Urol Clin North Am* 2007; **34**:35–42.

10. Gilstrap LC, Ramin SM. Urinary tract infections during pregnancy. *Obstet Gynecol Clin North Am* 2001; **28**:581–91.

11. Kinlay J, O'Connell D, Kinlay S. Incidence of mastitis in breastfeeding women six months after delivery: a prospective cohort study. *Med J Aust* 1998; **169**: 310–312.

12. Female admissions (aged 16–50 years) to adult, general critical care units in England Wales and Northern Ireland, Reported as "Currently Pregnant" or "Recently Pregnant." January 1, 2007 to December 31, 2007, in ICNARC 2009. Available at www.rcoa.ac.uk/system/files/PUB-ICNARC-ObsReport.pdf (accessed June 2015).

13. Goodnight WH, Soper DE. Pneumonia in pregnancy. *Crit Care Med* 2005; **33**:S390–97.

14. Chen YH, Keller J, Wang IT, Lin CC, Lin HC. Pneumonia and pregnancy outcomes: a nationwide population-based study. *Am J Obstet Gynecol* 2012; **207**:288.e1–7.

15. Pierce M, Kurinczuk JJ, Spark P, Brocklehurst P, Knight M. Perinatal outcomes after maternal 2009/H1N1 infection: national cohort study. *BMJ* 2011; **342**:3412–21.

16. Knight M, Kenyon S, Brocklehurst P, et al. on behalf of MBRRACE-UK, eds. Saving lives, improving mothers' care: lessons learned to inform future maternity care from the UK and Ireland confidential enquiries into maternal deaths and morbidity 2009–12. National Perinatal Epidemiology Unit, University of Oxford, Oxford; 2014.

17. Centor R, Witherspoon J, Dalton H, et al. The diagnosis of strep throat in adults in the emergency room. *Med Decision Making* 1981; **1**:239–46.

18. Loughnan BA, Grover M, Nielson P. Maternal death due to extended spectrum β-lactamase-producing *E. coli:* a warning for the future? *Int J Obstet Anesth* 2010; **19**:327–30.

19. Moodley J, Pattinson R, Baxter C, Sibeko S, Abdool Karim Q. Strengthening HIV services for pregnant women: an opportunity to reduce maternal mortality rates in Southern Africa/sub-Saharan Africa. *BJOG* 2011; **118**:219–25.

20. Bonet M, Pileggi VN, Rijken MJ, et al. Towards a consensus definition of maternal sepsis: results of a systematic review and expert consultation. *Reprod Health* 2017; **14**:67.

21. Royal College of Obstetricians and Gynaecologists. Maternal collapse in pregnancy and the puerperium (Greentop Guideline No. 56), 2011. Available at www .rcog.org.uk/en/guidelines-research-services/guide lines/gtg56/ (accessed June 2015).

22. Levy, M.M., Evans, L.E., Rhodes, A. The Surviving Sepsis Campaign Bundle: 2018 update. *Intensive Care Med* 2018; **44**:925–928

23. Daniels R, Nutbeam T, McNamara G, et al. The Sepsis Six and the severe sepsis resuscitation bundle: a prospective observational cohort study. *Emerg Med J* 2011; **28**:507–12.

24. S.F. Wong, K.M. Chow, M. de Swiet. Severe Acute Respiratory Syndrome and pregnancy. *BJOG* 2003; **110**: 641–642.

Management of Thromboembolic Phenomena in Pregnancy

Ellile Pushpanathan and Pervez Sultan

Case Study

A 36-year-old gravida 1, para 2 parturient was booked for an elective cesarean delivery at 38 weeks' gestation. Body mass index (BMI) at her booking appointment was 29 kg/m^2. Her previous pregnancy resulted in an emergency cesarean delivery following prolonged fetal bradycardia. She developed chorioamnionitis post-operatively requiring 7-day in-patient IV antibiotic therapy.

At 27 weeks' gestation, following recent history of long-haul travel, she developed an acutely painful and swollen left calf. Duplex ultrasonography demonstrated a left popliteal deep vein thrombosis (DVT). Further investigation revealed no other medical cause for the thrombosis, and the patient was diagnosed with pregnancy-associated venous thromboembolism (VTE). Self-administered subcutaneous low-molecular-weight heparin (LMWH) therapy was subsequently started for the remainder of her pregnancy.

On preoperative visit, she was visibly distressed and anxious to leave the hospital soon after her procedure. She confirmed that she had no other medical history, medications, or allergies. Preoperative hematology investigations revealed normal hemoglobin (112 g/liter) and clotting profile. Her last therapeutic LMWH injection was 24 hours previously.

The anesthetist sited a 16-gauge IV cannula and performed a combined spinal-epidural, administering intrathecal heavy bupivacaine with opioid. No complications were encountered during anesthesia. She received 2 liters of warmed compound sodium lactate solution intraoperatively, and the estimated blood loss was approximately 1.4 liters. Near-patient testing (venous blood gas sample) revealed a postoperative hemoglobin level of 87 g/liter.

Following surgery, the patient remained anxious to go home as soon as possible and avoid the prolonged admission that she had previously experienced.

Key Points

- If a parturient has had an antenatal DVT, she remains at high risk of thrombotic events after cesarean delivery.
- The need for prompt therapeutic anticoagulation postoperatively must be balanced against risks of bleeding and signs of blood loss.
- Patient choices must be accommodated if medically safe to do so.

Discussion

Venous thromboembolism, encompassing deep vein thrombosis (DVT) and pulmonary embolism (PE), is the leading cause of direct maternal deaths within the United Kingdom, with an estimated mortality of 1.08 per 100,000 pregnancies.[1] VTE is estimated to affect 0.5–3 of every 1,000 pregnancies.[2] Prompt diagnosis and early treatment are vital to improve VTE-related mortality within this patient cohort.[3]

Pregnancy itself is a significant risk factor for development of VTE, with parturients 10 times more likely to develop VTE than age-matched non-pregnant women.[3] The most common time for a parturient to develop VTE is the puerperium (6 weeks following delivery).[3] Table 48.1 summarizes the risk factors for development of VTE in pregnancy. The patient in this Case Study has multiple risk factors, including: advanced maternal age, high BMI, and recent immobilization, and is therefore deemed high risk of developing VTE.

Diagnosis of VTE in Pregnancy

The Royal College of Obstetricians and Gynaecologists (RCOG) recognizes that due to the presence of limited evidence surrounding management of VTE in pregnancy, recommendations are often extrapolated from nonpregnant women. Therefore, the RCOG provides

Table 48.1 Risk Factors for Development of VTE in Pregnancy

Age ≥ 35 years	Immobilization	Cesarean delivery
BMI prenatal > 25 kg/m^2	Parity ≥ 3	Surgical history
BMI at delivery > 25 kg/m^2	Transfusion	Gestational diabetes
Multiple pregnancy	Smoking	Assisted reproduction
Preeclampsia	Heart disease	

suggestions from which it is recommended that each hospital develop its own policies.

Diagnosis of Deep Vein Thrombosis

For diagnosis of DVT, compression duplex ultrasound is considered to be the "gold standard" investigation. This should be repeated after 7 days in the event of an inconclusive result with ongoing clinical suspicion.

Diagnosis of Pulmonary Embolism

All possible cases of PE should be investigated primarily with a chest radiograph because this can diagnose other common causes of dyspnea while minimizing radiation dose to the fetus. Follow-up investigations include either a ventilation-perfusion (VQ) scan or computerized tomographic pulmonary angiography (CTPA), with the choice of investigation depending on local policy. D-dimer levels are usually elevated by term and during the postnatal period; therefore, it is not deemed to be a useful investigation during pregnancy.[4]

The British Thoracic Society recommends CTPA as a first-line investigation in the nonpregnant population for suspected PE. However, during pregnancy, maternal breast tissue becomes more sensitive to radiation. Following a CTPA, the lifetime risk of breast cancer increases by 13.6 percent within the pregnant population.[5] CTPA does, however, expose the fetus to a lower dose of radiation than a VQ scan and can also accurately diagnose other respiratory conditions. The RCOG recommends avoiding CTPA, particularly in the presence of risk factors for breast cancer, including familial history and previous CTPA.

VQ scans do not pose the same risks to maternal breast tissue as CTPA, and these risks can be further mitigated by omitting the ventilation aspect of the scan. VQ scans do, however, subject the fetus to a higher radiation dose than CTPA. Risk-benefit analysis must be considered prior to exposing the fetus to any radiation because it is associated with prenatal death, intrauterine growth restriction, organ malformation, mental retardation, and childhood cancer.[6] Despite these risks, VQ scan remains the preferred investigation for PE in most units in view of the substantial maternal risk of breast cancer associated with CTPA.[7]

Management of VTE in Pregnancy

As pregnant women are at high risk of VTE, it is recommended that all suspected cases of VTE be treated empirically with LMWH until definitive investigation. Peripartum VTE investigation and management strategies are summarized in Table 48.2.

LMWH is preferred to unfractionated heparin (UFH) because it does not cross the placenta, is effective at preventing VTE recurrence in the pregnant population, and is associated with a decreased risk of bleeding compared with UFH.[8–11]

Maintenance anticoagulation therapy during pregnancy is usually achieved with subcutaneous therapeutic-dose LMWH injections. Vitamin K antagonists such as warfarin are contraindicated during pregnancy because of significant risks of fetal teratogenicity. Limited safety data during pregnancy are available for the newer oral anticoagulant agents such as dabigatran and rivaroxaban. However, administration during pregnancy is not advised because their small molecular size may result in fetal exposure following drug transfer across the placenta.[7]

Increased renal clearance of enoxaparin during pregnancy results in the need for twice-daily dosing rather than the usual once-daily regimen.[12] The two most commonly used LMWH agents are enoxaparin 1 mg/kg twice daily and dalteparin 100 units/kg once daily. Tinzaparin 175 units/kg may also be used, but long-term outcome data among parturients with VTE are lacking compared with enoxaparin and dalteparin.[8] In order to determine the dose of LMWH to be administered, most institutions recommend the use of either the maternal weight at 12 weeks' gestation or the most recent weight recorded. The recommended duration of therapy is also greater in the pregnant population, with treatment usually recommended for the remainder of pregnancy and at least 6 weeks postnatally. The total treatment time should be at least 3 months.

Anticoagulation therapy may be changed to oral medication from the third day postpartum because warfarin is not contraindicated during breastfeeding.[2]

Table 48.2 Diagnosis and Management of VTE during Pregnancy and Postpartum

	First trimester	Second trimester	Third trimester	Delivery to 3 days after deliver	Three days to 6 weeks after birth	More than 6 weeks after birth
Investigation	DVT: duplex ultrasound (USS) PE: chest radiograph (CXR), VQ scan, or CTPA					DVT: USS, D-dimer PE: D-dimer, CXR, CTPA
Treatment	Enoxaparin[a] or dalteparin[c]			Antenatal regime or enoxaparin[b] or Dalteparin[d]	Enoxaparin[b] Or dalteparin[d] and WLR; stop LMWH when therapeutic	Enoxaparin[b] or dalteparin[d] And WLR; stop LMWH when therapeutic
Duration of treatment	For the duration of pregnancy, 6 weeks after birth, and for at least 3 months					If no thrombophilia: Distal DVT 6 weeks Proximal DVT/PE 3 months

Note: WLR = warfarin loading regime.

[a] Enoxaparin 1 mg/kg twice daily.

[b] Enoxaparin 1.5 mg/kg once daily.

[c] Dalteparin 100 units/kg twice daily.

[d] Dalteparin 10,000–18,000 units once daily.

It is not known if rivaroxaban, dabigatran, or apixaban is passed into breast milk; therefore, these drugs are currently not recommended during breastfeeding.[13] In the postpartum period, renal clearance resumes to prepregnancy levels, so women may convert to a once-daily LMWH dosing regimen.[12]

In cases of massive life-threatening VTE, the choice of treatment is either IV UFH (currently recommended as first line), thrombolytic therapy, thoracotomy, or surgical embolectomy based on the urgency of the clinical situation and anatomic site of the VTE.

The indications for use of inferior vena caval (IVC) filters are contentious depending on which authority is consulted. However, one absolute indication for IVC filter placement is the diagnosis of VTE in patients who have contraindications to anticoagulation. Relative indications include iliocaval DVT, free-floating proximal DVT, and massive PE.[14]

Clinicians should be aware that pregnancy-associated increases in fibrinogen and factor VIII levels can lead to apparent heparin resistance and result in lower than expected activated partial thromboplastin time (aPTT) levels when UFH treatment is monitored. If suspected, then senior hematologists should be involved. Routine monitoring of LMWH treatment with peak anti-Xa activity is not advised.[3]

Anesthesia in the Parturient with VTE

Parturients receiving treatment doses of anticoagulation for VTE carry an increased risk of epidural hematoma and subsequent risk of cord compression if neuraxial anesthesia is employed. Therefore, it is widely accepted that anticoagulation is an absolute contraindication to neuraxial anesthesia.[15]

However, general anesthesia in the pregnant population carries greater risks both to the mother and to the fetus than neuraxial anesthesia.[1] Neuraxial anesthesia therefore should be offered for both labor analgesia and appropriate surgical procedures if sufficient time has lapsed between the last dose of LMWH and the procedure. Table 48.3 summarizes the recommendations regarding neuraxial anesthesia placement and epidural catheter removal in relation to timings of anticoagulation therapy.

With regard to spontaneous labor, it should be noted that women receiving therapeutic LMWH are instructed to stop administering injections once contractions commence. This is to both reduce the degree of postpartum hemorrhage and to allow sufficient time to pass after anticoagulation so that neuraxial anesthesia may be offered as an analgesic option.

A commonly employed anticoagulation regimen (or *bridging plan*) between treatment and surgery for

Table 48.3 Regional Anesthesia Administration during Anticoagulation: Recommendations from the Association of Anaesthetists of Great Britain and Ireland, Obstetric Anaesthetists' Association, and Regional Anaesthesia UK Joint Guideline

	Advised time interval between heparin administration and neuraxial block or epidural catheter removal	Advised time interval between epidural catheter removal or neuraxial block and next dose of heparin
LMWH prophylactic	12 hours	4 hours
LMWH therapeutic	24 hours	a
UFH (IV) treatment	4 hours	4 hours
UFH (SC) prophylaxis	4 hours	1 hour
Aspirin	No contraindication	

[a] Depending on clinical scenario, consider indications for anticoagulation, risk of hemorrhage, and local guidelines and protocols. For example, suggested regime at University College London Hospital: 5000 units Dalteparin 6 hours following epidural catheter removal, 5,000 units twice daily on day 1 after surgery, and once daily therapeutic dose on day 2 postoperatively.

Source: Association of Anaesthetists of Great Britain and Ireland.[17]

women diagnosed with VTE undergoing elective cesarean delivery is administration of a thromboprophylactic dose (rather than therapeutic dose) the evening prior to surgery. In this way, there is a 12-hour interval between last LMWH dose and regional anesthesia, which minimizes the risk of epidural hematoma and excessive surgical bleeding.

For urgent surgical cases, it is advisable to delay surgery as much as clinically permissible in order to allow the risk of LMWH-associated bleeding to subside. In the presence of acute hemorrhage, the action of LMWH may be 60–80 percent reversed with the use of IV protamine sulfate. The dose of protamine sulfate is calculated based on LMWH dose administered in the preceding 8 hours (1 mg protamine sulfate per 1 mg enoxaparin/100 units dalteparin/100 units tinzaparin). Peak anti-Xa levels may be measured every 3 hours to guide therapy.[16]

In more complicated cases, for example, patients with a caval DVT or free-floating proximal DVT (where the risk of further embolic events is high), senior hematologic opinion should be sought prior to surgery.

Postoperative Anticoagulation for Parturients on Therapeutic LMWH

Despite preoperative omission of anticoagulation, postoperative bleeding remains a major concern for patients receiving treatment for VTE. In patients receiving LMWH, rather than unfractionated heparin (UFH), the incidence of postoperative wound hematoma is higher, at approximately 2 percent.[3] In order to enable rapid detection of postoperative hemorrhage, the RCOG recommends for obstetricians to close the surgical wound with interrupted sutures or staples and employ wound drains.

In the presence of low predicted postoperative hemorrhage risk following cesarean delivery, the RCOG recommends omission of therapeutic dose LMWH 24 hours prior to surgery, administration of thromboprophylactic dose 12 hours before surgery and greater than 3 hours following surgery. Therapeutic anticoagulation may commence 6–8 hours after surgery following obstetric surgical review and consultation with the relevant hematologist and anesthetist, but the plan must be tailored according to indication for anticoagulation and risk of hemorrhage.

If heparin therapy is deemed to be essential, in the presence of high predicted postoperative hemorrhage risk, the use of IV UFH is recommended until the risk of hemorrhage resolves. IV UFH is particularly advantageous in this scenario because it has a shorter half-life than LMWH and can be completely reversed with protamine sulfate. If there is a high predicted postoperative hemorrhage risk where heparin treatment is not deemed essential, heparin should not be administered until the risk of hemorrhage resolves.

Learning Points

- Regional anesthesia may be offered 24 hours after therapeutic LMWH and 12 hours following thromboprophylactic LMWH doses.

- In emergency situations, IV protamine sulfate can be used to partially reverse the action of LMWH prior to surgery.
- Thromboprophylactic or therapeutic LMWH can be given 4 hours following epidural catheter removal.
- If the risk of hemorrhage is low following cesarean delivery, thromboprophylactic LMWH can be given 3 hours following surgery (4 hours if epidural catheter is removed) and therapeutic regimen restarted 6–8 hours later.
- If the risk of hemorrhage is high following cesarean delivery, IV UFH infusion should be considered until the risk of hemorrhage resolves.
- Treatment and prophylactic doses of LMWH are associated with an increased incidence of postoperative wound hematoma

References

1. Knight M, Kenyon S, Brockhurst P, et al. on behalf of MBRRACE-UK. Saving Lives, Improving Mother's Care: Lessons Learned to Inform Future Maternity Care in the UK and Ireland. Confidential enquiries into maternal deaths and morbidity 2009–2012. National Perinatal Epidemiology Unit, University of Oxford, Oxford; 2014.

2. Snow V, Qaseem A, Barry P, et al. Management of venous thromboembolism: a clinical practice guideline from the American College of Physicians and the American Academy of Family Physicians. *Ann Intern Med* 2007; **146**:204–10.

3. Greer I, Thomson, A. *The Acute Management of Thrombosis and Embolism during Pregnancy and the Puerperium.* Green Top Guideline No. 37b, Royal College of Obstetricians and Gynaecologists, London, 2010.

4. Francalanci I, Comeglio P, Alessandrello Liotta A, et al. D-dimer plasma levels during normal pregnancy measured by specific ELISA. *Int J Clin Lab Res* 1997; **27**:65–67.

5. Remy-Jardin M, Remy J. Spiral CT angiography of the pulmonary circulation. *Radiology* 1999; **212**: 615–36.

6. Chaparian A, Aghabagheri M. Fetal radiation doses and subsequent risks from xray examinations: should we be concerned? *Iran J Reprod Med* 2013; **11**:899–904.

7. Greer I. Thrombosis in pregnancy: updates in diagnosis and management. *Hematol Am Soc Hematol Educ Prog* 2012; **2012**:203–7.

8. Greer I, Nelson-Piercy C. Low-molecular-weight heparins for thrombophylaxis and treatment of venous-thromboembolism in pregnancy. *Blood* 2005; **106**:401–7.

9. Forestier F, Daffos F, Capella-Pavlovsky M. Low molecular weight heparin (PK 10169) does not cross the placenta during the second trimester of pregnancy: study by direct fetal blood sampling under ultrasound. *Thromb Res* 1984; **34**:557–60.

10. Forestier F, Daffos F, Rainaut M, Toulemonde F. Low molecular weight heparin (CY 216) does not cross the placenta during the third trimester of pregnancy. *Thromb Haemostat* 1987; **57**:234.

11. Brill-Edwards P, Ginsberg J, Gent M, et al. Safety of withholding heparin in pregnant women with a history of venous thromboembolism. *N Engl J Med* 2000; **343**: 1439–44.

12. Casele H, Laifer S, Woelkers DA, Venkataramann R. Changes in the pharmacokinetics of the low molecular weight enoxaparin sodium during pregnancy. *Am J Obstet Gynecol* 1999; **181**:1113–17.

13. Bates S, Greer I, Middeldorp S, et al. Thrombophilia, antithrombotic therapy, and pregnancy: antithrombotic therapy, and prevention of thrombosis. *Chest* 2012; **141**:e691s–736s.

14. Bilger A, Pottecher J, Greget M, Boudier E, Diemunsch P. Extensive pulmonary embolism after severe postpartum haemorrhage: management with an inferior vena cava filter. *Int J Obstet Anaesth* 2014; **23**(4):390–93.

15. Checketts M, Wildsmith J. Central nerve block and thrombophylaxis: is there a problem?. *Br J Anaesth* 1999; **82**:164–67.

16. Cushman M, Lim W, Zakai NA. *Clinical Practice Guide on Anticoagulant Dosing and Management of Anticoagulant Associated Bleeding Complications in Adults.* Washington, DC: American Society of Hematology; 2011.

17. Association of Anaesthetists of Great Britain and Ireland, Obstetric Anaesthetists' Association, Regional Anaesthesia UK. Regional anaesthesia in patients with abnormalities in coagulation, 2011. Available at www .aagbi.org/sites/default/files/RAPAC%20for%20consul tation.pdf (accessed February 1, 2015).

Pandemic Flu

Sioned Phillips and Frank Schroeder

Case Study

A previously well 32-year-old woman presented to the Emergency Department at 37 weeks' gestation with a two-day history of cough, fever, and general malaise; an increase in shortness of breath had prompted her to come to hospital.

On arrival, she was dyspneic with oxygen saturation of 88 percent on room air and grossly tachypoeic. Despite the administration of 15 liters of oxygen via a facemask, she remained hypoxemic ($PaO_2 = 60$ mmHg/8 kPa). She was tachycardic but normotensive and pyrexial. Her temperature was measured as 38.3°C. Chest radiography showed right lower lobe infiltrates. A nasopharyngeal swab was taken and subsequently confirmed the presence of H1N1 influenza A virus (RT-PCR test); co-amoxiclav, clarithromycin, and oseltamivir (Tamiflu) were started.

While being assessed in the Emergency Department, the patient's condition deteriorated rapidly, with worsening respiratory distress, hypoxia, and tachycardia. Cardiotocography identified fetal distress requiring an emergency cesarean delivery. The procedure was performed under general anesthesia following a rapid-sequence induction. Invasive monitoring was started, including arterial and central pressure monitoring. Following delivery, the patient remained sedated and ventilated owing to her high oxygen requirements and was transferred to the ICU.

Despite controlled ventilation with high inspiratory oxygen fractions ($FiO_2 = 0.9$), her oxygenation could not be improved ($PaO_2 = 45$ mmHg/6 kPa). A second chest radiograph showed bilateral infiltrates consistent with acute respiratory distress syndrome (ARDS). The patient also rapidly developed signs of distributive shock and renal failure, for which she was treated with vasopressors (norepinephrine and vasopressin) and renal replacement therapy (continuous venovenous diahemofiltration [CVVDH]). A trial of high-frequency oscillation ventilation (HFOV) was started, and over a period of 72 hours the patient's respiratory condition improved; conventional ventilation with low tidal volumes (6 ml/kg of body weight) was reinstated after another 48 hours. Her condition continued to improve, and a week after her admission to the Emergency Department, she was able to be extubated and discharged to normal ward care.

Key Points

- Pregnant women who are infected with H1N1 influenza A and show signs of acute respiratory distress or failure can deteriorate rapidly and may require ventilation and delivery of the premature fetus.
- Antiviral agents should be administered as soon as influenza is suspected.
- Appropriate timing of delivery needs to be determined by a multidisciplinary team of senior clinicians.
- Prompt and aggressive intensive care therapy with appropriate organ support should be instigated as soon as indicated.
- Influenza poses significant risk for pregnant women and their fetuses, and pregnant women should therefore be offered the seasonal and specific vaccines.

Discussion

Influenza is an RNA virus that is classified into either A, B, or C types; types A and B infect humans and are known to cause seasonal epidemics. Type A can also cause pandemics. Influenza A is characterized by its surface antigens: hemagglutinin (H) and neuraminidase (N). The different types of the surface antigens (e.g., H1, H2, N1, N2) are used to describe the subtype of the influenza A virus. These two surface antigens may undergo mutations, causing antigenic drift. It is this process that requires the annual modifications of the vaccine.[1]

Pregnant women who are infected with the H1N1 virus carry an increased risk of morbidity and mortality from pandemic influenza. This chapter focuses on the results of the pandemic caused by the influenza A subtype H1N1 in 2009–10.

Women are at higher risk of contracting the H1N1 virus and developing a severe respiratory infection through the antenatal period and for up to 2 weeks following delivery. A UK study from the pandemic in 2009 showed that pregnant women with H1N1 were three times more likely to be admitted to hospital than nonpregnant women.[2] Similar data from the United States show that pregnant women were four times more likely than the general population to be admitted if infected with H1N1.[3]

Pregnant women are at higher risk from viral infections due to pregnancy-related physiologic and immunologic changes. Increased heart rate and oxygen consumption and decreased lung capacity all lead to decreased cardiovascular reserve. Pregnant women have a lower oncotic pressure, which may predispose them to a higher risk of pulmonary edema and respiratory compromise. There is a decrease in cell-mediated immunity with normal levels of humoral immunity.[4] It is the T-helper cells of the cell-mediated immune system that facilitate the apoptosis of host cells infected with a virus.

The influenza vaccine is an inactivated vaccine, which may be mono- or multivalent. The inactivated pathogens provide prophylactic protection against the virus by eliciting both antibodies and cytotoxic T-lymphocytes.[5] The inactivation of the pathogen by either chemical exposure or heat denaturation renders the virus dead and noninfectious; it is therefore safe in pregnancy.[5] The valency of the vaccine describes the number of antigens to which the vaccine will convey immunity. A monovalent vaccine is a vaccine against a single strain (e.g., H1N1), whereas a multivalent vaccine will provide immunity against two or more strains of the same microorganism.[5] For example, the influenza vaccine may contain both the seasonal and pandemic strain of influenza.

The influenza vaccine is considered to be safe in pregnancy and provides excellent protection to both mother and fetus. It should be offered to all pregnant women.[6]

Presentation

The presentation of H1N1 consists of (in order of frequency) fever, cough, breathlessness, headache, sore throat, and nausea and vomiting.[2] Clinical signs include tachycardia, tachypnea, fever > 38°C, oxygen saturations < 94 percent on room air, and systolic hypotension.[2] Pregnant women are more likely to present with dyspnea as the predominant symptom.[3] One study has shown that the independent prognostic indicators for the severity of infection were levels of C-reactive protein (CRP) greater than 100 mg/liter and radiologic signs of pneumonia.[2] Patients may go on to develop ARDS and multiorgan failure, requiring higher levels of intensive care therapy.

Management

Once an infection with H1N1 virus or other types of influenza is suspected, a rapid and coordinated approach of different senior specialists is mandatory. The examination of the woman should be initiated with an assessment of the patient's airway, breathing, and circulation (ABC), keeping in mind that resuscitation of the mother is very likely to also improve the fetal condition. Adequate maternal oxygenation and ventilation, as well as a sufficient blood pressure, should be key goals in the initial resuscitation phase. It is important to appreciate the physiologic changes in pregnancy when managing the critically ill parturient. For example, the higher partial pressure of oxygen in the blood usually seen in pregnancy must be maintained to provide adequate oxygenation of the mother and the fetus. It cannot be overstated that aggressive management of the mother is the best way to improve fetal outcome.

Diagnosis

All women should be tested as soon as an infection with influenza is suspected. A rapid antigen test is available and will produce results within 30 minutes. This test has been shown to have a false-positive rate of 38 percent.[7] However, any woman with suspected pandemic influenza should be managed as if infected until a RT-PCR test (results 6–10 hours) or viral cultures (results 3–10 days) prove otherwise.[8]

Treatment

Oseltamivir (Tamiflu) and zanamivir (Relenza) are neuraminidase inhibitors that are used for the treatment of influenza. Treatment duration is usually between 5 and 10 days depending on the severity of disease. Zanamivir is an inhaled drug and is contraindicated in chronic respiratory disease because it may cause bronchospasm.[9] A meta-analysis has shown that oseltamivir reduces the time of clinical symptoms as well as the incidence of lower respiratory tract complications and hospital admissions.[10]

Antiviral drugs work best when given as close as possible to the onset of symptoms (or at least within the first 48 hours of the onset of symptoms). Early administration of antiviral drugs after admission to hospital for presumed influenza can prevent respiratory failure and death.[11]

Infection Control Guidance

The Centers for Disease Control and Prevention in the United States has issued infection control guidance for the management of pregnant or peripartum patients. They recommend:[12]

- All suspected or confirmed cases must be managed in isolation rooms.
- Standard precautions must be taken using gloves, gowns, and hand hygiene.
- Respiratory hygiene and cough etiquette are necessary (education, cover mouth and nose on sneezing).
- Hand hygiene after contact with respiratory secretions is required.
- Droplet precautions (facemask) are required.
- Spatial separation of patients who are febrile with respiratory illness is necessary.

These precautions should be continued for 7 days after the onset of the illness or 24 hours since last symptoms (fever, respiratory symptoms).

Following delivery, the mother and baby should be separated until the mother:

- Has received 48 hours of antiviral treatment,
- Has been apyrexial for 24 hours (without antipyretics), and
- Is able to control her cough and respiratory secretions.

For local implementation of these guidelines, close cooperation with the microbiology and/or infection control team is paramount.

Timing of Delivery

Frequently, the critically ill parturient will go into spontaneous labor and so negate the decision regarding time of delivery. However, if this is not the case, a multidisciplinary team decision on when to deliver is required, depending on the mother's clinical state. Early versus late delivery will not be an easy decision

because each may have benefits to the mother or fetus. The gestational age of the unborn fetus and the availability of neonatal care units may have an influence on decision-making.

Intensive Care Management

Ventilation

There are limited data regarding ventilation in the parturient owing to its relatively rare occurrence. Many women who need ventilation may also require assisted or operative delivery at some point. It may be intuitive that delivery will improve ventilation and oxygenation, but there is no conclusive evidence to support this approach.

A retrospective case review of 10 pregnant women, all in respiratory distress and requiring intubation and ventilation, looked at the effect of a cesarean delivery on maternal respiratory mechanics.[13] Although early delivery decreased the median fraction of the inspired oxygen concentration by 28 percent, all the other ventilator settings, such as respiratory rate, positive end-expiratory pressure (PEEP), tidal volume, peak airway pressure, and plateau pressure, remained unchanged. According to the authors, these results need to be interpreted with caution because the decrease in oxygen concentration occurred from immediately after delivery to up to 24 hours after delivery, and therefore a cause-and-effect relationship may not apply. In conclusion, delivery of the fetus does not necessarily provide a benefit to maternal oxygenation.

Chest wall compliance will decrease in pregnancy, especially in the third trimester. Therefore, plateau pressures outside the normally accepted limits (i.e., 35 cmH_20) can be required to maintain adequate tidal volumes. The administration of PEEP may be necessary to avoid collapse of basal lung segments, which can worsen hypoxia. A maternal arterial PaO_2 of 67mmHg is often quoted as the minimum oxygen concentration required to provide satisfactory fetal oxygenation.[14]

The standard ventilator care bundle[15] should be implemented. The 30-degree head-up tilt may have even more beneficial effects for the parturient because it should increase the functional residual capacity and also decrease esophageal reflux, which could lead to aspiration and ventilator-associated pneumonia.[14]

Some ICUs advocate performing a (percutaneous) tracheostomy early (within 1 week of ventilation).

However, tracheostomies can only be safely performed once the patient's oxygenation has already improved, and frequently, sometimes surprisingly, a very rapid recovery can be seen in this group of ICU patients. The procedure itself can also be associated with significant morbidity: complications can occur during the procedure (e.g., vascular injury) and/or after the patient has recovered from her illness (e.g., tracheal stenosis). There is also the cosmetic aspect of a tracheostomy scar in these often very young female patients.

Nonconventional strategies to improve oxygenation and decrease mortality in the general population such as nitric oxide, high-frequency oscillation ventilation (HFOV), and extracorporeal membrane oxygenation (ECMO) have not been well studied in the pregnant population. However, during the 2009 pandemic, ECMO and HFOV were frequently used when maternal oxygenation was at a critical level and conventional ventilation failed to improve the situation.

High-Frequency Oscillation Ventilation

When HFOV is applied via an endotracheal tube, small tidal volumes are delivered to the lungs with very high frequencies and relatively high airway pressures, thus reducing expansion and recoiling of alveoli. During HFOV, the lungs are exposed to fewer sheer forces and therefore experience less secondary damage to the small airways. There is no clear evidence that HFOV improves outcome. The OSCAR[16] trial showed no difference in in-hospital mortality, and the OSCILLATE[17] trial even showed a negative influence and an increase in mortality in patients ventilated with HFOV. However some centers in the United Kingdom have used HFOV for pregnant women with ARDS very successfully and with very good outcomes.

Extracorporeal Membrane Oxygenation

Extracorporeal membrane oxygenation (ECMO) may be the last resort to oxygenate a patient's lungs when conventional ventilation and HFOV are failing. ECMO is a technique derived from cardiopulmonary bypass in which deoxygenated blood is removed from the patient via a large vein and transported to a pump and membrane system allowing oxygenation and the removal of carbon dioxide. The oxygenated blood is then returned to the patient via either a vein or an artery. There have been case reports advocating the use of ECMO in pregnant women with severe respiratory disease.[18] However, there are problems associated with this technique in the parturient; femoral vascular access may be difficult to achieve, and poor flow through catheters can occur because of the presence of the gravid uterus. There is also the risk of severe hemorrhage because the patient will need to be systemically anticoagulated while being treated with ECMO. Pregnant patients who suffer severe influenza infections and (rapidly) develop respiratory failure should always be discussed with a local ECMO center.

Sepsis Management

The Surviving Sepsis care bundle should be implemented for the septic pregnant patient (discussed in Chapter 47). Pregnant women with influenza may present with sepsis and distributive shock as the predominant signs and relatively mild chest symptoms. It is important to administer broad-spectrum antibiotics as part of the initial management. Initially, the difference between viral and bacterial pneumonia may not be entirely clear. However, there is also the risk of secondary bacterial pneumonia following initial H1N1 viral infection.

Steroids may have a role in treatment. Although the evidence for steroids in sepsis and ARDS does not show significant improvement in outcomes, IV steroids are still used in severe septic shock when high-dose vasopressors are required. If steroids are considered to form part of the ICU therapy, the neonatal and obstetric teams should be involved in the treatment decisions.

Thromboembolic Prophylaxis

Thromboembolic prophylaxis is paramount in the pregnant patient because pregnancy itself is a major risk factor for thromboembolic events, especially when the pregnant patient becomes critically ill. Pharmacologic and mechanic antithrombotic measures should be taken.

Maternal Outcomes

During the 2009 H1N1 pandemic, in the United States there were 56 deaths among 953 pregnant patients with confirmed or suspected H1N1 infections; most maternal deaths occurred in the third trimester (36 [64.3 percent]). Women with other comorbidities were more likely to be hospitalized (55.3 percent), admitted to the ICU (62.8 percent), and die (78.3 percent).[19] The most common comorbidity in women who died was asthma (43.5 percent).[19] Other significant comorbidities were hypertension, obesity, pregestational or gestational diabetes, and anemia. In a UK study,[20] obesity and asthma were the most frequent risk factors for admission to hospital; obesity was also an independent risk factor for ICU admission.

Perinatal Outcomes

Perinatal outcomes were assessed in the United Kingdom during the 2009 H1N1 pandemic, and the mortality rate was higher in infants born to infected versus noninfected, mothers.[20] A significant proportion of infants born to infected mothers (23 percent) was admitted to a neonatal ICU, and eight infants were born with congenital abnormalities. However, only one (cephalic abnormality) was considered to be associated with the H1N1 infection.[20] Systematic follow-up examinations of babies born to mothers with H1N1 infections were not carried out, and exact data for the outcome of these infants are therefore unknown.

Learning Points

- Pregnant women carry an increased risk of morbidity and mortality if infected with influenza and should be offered the seasonal and specific vaccine.
- Influenza can be diagnosed using rapid antigen testing or viral swabs from the respiratory tract.
- Any woman suspected of having influenza should receive antiviral agents as soon as possible to decrease the risk of severe disease.
- Risk factors for pregnant women with severe disease are chronic respiratory disease, cardiovascular disease, obesity, and diabetes.
- Best practice should be followed by all teams (obstetric, anesthetic, intensive care, and medicine) when caring for the critically ill parturient.
- Women may develop respiratory and multiorgan failure requiring ICU management. Ventilation may be difficult and require nonconventional methods.
- *The fetus will have far less chance of survival if the mother is not promptly and aggressively treated with therapies that improve the maternal physiology.*

References

1. Rasmussen SA, Jamieson DJ, Bresee JS. Pandemic influenza and pregnant women. *Emerg Infect Dis* 2008; **14**:95–100.

2. Nguyen-Van-Tam JS, Openshaw PJM, Hashim A. Risk factors for hospitalization and poor outcome with pandemic A/H1NI influenza: United Kingdom first wave (May–September 2009). *Thorax* 2010; **65**:645–51.

3. Jamieson DJ, Honein MA, Rasmussen SA, et al; Novel Influenza A (H1N1) Pregnancy Working Group: H1N1 2009 influenza virus infection during pregnancy in the USA. *Lancet* 2009; **374**(9688):451–58.

4. Jamieson DJ, Regan NT, Rasmussen SA. Emerging infections and pregnancy. *Emerg Infect Dis* 2006; **12**:1638–1643.

5. Davies DH, Halablab MA, Clarke J, Cox FEG, Young TWK. *Infection and Immunity*. London: Taylor and Francis; 1999.

6. Centers for Disease Control and Prevention (CDC). *Seasonal Influenza Vaccination Resources for Health Professionals*. Available at www.cdc.gov/flu/professionals /vaccination/index.htm (accessed April 4, 2015).

7. Louie JK, Acosta MPH, Jamieson DJ, Honein MA. Severe 2009 H1N1 influenza in pregnant and postpartum women in California. *N Engl J Med* 2010; **362**:27–35.

8. Centers for Disease Control and Prevention (CDC). *Rapid Diagnostic Testing for Influenza: Information for Health Care Professionals*. Available at www.cdc.gov/fl u/professionals/diagnosis/rapidclin.htm (accessed January 13, 2015).

9. Centers for Disease Control and Prevention (CDC). *Influenza Antiviral Medications Summary for Clinicians*. Available at www.cdc.gov/flu/professionals/antivirals /summary-clinicians.htm (accessed August 20, 2014).

10. Dobson J, Whitely R, Pocock J, Monto A. Oseltamivir treatment for influenza in adults: a meta-analysis of random controlled trials. *Lancet* 2015; **385**:1729–37. doi: 10.1016/S0140-6736(14)62449–1.

11. Siston AM, Rasmussen SA, Honein MA, et al. Pandemic 2009 influenza A (H1N1) virus illness among pregnant women in the United States. *JAMA* 2010; **303**(15):1517.

12. Centers for Disease Control and Prevention (CDC). *Seasonal Influenza: Guidance for the Prevention and Control of Influenza in the Peri- and Postpartum Settings*. Available at www.cdc.gov/flu/professionals /infectioncontrol/peri-post-settings.htm (accessed August 19, 2014).

13. Tomlinson MW, Caruthers TJ, Whitty JE, Gonick B. Does delivery improve maternal condition in the

respiratory-compromised gravida? *Obstet Gynecol* 1998; **91**:108–11.

14. Van De Velde M, Scholefield H, Plante LA. *Maternal Critical Care: A Multidisciplinary Approach* Cambridge: Cambridge University Press; 2013.

15 Department of Health (UK). High Impact Intervention Care Bundle to Reduce Ventilation-Associated Pneumonia, 2011. Available at http://webarchive .natio nalarchives.gov.uk/20120118171705/http://hcai.dh.gov .uk/files/2011/03/2011-03-14-HII-Ventilator-Associate d-Pneumonia-FINAL.pdf (accessed October 23, 2018).

16. Young D, Lamb SE, Shah S, et al. OSCAR Study Group: High-frequency oscillation for acute respiratory distress syndrome. *N Engl J Med* 2013; **368**(9):806–13.

17. Ferguson ND, Cook DJ, Guyatt GH, et al. OSCILLATE Trial Investigators: high- frequency oscillation in early acute respiratory distress syndrome. *N Engl J Med* 2013; **368**(9):795–805.

18. King PT, Rosalion A, McMillian J, et al. Extra corporeal membrane oxygenation in pregnancy. *Lancet* 2000; **356**:45–46.

19. Yates L, Pierce M, Stephens S, et al. Influenza A/H1N1v in pregnancy: an investigation of the characteristics and management of affected women and the relationship to pregnancy outcomes for mother and infant. *Health Technol Asses* 2010 **14**:34,109–182.

20. Pierce M, Kurinczuk J, Spark P, Brocklehurst P, Knight M. Perinatal outcomes after maternal 2009/H1N1 infection: national cohort study *BMJ* 2011; **342**:d3214.

Reference Ranges in Pregnancy

Samantha Wilson and Samantha Allen

Anesthesia: Bromage Scoring System for Lower Limb Motor Block

Grade	Criteria
I	Free movement of legs and feet
II	Able to flex knees with free movement of feet
III	Unable to flex knees with free movement of feet
IV	Unable to move legs or feet

Source: Data from Bromage.[1]

Biochemistry and Liver Function Tests

	Nonpregnant adult	First trimester	Second trimester	Third trimester	References
Alanine transaminase (units/liter)	7–41	3–30	2–33	2–25	2–5
Albumin (g/dl)	4.1–5.3	3.1–5.1	2.6–4.5	2.3–4.2	5–8
Alkaline phosphatase (units/liter)	33–96	17–88	25–126	38–229	2–6
Alpha-1-antitrypsin (mg/dl)	100–200	225–323	273–391	327–487	2
Amylase (units/liter)	20–96	24–83	16–73	15–81	1, 2, 9, 10
Anion gap (mmol/liter)	7–16	13–17	12–16	12–16	2
Aspartate transaminase (units/liter)	12–38	3–23	3–33	4–32	1–4
Bicarbonate (mmol/liter)	22–30	20–24	20–24	20–24	2
Bilirubin, total (mg/dl)	0.3–1.3	0.1–0.4	0.1–0.8	0.1–1.1	1, 4
Bilirubin, unconjugated (mg/dl)	0.2–0.9	0.1–0.5	0.1–0.4	0.1–0.5	3, 5
Bilirubin, conjugated (mg/dl)	0.1–0.4	0–0.1	0–0.1	0–0.1	5
Bile acids (mmol/liter)	0.3–4.8	0–4.9	0–9.1	0–11.3	5,11
CA-125 antigen (units/ml)	7.2–27.0	2.2–26.8	12–25.1	16.8–43.8	12–14
Calcium, ionized (mg/dl)	4.5–5.3	4.5–5.1	4.4–5.0	4.4–5.3	3, 7, 15, 16
Calcium, total (mg/dl)	8.7–10.2	8.8–10.6	8.2–9.0	8.2–9.7	2, 3, 6, 8, 15–17
Ceruloplasmin (mg/dl)	25–63	30–49	49–53	43–78	3, 18
Chloride (mEq/liter)	102–109	101–105	97–109	97–109	2, 3, 19
Creatinine (mg/dl)	0.5–0.9	0.4–0.7	0.4–0.8	0.4–0.9	2, 3, 20

(cont.)

	Nonpregnant adult	First trimester	Second trimester	Third trimester	References
Gamma-glutamyl transpeptidase (units/liter)	9–58	2–23	4–22	3–26	2–5
Lactate dehydrogenase (units/liter)	115–221	78–433	80–447	82–524	2–4, 8
Lipase (units/liter)	3–43	21–76	26–100	41–112	9
Magnesium (mg/dl)	1.5–2.3	1.6–2.2	1.5–2.2	1.1–2.2	2, 3, 6–9, 15, 17
Osmolality (mOsm/kgH$_2$O)	275–295	275–280	276–280	278–280	17, 21
Phosphate (mg/dl)	2.5–4.3	3.1–4.6	2.5–4.6	2.8–4.6	2, 3, 6, 7, 22
Potassium (mEq/liter)	3.5–5.0	3.6–5.0	3.3–5.0	3.3–5.1	2, 3, 7, 8, 17, 19, 23
Prealbumin (mg/dl)	17–34	15–27	20–27	14–23	3
Protein, total (g/dl)	6.7–8.6	6.2–7.6	5.7–6.9	5.6–6.7	3, 7, 8
Sodium (mEq/liter)	136–146	133–148	129–148	130–148	2, 3, 7, 8, 17, 19, 23
Urea nitrogen (mg/dl)	7–20	7–12	3–13	3–11	2, 3, 19
Uric acid (mg/dl)	2.5–5.6	2.0–4.2	2.4–4.9	3.1–6.3	2, 3, 21

Cardiac Function Tests
Cardiac Function

	Nonpregnant adult	First trimester	Second trimester	Third trimester	References
Cardiac output (liters/min)	4.8–6.8	5.6–9.7	5.5–9.9	4.8–8.7	24–28
Cardiac index (liters/min/m^2)	2.6–4.2	3.2–4.6	3.1–4.7	2.5–4.4	25, 28
Stroke volume (ml)	79–90	77.5–107.6	70.3–107.6	54–99	25, 28, 29
Stroke index (ml/m^2)		46–62	39–62	30–42	25
Systemic vascular resistance (dynes/cm^5)	700–1600	747–1485	692–1201	1034–1201	25, 27, 30

Echocardiography

	Nonpregnant adult	First trimester	Second trimester	Third trimester	References
Intraventricular septal dimension (cm)	0.7–0.9	0.63–0.83	0.65–0.85	0.66–0.9	28–32
Posterior ventricular wall dimension (cm)	0.75–0.9	0.56–0.8	0.59–0.9	0.59–0.9	28–32
	116–143	108–167	115–150	128–162	28, 30–32

(cont.)

	Nonpregnant adult	First trimester	Second trimester	Third trimester	References
Left ventricular mass (g)					
Left ventricular mass index (g/m²)	40–78	53–79	58–82	60–88	28, 30–32
E/A ratio (This is an indicator of diastolic performance. Early (E) to late (A) ventricular filling velocities)	1.4–1.75	1.6	1.4	1.3	28, 30
Left ventricular diastolic diameter (cm)	4.3–4.8	4.3–4.6	4.4–4.9	5.1	29, 30
Left ventricular systolic diameter (cm)	2.8–3.1	2.8–2.9	2.8–3.4	2.8–3.3	29, 30
Left ventricular fractional shortening (%)	35–36	35–37	3.5	35,36	29, 30
Left ventricular ejection fraction (%)	60–73	61–75	61–63	60–73	29, 30

Cardiac Function: Blood Tests

	Nonpregnant adult	First trimester	Second trimester	Third trimester	References
Atrial natriuretic peptide (pg/ml)	Not reported	Not reported	28.1–70.1	Not reported	33
B-type natriuretic peptide (pg/ml)	<167 (age and gender specific)	18.4	13.5–29.5	15.5–46	33–35
Creatine kinase (units/liter)	39–238	27–83	25–75	13–101	3, 37
Creatine kinase – MB (units/liter). This is a cardiac marker of myocardial injury e.g. MI	<6	Not reported	Not reported	1.8–2.4	36
Troponin-I (mg/ml)	0–0.8	Not reported	Not reported	0–0.064	37, 38

Caring for the Acutely Unwell Parturient
Management of Anaphylaxis
Immediate Management

1. Use the ABC approach (airway, breathing, circulation). Team working enables several tasks to be accomplished simultaneously.
2. Remove all potential causative agents (including IV colloids, latex, and chlorhexidine), and maintain anesthesia, if necessary, with an inhalational agent.
3. Call for help, and note the time.
4. Maintain the airway and administer oxygen 100%. Intubate the trachea if necessary, and ventilate the lungs with oxygen.
5. Elevate the patient's legs if there is hypotension.
6. If appropriate, start cardiopulmonary resuscitation immediately according to Advanced Life Support Guidelines.
7. Administer epinephrine intravenously. An initial dose of 50 μg (0.5 ml of 1:10,000 solution) is

appropriate (adult dose). Several doses may be required if there is severe hypotension or bronchospasm.

8. If several doses of epinephrine are required, consider starting an IV infusion of epinephrine (it has a short half-life).

9. Administer saline 0.9% or lactated Ringer's solution at a high rate via an IV cannula of an appropriate gauge (large volumes may be required).[39]

Secondary Management

1. Administer chlorphenamine 10 mg IV (adult dose).
2. Administer hydrocortisone 200 mg IV (adult dose).
3. If the blood pressure does not recover despite an epinephrine infusion, consider administration of an alternative IV vasopressor based on the training and experience of the anesthetist, for example, metaraminol.
4. Treat persistent bronchospasm with an IV infusion of salbutamol. If a suitable breathing system connector is available, a metered-dose inhaler may be appropriate. Consider giving IV aminophylline or magnesium sulfate.
5. Arrange transfer of the patient to an appropriate critical care area.
6. Take blood samples (5–10 ml clotted blood) for mast cell tryptase as follows:

    a. Initial sample as soon as feasible after resuscitation has started – do not delay resuscitation to take the sample.
    b. Second sample at 1–2 hours after the start of symptoms.
    c. Third sample either at 24 hours or in convalescence (e.g., in a follow-up allergy clinic). This is a measure of baseline tryptase levels because some individuals have a higher baseline level.
    d. Ensure that the samples are labeled with the time and date.[39]

Local Anesthetic Toxicity
Clinical Features

Neurologic features	Cardiovascular features
Sudden change in mental state	Sinus bradycardia
Loss of consciousness	Asystole
Agitation	Conduction abnormalities
Tonic-clonic seizures	Ventricular tachyarrhythmia

Source: Data from AAGBI Safety Guideline: Management of Severe Local Anaesthetic Toxicity.[40]

Immediate Management

1. Stop injecting the local anesthetic.
2. Call for help.
3. Maintain the airway, and if necessary, secure it with a tracheal tube.
4. Give 100% oxygen, and ensure adequate lung ventilation (hyperventilation may help by increasing plasma pH in the presence of metabolic acidosis).
5. Confirm or establish IV access.
6. Control seizures: give a benzodiazepine, thiopental, or propofol in small incremental doses.
7. Assess cardiovascular status throughout.
8. Consider drawing blood for analysis, but do not delay definitive treatment to do this.

Treatment
In Circulatory Arrest

1. Start cardiopulmonary resuscitation (CPR) using standard protocols.
2. Manage arrhythmias using the same protocols, recognizing that arrhythmias may be very refractory to treatment
3. Consider the use of cardiopulmonary bypass if available.

Without Circulatory Arrest

1. Use conventional therapies to treat
    a. Hypotension
    b. Bradycardia
    c. Tachyarrhythmia
2. Consider IV lipid emulsion (following the regimen below).

Intravenous Lipid Emulsion Protocol

Immediately	Give an initial IV bolus injection of 20% lipid emulsion at 1.5 ml/kg over 1 minute *and*
	Start an IV infusion of 20% lipid emulsion at 15 ml/kg per hour.
After 5 minutes	Give a maximum of two repeat boluses (same dose) if • Cardiovascular stability has not been restored *or* • An adequate circulation deteriorates Leave 5 minutes between boluses. A maximum of three boluses can be given (including the initial bolus) *and* Continue infusion at same rate, *but*

277

(cont.)

> Double the rate to 30 ml/kg per hour at any time after 5 minutes *if*
>
> - Cardiovascular stability has not been restored or
> - An adequate circulation deteriorates
>
> Continue infusion until stable and adequate circulation restored or maximum dose of lipid emulsion given.

Follow-Up

1. Arrange safe transfer to a clinical area with appropriate equipment and suitable staff until sustained recovery is achieved.
2. Exclude pancreatitis by regular clinical review, including daily amylase or lipase assays for two days.
3. Report cases as follows:
   - Within the United Kingdom to the National Patient Safety Agency (via www.npsa.nhs.uk).
   - Within the Republic of Ireland to the Irish Medicines Board (via www.imb.ie).
4. If lipid has been given, please also report its use to the International Registry at www.lipidregistry .org. Details may also be posted at www.lipidrescue.org.

SPOILT Acronym for Intrauterine Resuscitation

*S*yntocinon – turn off.

*P*ressure – correct hypotension.

*O*xygen – give oxygen.

*I*V – infuse 1 liter of crystalloid.

*L*eft lateral position – adopt the full left lateral position.

*T*ocolysis – e.g., terbutaline.[41]

	Class I	Class II	Class III	Class IV
Blood loss (ml)[a]	Up to 750	750–1500	1500–2000	>2000
Blood loss (% blood volume)	Up to 15%	15–30%	30–40%	>40%
Heart rate (beats/min)	<100	>100	>120	≥140
Blood pressure	Normal	Normal	Decreased	Decreased
Pulse pressure	Normal/ increased	Decreased	Decreased	Decreased

(cont.)

	Class I	Class II	Class III	Class IV
Capillary refill	Normal	Decreased	Decreased	Decreased
Respiratory rate (breaths/min)	14–20	20–30	30–35	>35
Urine output (ml/h)	30 or more	20–30	5–15	Negligible
Mental state	Slightly anxious	Anxious	Anxious, confused	Confused, lethargic
Fluid replacement recommended	Crystalloid	Crystalloid	Crystalloid and blood	Crystalloid and blood

[a] These numbers relate to a parturient of average size and will vary with absolute blood volume.

Classification of Shock (Modified from ATLS)

Protocol for Management of Postpartum Hemorrhage (PPH)

Minor – Blood loss 500–1000 ml with no clinical signs of shock

1. Alert midwife in charge.
2. Alert first-line obstetric and anesthetic staff trained in PPH management.
3. Insert 14-gauge cannula, and& consider taking bloods for group and screen, full blood count, and coagulation screen including fibrinogen.
4. Start giving warmed crystalloids intravenously.
5. Record pulse and blood pressure every 15 minutes.
6. Reassess the situation and keep patient and partner informed.
7. Identify the cause of the bleeding and manage accordingly.

Major – Blood loss more than 1000 ml and continuing to bleed or with clinical signs of shock

1. Alert midwife in charge *and* an experienced midwife.
2. Call obstetric middle grade and alert the consultant.
3. Call anesthetic middle grade and alert the consultant.
4. Alert consultant clinical hematologist on call.
5. Alert blood transfusion laboratory.
6. Call ancillary staff to enable delivery of specimens and blood.
7. Alert one team member to document all events, timings, drugs given, etc.

8. Assess patient using ABCs and administer oxygen via facemask at 10–15 liters/min.
9. Insert 2 × 14-gauge cannulas and take bloods for crossmatch (4 units minimum), full blood count, coagulation screen including fibrinogen, renal and liver function to check baseline.
10. Lie patient flat and try to keep warm.
11. Monitor temperature every 15 minutes. Continuously monitor pulse, blood pressure, and& respiratory rate.
12. Insert a Foley catheter to measure urine output.
13. Consider arterial line insertion.
14. Start giving warmed crystalloids rapidly until blood is available. Blood filters should not be used because they slow the rate of fluid administration.
15. Blood products given include red cells, fresh frozen plasma, platelets, fibrinogen concentrate, and cryoprecipitate. Administration guided by blood test results including thromboelastometry as available.
16. Identify and treat the cause of bleeding as appropriate.
17. Reassess the situation and consider transfer and admission to high-dependency or intensive care unit when stable.[42]

Fetal and Neonatal Assessment
Apgar Score
The Apgar score is assessed at 1 and 5 minutes after delivery. Initial resuscitation measures should not be delayed in order to assess the Apgar score at 1 minute. A score of 3 is critically low; a score of 7–9 at 5 minutes is normal.[43]

	Score 0	Score 1	Score 2
Activity (tone)	Limp	Some flexion	Active motion
Pulse	Absent	<100/min	>100/min
Grimace (reflex irritability)	No response	Grimace	Cry or active withdrawal
Appearance (skin color)	Blue	Peripherally blue and centrally pink	Pink
Respiration	Absent	Weak cry or irregular respiration	Good cry

Fetal Blood Sampling Results
pH of 7.25 or above is normal.
pH of 7.21–7.24 is borderline.
pH of 7.20 or below is abnormal.[44]

Umbilical Cord Gases: Normal Ranges

	Venous blood	Arterial blood
pH	7.35 ± 0.05	7.28 ± 0.05
pCO_2 (mmHg)	38 ± 5.6	49 ± 8.4
pO_2 (mmHg)	29 ± 5.9	18 ± 6.2
Base excess (mEq/liter)	-4 ± 2	-4 ± 2
Bicarbonate (mmol/liter)	20 ± 2.1	22 ± 2.5

Note: Data presented as mean values ± standard deviation.
Source: Data from Yoemans et al.[45]

Electronic Fetal Monitoring: Cardiotocography

CTG feature	Baseline (beats/min)	Variability (beats/min)	Decelerations
Reassuring	110–160	5–25	None or early Variable decelerations with no concerning characteristics[a] for less than 90 minutes
Nonreassuring	100–109[b] or 161–180	<5 for more than 30–50 minutes or >25 for 15–25 minutes	Variable decelerations with no concerning characteristics[a] for 90 minutes or more *or* Variable decelerations with any concerning characteristics[a] in up to 50 percent of contractions for 30 minutes or more *or*

(cont.)

CTG feature	Baseline (beats/min)	Variability (beats/min)	Decelerations
Abnormal	<100 or >180	<5 for more than 50 minutes or >25 for more than 25 minutes or Sinusoidal	Variable decelerations with any concerning characteristics[a] in over 50 percent of contractions for less than 30 minutes or Late decelerations in over 50 percent of contractions for less than 30 minutes with no maternal or fetal clinical risk factors such as vaginal bleeding or significant meconium Variable decelerations with any concerning characteristics[a] in over 50 percent of contractions for 30 minutes (or less if any maternal or fetal clinical risk factors) or Late decelerations for 30 minutes (or less if any maternal or fetal clinical risk factors) or Acute bradycardia or a single prolonged deceleration lasting 3 minutes or more

[a] Regard the following as concerning characteristics of variable decelerations: lasting more than 60 seconds, reduced baseline variability within the deceleration, failure to return to baseline, biphasic (W) shape, no shouldering.

[b] Although a baseline fetal heart rate between 100 and 109 beats/min is a nonreassuring feature, continue usual care if there is normal baseline variability and no variable or late decelerations.

Source: Data from NICE Guideline: Intrapartum Care.[46]

CTG category	Features
Normal	All CTG features are reassuring
Suspicious	One nonreassuring and two reassuring CTG features
Pathologic	One abnormal or two nonreassuring CTG features
Need for urgent intervention	Acute bradycardia or a single prolonged deceleration for 3 minutes or more

Please refer to the 2017 NICE guidelines for detailed management based on the preceding CTG categories.

Hematology and Coagulation Tests
Hematology Blood Tests

	Nonpregnant adult	First trimester	Second trimester	Third trimester	References
Erythropoietin (units/liter)	4–27	12–25	8–67	14–222	47–49
Ferritin (mg/ml)	10–150	6–130	2–230	0–116	2–4, 47–51
Folate, red blood cell (ng/ml)	150–450	137–589	94–828	109–663	50, 52, 53
Folate, serum (ng/ml)	5.4–18	2.6–15	0.8–24	1.4–20.7	46, 50, 53–56
Hemoglobin (g/dl)	12–15.8	11.6–13.9	9.7–14.8	9.5–15	48–51, 56
Hematocrit (%)	35.4–44.4	31–41	30–39	28–40	3, 23, 47, 48, 50, 56, 57
Iron, total binding capacity (μg/dl)	251–406	278–403	Not reported	359–609	51

(cont.)

	Nonpregnant adult	First trimester	Second trimester	Third trimester	References
Iron, serum (µg/dl)	41–141	72–143	44–178	30–193	4, 7, 51
Mean corpuscular hemoglobin (pg/cell)	27–32	30–32	30–33	29–32	3
Mean corpuscular volume (× m^3)	79–93	81–96	82–97	81–99	9, 34, 56, 57
Platelets (× 10^9/liter)	165–415	174–391	155–409	146–429	3, 4, 9, 57–59
Mean platelet volume (µm^3)	6.4–11	7.7–10.3	7.8–10.2	8.2–10.4	3
Red blood cell count (× 10^6/mm^3)	4–5.2	3.42–4.55	2.81–4.49	2.71–4.43	3, 4, 9, 56, 57
Red cell distribution width (%)	<14.5	12.5–14.1	13.4–13.6	12.7–15.3	3
White blood cell count (× 10^3/mm^3)	3.5–9.1	5.7–13.6	5.6–14.8	5.9–16.9	3, 50, 56, 60
Neutrophils (× 10^3/mm^3)	1.4–4.6	3.6–10.1	3.8–12.3	3.9–13.1	3, 57, 58, 60
Lymphocytes (× 10^3/mm^3)	0.7–4.6	1.1–3.6	0.9–3.9	1–3.6	3, 57, 58, 60
Monocytes (× 10^3/mm^3)	0.1–0.7	0.1–1.1	0.1–1.1	0.1–1.4	3, 57, 60
Eosinophils (× 10^3/mm^3)	0–0.6	0–0.6	0–0.6	0–0.6	57, 60
Basophils (× 10^3/mm^3)	0–0.2	0–0.1	0–0.1	0–0.1	57, 60
Transferrin (mg/dl)	200–400	253–344	220–441	288–530	2, 3
Transferrin, saturation without iron (%)	22–46	Not reported	10–44	5–37	49
Transferrin, saturation with iron (%)	22–46	Not reported	18–92	9–98	49

Coagulation Blood Tests

	Nonpregnant adult	First trimester	Second trimester	Third trimester	References
Antithrombin, functional (%)	70–130	89–114	78–126	82–116	59, 61, 62
D-dimer (µg/ml)	0.22–0.78	0.05–0.99	0.32–1.29	0.13–1.7	59, 62–67
Factor V (%)	50–150	75–95	72–96	60–88	68
Factor VII (%)	50–150	100–146	95–153	149–211	59
Factor VIII (%)	50–150	90–210	97–312	143–353	59, 68
Factor VIII (%)	50–150	90–210	97–312	143–353	59, 68
Factor IX (%)	50–150	103–172	154–217	164–235	59
Factor XI (%)	50–150	80–127	82–144	65–123	59
Factor XII (%)	50–150	78–124	90–151	129–194	59
Fibrinogen (mg/dl)	211–496	244–510	291–538	301–696	3, 59, 62, 63, 65–67
Homocysteine (mmol/liter)	4.4–10.8	3.34–11	2–26.9	3.2–21.4	50, 52–55

(cont.)

	Nonpregnant adult	First trimester	Second trimester	Third trimester	References
International normalized ratio (INR)	0.9–1.04	0.86–1.08	0.83–1.02	0.80–1.09	61, 66
Partial thromboplastin time, activated (s)	26.3–39.4	23–38.9	22.9–38.1	22.6–35	3, 59, 61, 66
Plasminogen activator inhibitor-1 (PAI-1) antigen (pg/ml)	17.3+/−5.7	17.7+/−1.9	Not reported	66.4+/−4.9	67
PAI-1 activity (arbitrary units)	9.3+/−1.9	9+/-0.8	Not reported	31.4+/−3	67
Prothrombin time (s)	12.7–15.4	9.7–13.5	9.5–13.4	9.6–12.9	3, 59, 66
Protein C, functional (%)	70–130	78–121	83–133	67–135	61, 68, 69
Protein S, total (%)	70–140	39–105	27–101	33–101	59, 68, 69
Protein S, free (%)	70–140	34–133	19–113	20–65	68, 69
Protein S, functional activity (%)	65–140	57–95	42–68	16–42	68
Tissue plasminogen activator (ng/ml)	1.6–13	1.8–6	2.36–6.6	3.34–9.2	59, 61, 67
Tissue plasminogen activator inhibitor-1 (ng/ml)	4–43	16–33	36–55	67–92	59
von Willibrand factor antigen (%)	75–125	62–318	90–247	84–422	62, 70, 71
ADAMTS-13, von Willibrand cleaving protease	40–170	40–160	22–135	38–105	62, 71

Thromboelastography (TEG) in the Term Parturient

	Pregnant (preoperative) n = 50, mean (2 SD)	Pregnant (postoperative) n = 50, mean (2 SD)	Nonpregnant reference, mean (2 SD)
R time (min)	7 (1–13)	6.6 (2.4–10.8)	4–8
K time (min)	2 (0.2–3.8)	1.8 (0.4–3.2)	0–4
MA (mm)	75.4 (64.6–86.2)	76.4 (66.8–86)	54–72
Alpha angle (degree)	64.8 (47.6–82)	67.3 (53.5–81.1)	47–74
Ly30 (%)	1.6 (0–8.8)	0.7 (0–4.9)	0–8
CI	1.2 (−5.4–7.8)	1.8 (−3.4–7.0)	−3–3

Source: Data from Macafee et al.[72]

ROTEM Thromboelastometry in the Obstetric Population

Test		Pregnant Median (95% reference limits)	Control (nonpregnant) Median (95% reference limits)
INTEM	CT (s)	140 (86–168)	151 (113–266)
	CFT (s)	48 (33–108)	54 (35–120)
	Alpha angle (degree)	81 (71–83)	79 (63–83)
	MCF (mm)	71 (55–79)	64 (57–73)
EXTEM	CT (s)	47 (31–80)	48 (30–91)
	CFT (s)	50 (43–86)	61 (37–104)
	Alpha angle (degree)	80 (64–83)	78 (66–83)
	MCF (mm)	73 (66–92)	66 (53–74)
FIBTEM	CT (s)	49 (20–95)	48 (29–92)
	CFT (s)	N/A	N/A
	Alpha angle (degree)	78 (33–86)	69 (16–81)
	MCF (mm)	25 (15–38)	17 (11–37)

Source: Data from Armstrong et al.[73]

Lipids

	Nonpregnant adult	First trimester	Second trimester	Third trimester	References
Cholesterol, total (mg/dl)	<200	141–210	176–299	219–349	3, 74–76
High-density lipoprotein cholesterol (mg/dl)	40–60	40–78	52–87	48–87	3, 74–76
Low-density lipoprotein cholesterol (mg/dl)	<100	60–153	77–184	101–224	3, 74–76
Very-low-density lipoprotein cholesterol (mg/dl)	6–40	10–18	13–23	21–36	75
Triglycerides (mg/dl)	<150	40–159	75–382	131–453	2, 3, 74–76
Alipoprotein A-I (mg/dl)	119–240	111–150	142–253	145–262	2, 75, 78
Alipoprotein B (mg/dl)	52–163	58–81	66–188	85–238	2, 75, 78

Metabolic and Endocrine Tests
Blood Tests

	Nonpregnant adult	First trimester	Second trimester	Third trimester	References
Aldosterone (ng/dl)	2–9	6–104	9–104	15–101	79–81
Angiotensin-converting enzyme (units/liter)	9–67	1–38	1–36	1–39	18, 20
Alpha-fetoprotein (ng/ml)	0–8.5	Not reported	50–425	50–590	82, 83
Cortisol (µg/dl)	0–25	7–19	10–42	12–50	3, 81
Hemoglobin A1C (%)	4–6	4–6	4–6	4–7	15, 78, 84
Parathyroid hormone (pg/ml)	8–51	10–15	18–25	9–26	6
Parathyroid hormone-related protein (pmol/liter)	<1.3	0.7–0.9	1.8–2.2	2.5–2.8	6
Renin, plasma activity (ng/ml/h)	0.3–9	Not reported	7.5–54	5.9–58.8	19, 80
Thyroid-stimulating hormone (milli-int units/ml) American Thyroid Association recommendation	0.34–4.25	0.6–3.4 / 0.1–2.5	0.37–3.6 / 0.2–0.3	0.38–4.04 / 0.3–3	2, 3, 85 / 86
Thyroxine-binding globulin (mg/dl)	1.3–3	1.8–3.2	2.8–4	2.6–4.2	3
Thyroxine, free (ng/dl)	0.8–1.7	0.8–1.2	0.6–1	0.5–0.8	3, 85
Thyroxine, total (mcg/dl)	5.4–11.7	6.5–10.1	7.5–10.3	6.3–9.7	3, 8
Triiodothyronine, free (pg/ml)	2.4–4.2	4.1–4.4	4–4.2	Not reported	85
Triiodothyronine, total (ng/dl)	77–135	97–149	117–169	123–162	3

Blood Gas Analysis

	Nonpregnant adult	First trimester	Second trimester	Third trimester	References
pH	7.38–7.42 (arterial)	7.36–7.52 (venous)	7.4–7.52 (venous)	7.41–7.53 (venous) / 7.39–7.45 (arterial)	7, 88
pO_2 (mmHg)	90–100	93–100	90–98	92–107	87, 88
pCO_2 (mmHg)	38–42	Not reported	Not reported	25–53	87
Bicarbonate (HCO_3) (mEq/liter)	22–26	Not reported	Not reported	16–22	87

Neurology
Diagnostic Criteria for Dural Puncture Headache (International Headache Society)

A. Headache that gets worse within 15 minutes after sitting or standing and improves within 15 minutes after lying, with at least one of the following and fulfilling criteria B and C:

- Neck stiffness
- Tinnitus
- Hyperacusis
- Photophobia
- Nausea

B. Dural puncture has been performed.
C. Headache develops within 5 days of dural puncture.
D. Headache resolves either
  - Spontaneously within 1 week
  - Within 48 hours after effective treatment of the spinal fluid leak (usually by epidural blood patch)[89]

Grading System for Subarachnoid Hemorrhage (World Federation of Neurologic Surgeons)

This clinical grading system is intended to be a simple, reliable, and clinically valid way to grade a patient with subarachnoid hemorrhage. It offers less interobserver variability than some of the earlier classification systems.

Grade	Glasgow coma scale (GCS)	Motor deficit[a]
1	15	Absent
2	13–14	Absent
3	13–14	Present
4	7–12	Present or absent
5	3–6	Present or absent

[a] Where a motor deficit refers to a major focal deficit.
Source: Data from World Federation of Neurological Surgeons.[90]

Interpretation

- Maximum score of 15 has the best prognosis.
- Minimum score of 3 has the worst prognosis.
- Scores of 8 or above have a good chance for recovery.
- Scores of 3–5 are potentially fatal, especially if accompanied by fixed pupils or absent oculovestibular responses.

- Young children may be nonverbal, requiring a modification of the coma scale for evaluation.[90]

Glasgow Coma Scale = (Score for Eye Opening) + (Score for Best Verbal Response) + (Score for Best Motor Response)

Eye opening	Best verbal response	Best motor response
Eyes open spontaneously (4)	Orientated (5)	Obeys commands (6)
Eyes open to verbal command (3)	Confused (4)	Localizing pain (5)
Eyes open to pain (2)	Inappropriate words (3)	Withdrawal from pain (4)
No eye opening (1)	Incomprehensible sounds (2)	Flexion to pain (3)
	No verbal response (1)	Extension to pain (2)
		No motor response (1)

Chiari Malformations

These cerebellar malformations usually occur as a result of lack of space within the posterior cranial fossa, causing the cerebellum and brain stem to be pushed down through the foremen magnum and into the upper spinal canal. Four types are described.[91]

Type 1
Extension of the cerebellar tonsils into the foramen magnum without brain stem involvement. Most common and may be asymptomatic. Only acquired type.

Type 2 (Classic Chiari Malformation)
Extension of both cerebellum and brain stem into foramen magnum. Cerebellar vermis may be partially complete or absent. Usually accompanied by a myelomeningocele. Arnold-Chiari malformation specifically describes this type.

Type 3
Cerebellum, brain stem, and occasionally part of the fourth ventricle herniated through the foramen magnum and into the spinal cord. The herniated cerebellar tissue can also enter an occipital encephalocele. The most serious form of Chiari malformation. Associated with severe neurologic defects.

Type 4 (Cerebellar Hypoplasia)
Associated with an incomplete or underdeveloped cerebellum. Cerebellar tonsils in normal position but

285

parts of cerebellum are missing, and positions of the skull and spinal cord may be visible.

Obesity Classification

Body Mass Index range (kg/m²)	Classification
<18.5	Underweight
18.5 to <25	Healthy weight
25 to <30	Overweight
30 to <40	Obese
40+	Morbidly obese

Source: Data from Public Health England.[92]

Placental Abnormalities (Risk Factors)
Risk Factors for Placental Abruption

1. Abruption in previous pregnancy
2. Preeclampsia
3. Fetal growth restriction
4. Nonvertex presentation
5. Polyhydramnios
6. Increasing maternal age
7. Multiparity
8. Low BMI
9. Pregnancy following assisted reproduction techniques

10. Intrauterine infection
11. Premature rupture of membranes
12. Abdominal trauma
13. Smoking
14. Drug misuse (especially cocaine and amphetamine use in pregnancy)[93]

Risk Factors for Placenta Previa

1. Previous placenta previa
2. Previous cesarean delivery (risk increases with increasing numbers of previous cesarean deliveries)
3. Previous termination of pregnancy
4. Multiparity
5. Advanced maternal age (>40)
6. Multiple pregnancy
7. Smoking
8. Endometrial deficiency due to
   - Uterine scar
   - Endometritis
   - Manual removal of placenta
   - Curettage
   - Submucous fibroid
9. Assisted conception[93]

Renal Function Tests

	Nonpregnant adult	First trimester	Second trimester	Third trimester	References
Effective renal plasma flow (ml/min)	492–696	696–985	612–1170	595–945	94, 95
Glomerular filtration rate (GFR) (ml/min)	106–132	131–166	135–170	117–182	94–96
Filtration fraction (%)	16.9–24.7	14.7–21.6	14.3–21.9	17.1–25.1	94–96
Osmolarity, urine (mOsm/kg)	500–800	326–975	278–1066	238–1034	97
24-h albumin excretion (mg/24 h)	<30	5–15	4–18	3–22	97, 98
24-h calcium excretion (mmol/24 h)	<7.5	1.6–5.2	0.3–6.9	0.8–4.2	23
24-h creatinine clearance (ml/24 h)	91–130	69–140	55–136	50–166	23, 95
24-h creatinine excretion (mmol/24 h)	8.8–14	10.6–11.6	10.3–11.5	10.2–11.4	97
24-h potassium excretion (mmol/24 h)	25–100	17–33	10–38	11–35	23
24-h protein excretion (mg/24 h)	<150	19–141	47–186	46–185	98
24-hr sodium excretion (mmol/24 h)	100–260	53–215	34–213	37–149	21, 23

Week	Vital capacity (liters)				Inspiratory capacity (liters)				Exploratory reserve volume (liters)				Residual volume (liters)			
	Pregnancy			Postpartum	Pregnancy			Postpartum	Pregnancy			Postpartum	Pregnancy			Postpartum
	10	24	36	10	10	24	36	10	10	24	36	10	10	24	36	10
No cardiac disease	3.8	3.9	4.1	3.8	2.6	2.7	2.9	2.5	1.2	1.2	1.2	1.3	1.2	1.1	1.0	1.2
Mitral valve disease	2.9	2.7	2.6	3.1	2.0	1.9	2.0	2.1	0.9	0.8	0.6	1.0	1.3	1.2	1.1	1.4
Aortic valve disease	3.7	3.8	3.6	3.7	2.7	2.7	2.6	2.6	1.0	1.1	1.0	1.1	0.8	1.0	0.9	0.8
Emphysema	2.8	3.0	3.0	2.8	1.6	1.9	1.9	1.6	1.2	1.1	1.1	1.2	1.7	1.9	2.1	1.6
Pulmonary sarcoidosis	2.3	2.2	2.2	2.4	1.4	1.4	1.5	1.5	0.9	0.8	0.7	0.9	0.8	0.7	0.7	0.7

Source: Data from Gazioglu et al.[100]

Renal Transplant Recipients: Criteria for Considering Pregnancy

1. Good general health for approximately 2 years after transplantation
2. Good, stable allograft function (serum creatinine < 2 mg/dl, preferably <1.5)
3. No recent episodes of acute rejection and no evidence of ongoing rejection
4. Normal blood pressure on minimal antihypertensive regimen (one drug only)
5. Absence of or minimal proteinuria (<0.5 g/24 h)
6. Normal allograft ultrasound (absence of pelvicalyceal distension)
7. Recommended immunosuppression:
   - Prednisolone < 15 mg/day
   - Azathioprine < 2mg/day
   - Cyclosporine or tacrolimus at therapeutic levels
8. Mycophenolate mofetil and sirolimus are contraindicated and should be stopped 6 weeks before conception is attempted.[99]

Respiratory Function
Lung Volumes in Pregnancy and in Parturients with Cardiac Disease

Surgery
Classification for Operative Vaginal Delivery
Outlet

- Fetal scalp is visible without separating the labia.
- Fetal skull has reached pelvic floor.
- Sagittal suture is in the anteroposterior diameter or right or left occiput anterior or posterior position (rotation does not exceed 45 degrees).
- Fetal head is at or on the perineum.[101]

Low

Leading point of the skull (not caput) is at station plus 2 cm or more and not on the pelvic floor. Two subdivisions:

- Rotation of 45 degrees or less from the occipitoanterior position
- Rotation of more than 45 degrees including the occipitoposterior position[101]

Mid

Fetal head is no more than one-fifth palpable per abdomen. Leading point of the skull is above station plus 2 cm but not above the ischial spines. Two subdivisions:

- Rotation of 45 degrees or less from the occipitoanterior position
- Rotation of more than 45 degrees including the occipitoposterior position[101]

High

Not included in the classification because operative vaginal delivery is not recommended in this situation where the head is two-fifths or more palpable abdominally and the presenting part is above the level of the ischial spines.[101]

WHO Safer Childbirth Checklist

The World Health Organization (WHO) developed this checklist in response to the high mortality rate of pregnant women and neonates in the low-resource setting, most of which were preventable. This consists of 29 points addressing the major causes in low-income countries of

1. Maternal death: hemorrhage, hypertensive disorders, obstructed labor, infection
2. Intrapartum-related stillbirth: inadequate intrapartum management
3. Neonatal death: infection, asphyxia, prematurity

The checklist is divided into four sections, and the points covered in each section are summarized below.

Section	Points covered
1. On admission	Patient identity, basic monitoring, need for any treatment, including magnesium sulfate and antimicrobials
2. Just before pushing/cesarean delivery	Appropriate equipment for delivery present, need for any magnesium sulfate or antimicrobials
3. Soon after birth (within 1 hour)	Identify any maternal bleeding and manage appropriately, need for any further neonatal care
4. Before discharge	No further maternal bleeding, need for maternal or neonatal antimicrobials, establishing feeding in neonate

This checklist is currently being trialed in over 100 hospitals.[102]

Lucas Classification of Urgency of Cesarean Delivery

Grade	Definition
I Emergency	Immediate threat to life of woman or fetus
II Urgent	Maternal or fetal compromise that is not immediately life threatening
III Scheduled	Needing early delivery but no maternal or fetal compromise
IV Elective	At a time to suit the woman and maternity team

Source: Data from Lucas et al.[103]

Dupuis Classification for Emergency Cesarean Delivery

Red	Very urgent cesarean delivery for life-threatening maternal or fetal situation
Orange	Urgent cesarean delivery
Green	Nonurgent intrapartum cesarean delivery

Source: Data from Dupuis et al.[104]

Persistent Postoperative Pain: Diagnostic Criteria

1. Pain that develops after surgery
2. Pain of at least 2 months' duration
3. Other causes have been excluded[105]

Vitamins and Minerals

	Nonpregnant adult	First trimester	Second trimester	Third trimester	References
Copper (µg/dl)	70–140	112–199	165–221	130–240	3, 106, 107
Selenium (µg/dl)	63–160	116–146	75–145	71–133	3, 106
Vitamin A (retinol) (µg/dl)	20–100	32–46	35–44	29–42	3
Vitamin B_{12} (pg/ml)	279–966	118–438	130–656	99–526	50, 53
Vitamin C (mg/dl)	0.4–1	Not reported	Not reported	0.9–1.3	108
Vitamin D, 1,25-dihydroxy (pg/ml)	25–45	20–65	72–160	60–119	6, 15
Vitamin D 24,25-dihydroxy (ng/ml)	0.5–5	1.2–1.8	1.1–1.5	0.7–0.9	109
Vitamin D 25-hydroxy (ng/ml)	14–80	18–27	10–22	10–18	6, 109
Vitamin E (µg/ml)	5–18	7–13	10–16	13–23	3
Zinc (µg/dl)	75–120	57–88	51–80	51–80	3, 56, 106

References

1. Bromage PR. *Epidural Analgesia*. Philadelphia, PA: Saunders; 1978: 14.

2. Larsson A, Palm M, Hansson L-O, et al. Reference values for clinical chemistry tests during normal pregnancy. *BJOG* 2008; 115:874 [PMID: 18485166].

3. Lockitch G. *Handbook of Diagnostic Biochemistry and Hematology in Normal Pregnancy*. Boca Raton, FL: CRC Press; 1993.

4. Van Buul EJA, Steegers EAP, Jongsma HW, et al. Haematological and biochemical profile of uncomplicated pregnancy in nulliparous women; a longitudinal study. *Neth J Med* 1995; 46:73.

5. Bacq Y, Zarka O, Bréchot JF, et al. Liver function tests in normal pregnancy: a prospective study of 102 pregnant women and 102 matched controls. *Hepatology* 1996; 23:1030 [PMID: 8621129].

6. Ardawi MSM, Nasrat HAN, BA'Aqueel HS. Calcium-regulating hormones and parathyroid hormone-related peptide in normal human pregnancy and postpartum: a longitudinal study. *Eur J Endocrinol* 1997; 137:402 [PMID: 9368509].

7. Handwerker SM, Altura BT, Altura BM. Serum ionized magnesium and other electrolytes in the antenatal period of human pregnancy. *J Am Coll Nutr* 1996; 15:36 [PMID: 8632112].

8. Hytten FE, Lind T. *Diagnostic Indices in Pregnancy*. Summit, NJ, CIBA-GEIGY; 1975.

9. Karsenti D, Bacq Y, Bréchot JF, et al. Serum amylase and lipase activities in normal pregnancy: a prospective case-control study. *Am J Gastroenterol* 2001; 96:697 [PMID: 11280536].

10. Strickland DM, Hauth JC, Widish J, et al. Amylase and isoamylase activities in serum of pregnant women. *Obstet Gynecol* 1984; 63:389 [PMID: 6199704].

11. Carter J. Serum bile acids in normal pregnancy. *BJOG* 1991; 98:540 [PMID: 1873244].

12. Spitzer M, Kaushal N, Benjamin F. Maternal CA-125 levels in pregnancy and the puerperium. *J Reprod Med* 1998; 43:387.

13. Aslam N, Ong C, Woelfer B, et al. Serum CA-125 at 11–14 weeks of gestation in women with morphologically normal ovaries. *BJOG* 2000; 107:689.

14. Jacobs IJ, Fay TN, Stabile I, et al. The distribution of CA 125 in the reproductive tract of pregnant and non-pregnant women. *Br J Obstet Gynaecol* 1988; 95:1190.

15. Mimouni F, Tsang RC, Hertzbert VS, et al: Parathyroid hormone and calcitriol changes in normal and insulin-dependent diabetic pregnancies. *Obstet Gynecol* 1989; 74:49 [PMID: 2733941].

16. Pitkin RM, Gebhardt MP. Serum calcium concentrations in human pregnancy. *Am J Obstet Gynecol* 1977; 127:775 [PMID: 848531].

17. Shakhmatova EI, Osipova NA, Natochin YV. Changes in osmolality and blood serum ion concentrations in pregnancy. *Hum Physiol* 2000; 26:92.

18. Louro MO, Cocho JA, Tutor JC. Assessment of copper status in pregnancy by means of determining the specific oxidase activity of ceruloplasmin. *Clin Chim Acta* 2001; 312:123 [PMID: 11580917].

19. Dux S, Yaron A, Carmel A, et al. Renin, aldosterone, and serum-converting enzyme activity during normal and hypertensive pregnancy. *Gynecol Obstet Invest* 1984; 17:252 [PMID: 6329926].

20. Parente JV, Franco JG, Greene LJ, et al. Angiotensin-converting enzyme: serum levels during normal pregnancy. *Am J Obstet Gynecol* 1979; 135:586 [PMID: 228554].

21. Davidson JB, Vallotton MB, Lindheimer MD. Plasma osmolality and urinary concentration and dilution during and after pregnancy: evidence that lateral recumbency inhibits maximal urinary concentrating ability. *BJOG* 1981; 88:472 [PMID: 7236550].

22. Kato T, Seki K, Matsui H, et al. Monomeric calcitonin in pregnant women and in cord blood. *Obstet Gynecol* 1998; 92:241 [PMID: 9699759].

23. Singh HJ, Mohammad NH, Nila A. Serum calcium and parathormone during normal pregnancy in Malay women. *J Matern Fetal Med* 1999; 8:95 [PMID: 10338062].

24. Rang S, van Montfrans GA, Wolf H. Serial hemodynamic measurement in normal pregnancy, preeclampsia, and intrauterine growth restriction. *Am J Obstet Gynecol* 2008; 198(5):519.e1–9 [PMID: 18279824].

25. Moertl MG, Ulrich D, Pickel K, et al. Changes in haemodynamic and autonomous nervous system parameters measured non-invasively throughout normal pregnancy. *Eur J Obstet Gynecol Reprod Biol* 2009; 144(Suppl 1): S179-83 [PMID: 19285779].

26. Pandey AK, Das A, Srinivas C, et al. Maternal myocardial performances in various stages of pregnancy and post-partum. *Res J Cardiol* 2010; 3(1):9–16.

27. Lees M. Central circulatory responses in normotensive and hypertensive pregnancy. *Postgrad Med J* 1979; 55(643):311–14 [PMCID: PMC2425449].

28. Poppas A, Shroff SG, Korcarz CE, et al. Serial assessment of the cardiovascular system in normal pregnancy: role of arterial compliance and pulsatile arterial load. *Circulation* 1997; 95:2407–15.

29. Katz R, Karliner JS, Resnik R. Effects of a natural volume overload state (pregnancy) on left ventricular performance in normal human subjects. *Circulation* 1978; 58:434–41.

30. Mesa A, Jessurun C, Hernandez A, et al. Left ventricular diastolic function in normal human pregnancy. *Circulation* 1999; 99:511–17.

31. Savu O, Jurcuț R, Giușcă S, et al. Morphological and functional adaptation of the maternal heart during pregnancy. *Circ Cardiovasc Imaging* 2012; 5:289.

32. Vitarelli A, Capotosto L. Role of echocardiography in the assessment and management of adult congenital heart disease in pregnancy. *Int J Cardiovasc Imaging* 2011; 27:843.

33. Borghi CB, Esposti DD, Immordino V, et al. Relationship of systemic hemodynamics, left ventricular structure and function, and plasma natriuretic peptide concentrations during pregnancy complicated by preeclampsia. *Am J Obstet Gynecol* 2000; 183:140 [PMID: 10920322].

34. Resnik JL, Hong C, Resnik R, et al. Evaluation of B-type natriuetic peptide (BNP) levels in normal and preeclamptic women. *Am J Obstet Gynecol* 2005; 193:450–58.

35. Hamid RR, Larsson A, Pernow J, et al. Assessment of left ventricular structure and function in preeclampsia by echocardiography and cardiovascular biomarkers. *J Hypertens* 2009; 27:2257-64.

36. Leiserowitz GS, Evans AT, Samuels SJ, et al. Creatine kinase and its MB isoenzyme in the third trimester and the peripartum period. *J Reprod Med* 1992; 37:910 [PMID: 1460608].

37. Koscica KL, Bebbington M, Bernstein PS. Are maternal serum troponin I levels affected by vaginal or cesarean delivery? *Am J Perinatol* 2004; 21(1):31.

38. Shivvers SA, Wians FH, Keffer JH, et al. Maternal cardiac troponin I levels during labor and delivery. *Am J Obstet Gynecol* 1999; 180:122 [PMID: 9914590].

39. Association of Anaesthetists of Great Britain and Ireland (AAGBI) . *AAGBI Safety Guideline: Management of Suspected Anaphylaxis*, 2009. Available at www.aagbi.org/sites/default/files/Anaesth-web-laminate-final.pdf (accessed October 22, 2018).

40. Association of Anaesthetists of Great Britain and Ireland (AAGBI). *AAGBI Safety Guideline: Management of Severe Local Anaesthetic Toxicity*, 2010. Available at www.aagbi.org/sites/default/files/la_toxicity_2010_0.pdf (accessed October 22, 2018).

41. Thurlow JA, Kinsella SM. Intrauterine resuscitation: active management of fetal distress. *Int J Obstet Anaesth* 2002; 11:105.

42. *Greentop Guideline 52. Prevention and Management of PPH*, 2016. Available at https://obgyn.onlinelibrary .wiley.com/doi/epdf/10.1111/1471-0528.14178 (accessed October 22, 2018).

43. Apgar V. A proposal for a new method of evaluation of the newborn infant. *Can Res Anaesth Analg* 1953; 32(4):260–67.

44. *Intrapartum Care for Healthy Women and Babies: NICE Clinical Practice Guideline*, December 3, 2014. Available at www.nice.org.uk/guidance/cg190 (accessed October 18, 2018).

45. Yeomans ER, Hauth JC, Gilstrap LC III, Stckland DM. Umbilical cord pH, PCO_2 and bicarbonate following uncomplicated term vaginal deliveries. *Am J Obstet Gynecol* 1985; 151:798–800.

46. *NICE Guideline: Intrapartum Care*, February 2017. Available at www.nice.org.uk/guidance/cg190/chapter/Recommendations#monitoring-during-labour.

47. Beguin Y, Lipscei G, Thourmsin H, et al. Blunted erythropoietin production and decreased erythropoiesis in early pregnancy. *Blood* 1991; 78(1):89.

48. Bianco I, Mastropietro F, D'Aseri C, et al. Serum levels of erythropoietin and soluble transferrin receptor during pregnancy in non-β-thalassemic and β-thalassemic women. *Haematologica* 2000; 85:902 [PMID: 10980626].

49. Milman N, Graudal N, Nielsen OJ. Serum erythropoietin during normal pregnancy: relationship to hemoglobin and iron status markers and impact of iron supplementation in a longitudinal, placebo-controlled study on 118 women. *Int J Hematol* 1997; 66:159 [PMID: 9277046].

50. Milman N, Bergholt T, Byg KE, et al. Reference intervals for haematological variables during normal pregnancy and postpartum in 434 healthy Danish women. *Eur J Haematol* 2007; 79:39 [PMID: 17598837].

51. Romslo I, Haram K, Sagen N, et al. Iron requirement in normal pregnancy as assessed by serum ferritin, serum transferring saturation and erythrocyte protoporphyrin determinations. *Br J Obstet Gynaecol* 1983; 90:101 [PMID: 6824608].

52. Milman N, Byg KE, Hvas AM, et al. Erythrocyte folate, plasma folate and plasma homocysteine during normal pregnancy and postpartum: a longitudinal study comprising 404 Danish women. *Eur J Haematol* 2006; 76:200 [PMID: 16412135].

53. Walker MC, Smith GN, Perkins SL, et al. Changes in homocysteine levels during normal pregnancy. *Am J Obstet Gynecol* 1999; 180:660 [PMID: 10076144].

54. López-Quesada E, Vilaseca MA, Lailla JM. Plasma total homocysteine in uncomplicated pregnancy and in preeclampsia. *Eur J Obstet Gynecol Reprod Biol* 2003; 108:45 [PMID: 19899161].

291

55. Özerol E, Özerol I, Gökdeniz R, et al. Effect of smoking on serum concentrations of total homocysteine, folate, vitamin B_{12}, and nitric oxide in pregnancy: a preliminary study. *Fetal Diagn Ther* 2004; 19:145.

56. Qvist I, Abdulla M, Jägerstad M, et al. Iron, zinc and folate status during pregnancy and two months after delivery. *Acta Obstet Gynaecol Scand* 1986; 65:15 [PMID: 3716775].

57. Balloch AJ, Cauchi MN. Reference ranges for haematology parameters in pregnancy derived from patient populations. *Clin Lab Haematol* 1993; 15:7 [PMID: 8472501].

58. AzizKarim S, Khurshid M, Rizvi JH, et al. Platelets and leucocyte counts in pregnancy. *J Pak Med Assoc* 1992; 42:86.

59. Choi JW, Pai SH. Tissue plasminogen activator levels change with plasma fibrinogen concentrations during pregnancy. *Ann Hematol* 2002; 81:611 [PMID: 12454697].

60. Belo L, Santos-Silva A, Rocha S, et al. Fluctuations in C-reactive protein concentration and neutrophil activation during normal human pregnancy. *Eur J Obstet Gynecol Reprod Biol* 2005; 123:46 [PMID: 16260340].

61. Cerneca F, Ricci G, Simeone R, et al. Coagulation and fibrinolysis changes in normal pregnancy increased levels of procoagulants and reduced levels of inhibitors during pregnancy induce a hypercoagulable state, combined with a reactive fibrinolysis. *Eur J Obstet Gynecol Reprod Biol* 1997; 73:31 [PMID: 9175686].

62. Lattuada A, Rossi E, Calzarossa C, et al. Mild to moderate reduction of a von Willebrand factor cleaving protease (ADAMTS-13) in pregnant women with HELLP microangiopathic syndrome. *Haematologica* 2003; 88(9):1029.

63. Francalanci I, Comeglio P, Liotta AA, et al. D-Dimer concentrations during normal pregnancy, as measured by ELISA. *Thromb Res* 1995; 78:399 [PMID: 7660356].

64. Kline JA, Williams GW, Hernandez-Nino J. D-Dimer concentrations in normal pregnancy: new diagnostic thresholds are needed. *Clin Chem* 2005; 51:825 [PMID: 15764641].

65. Morse M. Establishing a normal range for D-dimer levels through pregnancy to aid in the diagnosis of pulmonary embolism and deep vein thrombosis. *J Thromb Haemost* 2004; 2:1202 [PMID: 15219216].

66. Liu XH, Jiang YM, Shi H, et al. Prospective, sequential, longitudinal study of coagulation changes during pregnancy in Chinese women. *Int J Gynaecol Obstet* 2009; 105(3):240.

67. Hale SA, Sobel B, Benvenuto A, et al. Coagulation and fibrinolytic system protein profiles in women with normal pregnancies and pregnancies complicated by hypertension. *Pregnancy Hypertens* 2012; 2:152.

68. Lefkowitz JB, Clarke SH, Barbour LA. Comparison of protein S functional and antigenic assays in normal pregnancy. *Am J Obstet Gynecol* 1996; 175:657 [PMID: 8828430].

69. Faught W, Garner P, Jones G, et al. Changes in protein C and protein S levels in normal pregnancy. *Am J Obstet Gynecol* 1995; 172:147 [PMID: 7847526].

70. Wickström K, Edelstam G, Löwbeer CH, et al. Reference intervals for plasma levels of fibronectin, von Willebrand factor, free protein S and antithrombin during third-trimester pregnancy. *Scand J Clin Lab Invest* 2004; 64:31 [PMID: 13035697].

71. Mannucci PM, Canciani MT, Forza I, et al. Changes in health and disease of the metalloprotease that cleaves von Willebrand factor. *Blood* 2001; 98(9):2730.

72. Macafee B, Campbell JP, Ashpole K, et al. Reference ranges for thromboelastography (TEG) and traditional coagulation tests in term parturient undergoing caesarean section under spinal anaesthesia. *Anaesthesia* 2012; 67:741–47.

73. Armstrong S, Fernando R, Ashpole K, et al. Assessment of coagulation in the obstetric population using ROTEM thromboelastometry. *Int J Obstet Anaesth* 2011; 20:293–98.

74. Belo L, Caslake M, Gaffney D, et al. Changes in LDL size and HDL concentration in normal and preeclamptic pregnancies. *Atherosclerosis* 2002; 162:425 [PMID: 11996963].

75. Desoye G, Schweditsch MO, Pfeiffer KP, et al. Correlation of hormones with lipid and lipoprotein levels during normal pregnancy and postpartum. *J Clin Endocrinol Metab* 1987; 64:704 [PMID: 3546352].

76. Jimenez DM, Pocovi M, Ramon-Cajal J, et al. Longitudinal study of plasma lipids and lipoprotein cholesterol in normal pregnancy and puerperium. *Gynecol Obstet Invest* 1988; 25:158 [PMID: 3391425].

77. Piechota W, Staszewski A. Reference ranges of lipids and apolipoproteins in pregnancy. *Eur J Obstet Gynecol Reprod Biol* 1992; 45:27 [PMID: 1618359].

78. Montelongo A, Lasunción MA, Pallardo LF, et al. Longitudinal study of plasma lipoproteins and hormones during pregnancy in normal and diabetic women. *Diabetes* 1992; 41:1651 [PMID: 1446807].

79. Elsheikh A, Creatsas G, Mastorakos G, et al. The renin-aldosterone system during normal and hypertensive pregnancy. *Arch Gynecol Obstet* 2001; 264:182 [PMID: 11205704].

80. Kim EH, Lim JH, Kim YH, et al. The relationship between aldosterone to renin ratio and RI value of the

uterine artery in the preeclamptic patient vs. normal pregnancy. *Yonsei Med J* 2008; 49(1):138.

81. Suri D, Moran J, Hibbard JU, et al. Assessment of adrenal reserve in pregnancy: defining the normal response to the adrenocorticotropin stimulation test. *J Clin Endocrinol Metab* 2006; 91:3866 [PMID: 16895954].

82. Kratz A, Pesce MA, Basner RC, Einstein AJ. Appendix: laboratory values of clinical importance, in Longo DL, Fauci AS, Kasper DL, et al. (eds.), *Harrison's Principles of Internal Medicine* (18th edn). New York, NY: McGraw-Hill; 2012, App. 1, p. A1.

83. Leek AE, Ruoss CF, Kitau MJ, Chard T. Maternal plasma alpha-fetoprotein levels in the second half of normal pregnancy: relationship to fetal weight, and maternal age and parity. *Br J Obstet Gynaecol* 1975; 82(8):669–73.

84. Radder JK, Van Roosmalen J. HbAIC in healthy, pregnant women. *Neth J Med* 2005; 63:256 [PMID: 16093576].

85. Price A, Obel O, Cresswell J, et al. Comparison of thyroid function in pregnant and non-pregnant Asian and western Caucasian women. *Clin Chim Acta* 2001; 208:91.

86. Stagnaro-Green A, Abalovich M, Alexander E, et al. Guidelines of the American Thyroid Association for the diagnosis and management of thyroid disease during pregnancy and postpartum. *Thyroid* 2011; 21:1081.

87. Fadel HE, Northrop G, Misenhimer HR, et al. Acid-base determinations in amniotic fluid and blood of normal late pregnancy. *Obstet Gynecol* 1979; 53:99 [PMID: 32503].

88. Spiropoulos K, Prodromaki E, Tsapanos V. Effect of body position on PaO_2 and $PaCO_2$ during pregnancy. *Gynecol Obstet Invest* 2004; 58:22 [PMID: 15028865].

89. International Headache Society. *Classification of Headache Disorders*, 2018. Available at http://ihs-classification.org/en/02_klassifikation/03_teil2/07.02.01_nonvascular.html (accessed October 312, 2018).

90. World Federation of Neurological Surgeons. *Grading System for Subarachnoid Haemorrhage*, 2011. Available at www.strokecenter.org/wp-content/uploads/2011/08/WWF_scale.pdf (accessed October 31, 2018).

91. National Institute of Neurological Disorders and Stroke. *Chiari Malformation Information Page*, 2016. Available at www.ninds.nih.gov/Disorders/All-Disorders/Chiari-Malformation-Information-Page (accessed October 31, 2018).

92. Public Health England. *Measurement of Obesity*, 2014. Available at http://webarchive.nationalarchives.gov.uk/20170110170040/https://www.noo.org.uk/NOO_about_obesity/measurement (last accessed October 31, 2018)

93. *RCOG Green Top Guideline 63: Risk Factors for Placental Abruption*, 2011. Available at www.rcog.org.uk/globalassets/documents/guidelines/gtg_63.pdf (accessed October 31, 2018).

94. Dunlop W. Serial changes in renal haemodynamics during normal human pregnancy. *Br J Obstet Gynaecol* 1981; 88:1 [PMID: 7459285].

95. Ezimokhai M, Davison JM, Philips PR, et al. Non-postural serial changes in renal function during the third trimester of normal human pregnancy. *Br J Obstet Gynaecol* 1981; 88:465 [PMID: 7236549].

96. Moran P, Baylis PH, Lindheimer J, et al. Glomerular ultrafiltration in normal and preeclamptic pregnancy. *J Am Soc Nephrol* 2003; 14:648 [PMID: 12595500].

97. Risberg A, Larsson A, Olsson K, et al. Relationship between urinary albumin and albumin/creatinine ratio during normal pregnancy and pre-eclampsia. *Scand J Clin Lab Invest* 2004; 64:17 [PMID: 15025425].

98. Higby K, Suiter CR, Phelps JY, et al. Normal values of urinary albumin and total protein excretion during pregnancy. *Am J Obstet Gynecol* 1994; 171:984 [PMID: 7943114].

99. Pregnancy in renal transplant recipients. *Nephrol Dial Transplant* 2002; 17(Suppl 4):50–55. Available at https://doi.org/10.1093/ndt/17.suppl_4.50 (accessed October 31, 2018).

100. Gazioglu K, Kaltreider NL, Rosen M, et al. Pulmonary function during pregnancy in normal women and in patients with cardiopulmonary disease. *Thorax* 1970; 25:445–50.

101. *Green Top Guideline 26: Operative Vaginal Delivery*, 2011. Available at www.rcog.org.uk/globalassets/documents/guidelines/gtg_26.pdf (accessed October 31, 2018).

102. World Health Organization. *WHO Safer Childbirth Checklist*, 2015. Available at www.who.int/patientsafety/implementation/checklists/childbirth-checklist/en/ (accessed October 31, 2018).

103. Lucas DN, Yentis SM, Kinsella SM, et al. Urgency of caesarean section: a new classification. *J R Soc Med* 2000; 93:346–50.

104. Depuis O, Sayegh I, Decullier E, et al. Red, orange and green caesarean sections: a new communication tool for on-call obstetricians. *Eur J Obstet Gynecol Reprod Biol* 2008; 140:206–11.

105. Macrae WA. Chronic post-surgical pain: 10 years on. *Br J Anaesth* 2008; 101:77–86.

293

106. Álvarez SI, Castañón SG, Ruata MLC, et al. Updating of normal levels of copper, zinc and selenium in serum of pregnant women. *J Trace Elem Med Biol* 2007; 21(S1):49.

107. Ilhan N, Ilhan N, Simsek M. The changes of trace elements, malondialdehyde levels and superoxide dismutase activities in pregnancy with or without preeclampsia. *Clin Biochem* 2002; 35:393 [PMID: 12270770].

108. Sharma SC, Sabra A, Molloy A, et al. Comparison of blood levels of histamine and total ascorbic acid in pre-eclampsia with normal pregnancy. *Hum Nutr Clin Nutr* 1984; 38C:3.

109. Reiter EO, Braunstein GD, Vargas A, et al. Changes in 25-hydroxyvitamin D and 24,25-dihydroxyvitamin D during pregnancy. *Am J Obstet Gynecol* 1979; 135:227 [PMID: 474676].

Index